A HANDBOOK OF MEDICAL LABORATORY TECHNOLOGY

SECOND EDITION

Editor

V.H. Talib

M.D.

Head of Department, Department of Clinical Pathology,
Safdarjang Hospital, New Delhi; and
Course Director, Medical Laboratory Technology
(Under Directorate General of Health Services,
Ministry of Health and Family Welfare, Government of India),
Safdarjang Hospital, New Delhi

Co-editor

S.R. Khurana

M.B.B.S., D.C.P.

Senior Medical Officer, Department of Clinical Pathology,
Safdarjang Hospital, New Delhi

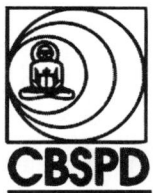

CBSPD

CBS Publishers & Distributors Pvt Ltd

New Delhi • Bengaluru • Chennai • Kochi • Kolkata • Lucknow • Mumbai
Hyderabad • Jharkhand • Nagpur • Patna • Pune • Uttarakhand

A Handbook of
Medical Laboratory
Technology

ISBN: 978-81-239-0677-5

Copyright © VH Talib

Second Edition: 1999
Reprint: 2000, 2002, 2003, 2004, 2006, 2007, 2008, 2009, 2011, 2012, 2013, 2014, 2015, 2017, 2019, 2022, 2023

First Edition: 1998
Reprint: 1991, 1993, 1995, 1996, 1998

Published by **Satish Kumar Jain** and produced by **Varun Jain** for

CBS Publishers & Distributors Pvt Ltd
4819/XI Prahlad Street, 24 Ansari Road, Daryaganj, New Delhi 110 002
Ph: 011-23289259, 23266861, 23266867   Fax: 011-23243014   Website: www.cbspd.com
e-mail: delhi@cbspd.com

Corporate Office: 204 FIE, Industrial Area, Patparganj, Delhi 110 092
Ph: 011-4934 4934   Fax: 011-4934 4935   e-mail: publishing@cbspd.com; publicity@cbspd.com

Branches

- **Bengaluru:** Seema House 2975, 17th Cross, KR Road, Banasankari 2nd Stage, Bengaluru 560 070, Karnataka, India
  Ph: +91-80-26771678/79   Fax: +91-80-26771680   e-mail: bangalore@cbspd.com
- **Chennai:** 7, Subbaraya Street, Shenoy Nagar, Chennai 600 030, Tamil Nadu, India
  Ph: +91-44-26680620, 26681266   e-mail: chennai@cbspd.com
  Fax: +91-44-42032115
- **Kochi:** 42/1325, 1326, Power House Road, Opp KSEB, Power House, Ernakulam Kochi 682 018, Kerala, India
  Ph: +91-484-4059061-65,67   Fax: +91-484-4059065   e-mail: kochi@cbspd.com
- **Kolkata:** 147, Hind Ceramics Compound, 1st Floor, Nilgunj Road, Belghoria, Kolkata-700056, West Bengal, India
  Ph: +91-9096713055/7798394118, 9836841399   e-mail: kolkata@cbspd.com
- **Lucknow:** Basement, Khushnuma Complex, 7 Meerabai Marg (Behind Jawahar Bhawan),Lucknow-226001, UP, India
  Ph: +0522-4000032   e-mail: tiwari.lucknow@cbspd.com
- **Mumbai:** PWD Shed, Gala no 25/26, Ramchandra Bhatt Marg, Next to JJ Hospital Gate no. 2, Opp. Union Bank of India, Noorbaug, Mumbai-400009, Maharashtra, India
  Ph: 022-66661880/89   e-mail: mumbai@cbspd.com

Representatives

• Hyderabad	0-9885175004	• Jharkhand	0-9811541605	• Nagpur	0-9421945513
• Patna	0-9334159340	• Pune	0-9923910676	• Uttarakhand	0-9716462459

Printed at SRK Graphics, Shahdara, Delhi, India

FOREWORD

This book is a cummulation of the cooperative efforts of the staff of department of Clinical Pathology, Blood Bank, Histopathology and Microbiology, Safdarjang Hospital, New Delhi. Although there are many authoritative and exhaustive books on the subject of Medical Laboratory Technology yet there is dearth of a hand book in the subject. I appreciate the great pains, hard labour and dedication by the Course Director, Medical Laboratory Technology course in writing & editing of this hand book for the benefit of all students including medical undergraduates, postgraduates and practioners.

There was a need for such a comprehensive hand book which deals at the same time with subjects of Haematology, Clinical Pathology, Biochemistry, Microbiology & Histopathology, Immunology and Blood Banking with standard methods & their interpretations.

Editor and contributers deserve credit for the excellent hard work and presentation of this hand book which is first of its kind from this country for Inservice Training Course of Medical Laboratory Technology and as well to all medical undergraduates and postgraduates. I hope the hand book will receive a warm welcome not merely because no Indian book exists in this field but because comprehensive contents presented in each field of Laboratory technology.

NIRMAN BHAVAN,
NEW DELHI

(G.K. VISHWAKARMA)
DIRECTOR GENERAL HEALTH SERVICES

December 22nd 1987.

CONTRIBUTORS

V.H. Talib
M.B.B.S., M.D., FIC (Path.) , FIMSA,
MCAIC, Delhi (India),
FIMSA, FRSH (London)
Head of Department of Laboratory Medicine
Safdarjung, New Delhi.

S.R. Khurana
M.B.B.S., D.C.P.
Chief Medical Officer
CGHS, Delhi.

Geeta Ashokraj
M.B.B.S., M.D., MNAMS (Morbid Anatomy)
Professor of Pathology (CIO) &
Professor and Therapist
Dharan, Nepal.

S.N. Haldar
M.B.B.S.
Ex-Head of Department Blood Bank &
Ex-Director CGHS
Nirman Bhawan, New Delhi.

Shashi Gupta
M.B.B.S., M.D.
Ex-Senior Resident
(Clinical Pathology)
Consultant Pathologist, New Delhi.

Neha Trivedi
M.D.
Senior Resident
Laboratory Medicine
Safdarjang Hospital, New Delhi.

Atul Goel
M.B.B.S., M.D.
Ex-Senior Resident
Department of Laboratory Medicine
Blood Bank and Transfusion Medicine
and Central Institute of Orthopaedics (CIO)
Safdarjang Hospital, New Delhi.

S.H. Talib
M.B.B.S., M.D. (Medicine)
Professor & Head, Medicine
FCAI Govt. Medical College
Aurangabad (MS).

S.K. Verma
M.B.B.S., M.D.
Senior Pathologist, Lab Medicine
Safdarjang Hospital, New Delhi.

S.K. Khurana
M.B.B.S., M.D.
Pathologist, Lab Medicine
Safdarjang Hospital, New Delhi.

Kaiser Saleem
M.B.B.S., M.D.
Senior Resident (Medicine)
Consultant Medicine
Raipur (MP).

PREFACE TO THE SECOND EDITION

The present edition of MLT Book is the second revision which had acquired an outstanding reputation. The book has been kept handy and comprehensive for the benefit of all students, technical staff, undergraduates, postgraduates and practitioners.

Few haematological and biochemical techniques have been revised and updated. Manual as well as automatic methods have been incorporated. Special techniques in the field of histocytochemistry have also been added. Ever since the publication of the first edition, 1987, the book is continuously in demand and has been appreciated both in India and abroad. Introduction to chapters of Quality Control, Automation is in accordance with revolutionary change in the trends and technologists related to modern medical laboratory diagnostics, specially of newer technology PCR and flowcytometry. A chapter on AIDS with reference to precautionary measures for working technical staff has been incorporated. Special indexes has been incorporated for easy use by all group of technical staff and medical officials.

I am fully confident that this book shall prove to be of immense value and help to one and all. I am grateful to all my contributors and my daughter Ambreen Talib and Saba Talib for their help in revising the book. Comments and suggestions shall be welcomed and appreciated.

(V.H. TALIB)

Head of Department
Department of Laboratory Medicine
Safdarjang Hospital, New Delhi

PREFACE TO THE FIRST EDITION

There is a great need and demand of the comprehensive book in the field of Medical laboratory technology. Medical diagnostic laboratory is a back bone not only to clinician but to the patient also. Better diagnosis does mean better patient care.

In preparing this handbook on technology, I have fully utilized the opportunity to include all branches of medical laboratory technology including Haematology, Clinical Pathology, Histopathology, Biochemistry, Microbiology, Blood Banking and Immunology. Most of the important and common tests are now included to make this book as much useful and complete as possible.

All students, technical staff, practitioners and individuals related to diagnostic and/or therapeutic medicine would find this book very useful.

I have tried my level best to bring this first edition up-to-date in confirmatory with limitations of a common laboratory in both urban and rural areas of our country. Being a hand book of laboratory technology, quite a few theoretical aspects have not been dealt due to limitations of space.

Inspite of this, there is still a chance of some omissions. I shall be grateful, if any such is brought to notice for consideration in the next edition.

I take the opportunity to thank my friends and colleagues who have contributed various chapters of this hand book, to whom I remain grateful.

(V.H.TALIB)

Department of Clinical Pathology
Safdarjang Hospital
New Delhi
July 30, 1988

CONTENTS

SECTION VI — HISTOPATHOLOGY

SECTION VII — BIOCHEMISTRY

SECTION VIII — BLOOD BANKING AND BLOOD TRANSFUSION

SECTION 1
HAEMATOLOGY

CHAPTER 1

PERIPHERAL BLOOD EXAMINATION

COLLECTION OF BLOOD

There are two ways of obtaining the samples
 i) From the Vein
 ii) From the Capillary
Venous blood is preferred because a number of investigations can be done and repeated on the same sample and because the examination can be done at leisure.

Venous Blood

Venous blood is obtained by venepuncture. Good light and a comfortable position for both the patient and the operator are necessary. Ideally, the patient should be lying down. In the adult, one of the veins in the antecubital fossa is chosen. Make the veins prominent by applying a tourniquet or a blood pressure cuff kept at the diastolic pressure; further the patient is asked to open and close his hand several times vigorously and then keep the fist clinched on a roll of bandage. Select the vein that is both visible and palpable and well fixed to the surrounding tissue (Fig. 1). Check all the equipment, the needle should be sharp (19–20 s.w.G.) patent

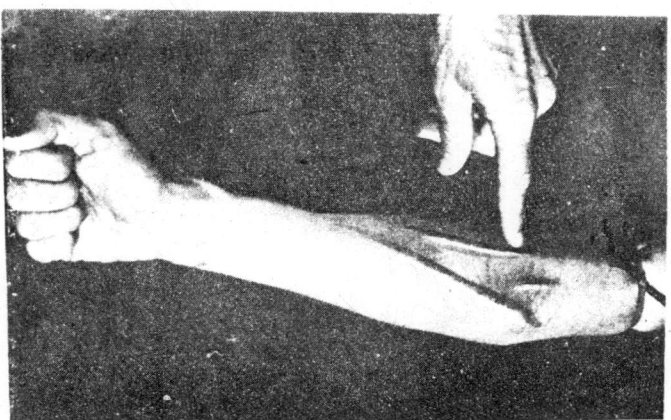

Fig. 1 Showing visible, palpable veins in antecubital fossa

and tight fitting; the syringe should be dry and with all the air expelled from it; and the bottle or the tube to receive the sample must be ready at hand. The patient is reassured and the part cleaned with clean gauge or cotton moistened with rectified spirit. The patient's forearm is grasped with left hand and to steady the vein, the thumb retracts downwards soft tissues below the site of the puncture. The needle is brought to the skin over the vein, the bevel of the needle turned up. If the vein is large and well fixed, the skin and the vein may be punctured with a single short thrust. If the vein is small or slippery the skin is punctured first and the vein next, the plunger is pulled back gently. When the blood starts flowing into the syringe, the tourniquet is released and after sufficient blood has been collected the needle is withdrawn. The punctured site is gently pressed with a swab of cotton or gauge moistened with spirit

for two minutes, the patient elevates the arm and is asked to maintain the pressure for a few minutes more to prevent a haematoma. Before emptying the syringe into the bottle, the needle must be removed. The contents are delivered slowly and mixed with the anticoagulant by gentle shaking for 1 minute.

Capillary Blood

Cappillary blood is obtained by pricking the skin. Only a few drops of blood can be collected in this manner. Blood is collected directly in appropriate pipettes and has to be manipulated immediately. Haemoglobin estimation, red cell count, leucocyte count, platelet count and reticulocyte count can be done with capillary blood. For preparing smears for a differential count, capillary blood without an anticoagulant is preferred.

In adult, capillary blood is obtained from the ball of the finger or the lobe of the ear; in infants, the sites are the ball of the thumb, the great toe or the heel.

Technique: Examine the site of the puncture to make sure that there is no oedema or congestion or that the site is not too cold or blood less. If the last, place the part in warm water to promote congestion. Both the patient and the operator should be seated comfortably and in good light. All the apparatus must be ready at hand before the site is punctured. The site chosen is cleaned with spirit and the part must be allowed to dry completely before the puncture is made. The point of the needle is touched to the skin and a bold quick prick is made. The prick must be deep enough (2–4 mm) to ensure a free flow of blood. The needle must be sharp and sterilized. Blood must flow spontaneously from the stab. The first drop is wiped off and the second one used for filling the pipette. Squeezing of the finger is not permissible as this will dilute the blood with the tissue fluid.

ANTICOAGULANTS

For various purposes a number of different anticoagulants are available. The anticoagulants in use are:
 (1) Disodium or dipotassium ethylenediamine tetra acetic acid (EDTA; Sequestrene);
 (2) Ammonium and potassium oxalate mixture;
 (3) Tri-sodium citrate;
 (4) Heparin and
 (5) Acid-Citrate-Dextrose Solution (A.C.D.)

(1) Ethylenediamine tetra acetic acid (EDTA)

The sodium and potassium salts of EDTA are powerful anticoagulants and they are the anticoagulants of choice for routine haematological work. EDTA acts by its chelating effect on the calcium molecules in blood. To achieve this requires a concentration of 1.2 mg (approximately 4μmol) of the anhydrous salt per ml of blood. The recommended concentration of the dipotassium salt is 1.50 ± 0.25 mg/ml of blood.

Excess of EDTA affects both red cells and leucocytes, causing shrinkage and degenerative changes. EDTA in excess of 2 mg/ml of blood may result in significant decrease in packed cell volume (PCV) and increase in mean cell haemoglobin concentration (MCHC). The platelets are also affected; excess of EDTA causes them to swell and then disintegrate, causing an artificially high platelet count as the fragments are large enough to be counted as morphologically normal platelets. Care must therefore be taken to ensure that the correct amount of blood is added, and that by repeated inversions of the container the anticoagulant is thoroughly mixed in the blood added to it. The dipotassium salt is very soluble (1650 g/l) and is to be preferred on this account to the disodium salt which is considerably less soluble (108 g/1). Rapid solution of the EDTA can be ensured by coating the container with a thin film of the salt.

The dilithium salt of EDTA is equally effective as an anticoagulant, and its use has the advantage that the same sample of blood can be used for chemical investigations. However, it is less soluble than the dipotassium salt (160 g/1).

EDTA is not suitable for use in the investigation of coagulation problems and should not be used in the estimation of prothrombin time.

(2) Ammonium and potassium oxalate mixture

This consists of a mixture of 2 parts of potassium oxlate and 3 parts of ammonium oxalate. Take 1% solution of pottassium oxalate 0.4 ml and 1% solution of ammonium oxalate 0.6 ml in a test tube. Evaporate to dryness in the incubator. This amount of oxalates is sufficient to prevent coagulation of 5 ml of blood.

(3) Trisodium citrate

0.109 mol/l trisodium citrate (32 g/l $Na_3C_6H_5O_7.2H_2O$) is the anticoagulant of choice in coagulation studies. Nine volumes of blood are added to 1 volume of the sodium citrate solution and immediately well mixed with it. Sodium citrate is also the anticoagulant most widely used in the estimation of the sedimentation rate (ESR); for this 4 volumes of venous blood are diluted with 1 volume of the sodium citrate solution.

(4) Heparin

This may be used at a concentration of 15 ± 2.5 iu per ml of blood. Heparin is an effective anticoagulant and does not alter the size of the red cells; it is a good dry anticoagulant when it is important to reduce to a minimum the chance of lysis occuring after blood has been withdrawn. However, heparinized blood should not be used for making blood films as it gives a faint blue coloration to the background when the films are stained by Romanowsky dyes. This is especially marked in the presence of abnormal proteins. Heparin is the best anticoagulant to use for osmotic fragility tests; otherwise it is inferior to EDTA for general use and should not be used for leucocyte count as it tends to cause the leucocytes to clump.

(5) Acid-Citrate-Dextrose solution (ACD)

This is preferred for blood transfusions, for preserving red cells, for enzyme studies, and for the study of haemolytic processes. A standard preparation consists of sodium citrate 1.32 gm, citric acid 0.48 gm, dextrose 1.40 gm, and distilled water to 100 ml. One ml of ACD solution is sufficient to prevent coagulation of 4 ml of blood.

Mode of action of Anticoagulants

EDTA and sodium citrate remove calcium which is essential for coagulation. Calcium is either precipitated as insoluble oxalate (crystals of which may be seen in oxalated blood) or bound in a non-ionized form. Heparin works in a different way; it neutralizes thrombin by inhibiting the interaction of several clotting factors in the presence of a plasma co-factor, antithrombin III. Sodium citrate or heparin can be used to render blood incoagulable before transfusion. For better longterm preservation of red cells for certain tests and for transfusion purposes citrate is used in combination with dextrose in the form of acid-citrate-dextrose (ACD), citrate-phosphate-dextrose (CPD) or Alsever's solution.

Effects of Anticoagulants of Blood Cell Morphology

If blood is allowed to stand in the laboratory before films are made, degenerative changes occur. The changes are not solely due to the presence of an anticoagulant for they also occur in defibrinated blood.

Irrespective of anticoagulant, films made from blood which has been standing for not more than 1 hr at room temperature (18–25°C) are not easily distinguished from films made immediately after collection of the blood. By 3 hr changes may be discernible and by 12–18 hr these become striking. Some but not all neutrophils are affected: their nuclei may stain more homogeneously than in fresh blood, the nuclear lobes may become separated and the cytoplasmic margin may appear ragged or less well defined; small vacuoles appear in the cytoplasm. Some or many of the large mononuclears develop marked changes; small vacuoles appear in the cytoplasm and the nucleus undergoes irregular lobulation which may almost amount to disintegration. Some of the lymphocytes, too, undergo a similar type of change; a few vacuoles may be seen in the cytoplasm and the nucleus may undergo major budding so as to give rise to nuclei with two or three lobes. Other lymphocyte nuclei may stain more homogeneously than usual.

The red cells (of normal blood at least) are little affected by standing for up to 6 hr at room temperature (18–25°C). Longer periods lead to progressive crenation and sphering.

The cells in defibrinated blood undergo degenerative changes at about the same rate as those in EDTA blood.

All the above changes are retarded but not abolished in blood kept at 4°C. Their occurrence underlines the importance of making films as soon as possible after withdrawl. But delay of up to 1–3 hr or so is certainly permissible.

The practice of making films of blood before it is added to the anticoagulant (e.g. at the bedside) is to be commended, especially when screening for lead toxicity, as the granules of punctate basophilia may not stain in anticoagulated blood. In fresh blood films, however, the platelets usually clump and it is less easy to estimate the platelet count from inspection of the film. Such films are nevertheless of particular value in investigating patients suspected of suffering from purpura, as in certain rare conditions, the absence of platelet clumping is a useful pointer to the diagnosis.

ESTIMATION OF HAEMOGLOBIN CONCENTRATION

Haemoglobin is a chromoprotein consisting of the colorless globin molecule attached to four red colored haem molecules. The globin molecule consists of two alpha polypeptide chains and two beta polypeptide chains. Haem is a metal complex containing an iron atom in the centre of a porphyrin structure. Haemoglobin is formed in developing erythrocytes (normoblasts) in the marrow.

The biosynthesis of haemoglobin involves the triad of manufacture of haem, manufacture of globin and iron metabolism. Methods for estimation of haemoglobin are as follows:

(1) Cyanmethaemoglobin method

Principle: Potassium ferricyanide converts Hb from ferrous to ferric state to form meth-Hb. The resulting meth-Hb combines with potassium cyanide to produce the stable pigment cyanmeth Hb. Cyanmeth-Hb represents the sum of Oxy-Hb, Carboxy-Hb and meth-Hb.

Apparatus: Photoelectric colorimeter with filter 540 nm, test tubes, 5 ml pipettes and $20\mu l$ micropipette (an accurately calibrated Sahli's pipette may be used).

Precaution: Do not pipette reagent by mouth. This reagent is poisonous. The concentration of KCN in Hb diluting reagent is 50 mg/litre. The lethal dose of Hb diluting reagent is about 4,000 mgm/litre.

Reagent Drabkin's solution: Dissolve 5 gms of sodium bicarbonate in distilled water first. Add 0.250 gm of potassium cyanide KCN in the solution, add 1 litre of distilled water. Then add 1.0 gm of potassium ferricyanide $K_4Fe(CN)_6$ in the solution. Shake well, make final volume with distilled water to 5 litres.

Interfering substance: Gross lipemia may result in a positive error of upto 3 g/dl.

Calibration curve: Hb standard for the cyanmeth-Hb method is used for calibrating. Into three clean and dry test tubes add solutions as described below:
1. Pipette 5 ml of Hb standard in the first tube (60 mg/100 ml)
2. Into the second test tube pipette exactly 2.5 ml of Hb standard and add in the same tube exactly 2.5 ml of Hb diluting reagent. Stopper the tube and mix by repeated inversion, this is 1:1 dilution of standard, (30 mg cyanmeth Hb per 100 ml).
3. In the third test tube add 5.0 ml of Hb diluting reagent which serves as a blank.

Measurement of Optical Density/Transmittance

1. Set the wavelength of Photoelectric colorimeter at 540nm, pour the blank (test tube no. 3) into the cuvette. Set the optical density to zero or transmission at 100 per cent.
2. Pour the diluted Hb standard (test tube no. 2) into the cuvette and record the optical density or per cent transmission (cyanmeth-Hb standard)
3. Pour the undiluted Hb standard into the cuvette and record the optical density or per cent transmission.
4. If per cent transmission is determined, convert the reading to optical density.
5. Plot a graph Hb in mg/dl on horizontal axis and optical density on the vertical axis.
6. The value of cyanmeth-Hb in mg/dl is given on each vial. Half of this value will give the concentration of cyanmeth-Hb in the tube containing 1:1 dilution of Hb standard.
7. The equivalent g/dl Hb conc. in the undiluted and diluted standard can be calculated as shown below:
   Equivalent g/dl Hb value of undiluted standard
   — g/dl Hb value of undiluted standard × dilution factor.
   — 0.06 × 251 (if the conc. of Hb standard is 60 mg/dl).
   — 15.06 equivalent g/dl Hb value of 1:1 diluted standard.
   — g/dl Hb value of diluted standard × dilution factor.
   — 0.03 × 251 (Half conc. of the Hb standard 60 mg/dl).
   — 7.53 = 7.5

Note: The mg/dl Hb value (printed on the label) divided by 1000 gives the g/dl Hb.

The procedure using 0.02 ml of whole blood in 5 ml of Hb diluting reagent, the dilution factor is 251. Alternatively the procedure using 0.02 ml of whole blood in 6 ml of Hb diluting reagent, the dilution factor is 301.

8. Draw a straight line connecting the two plotted points on the graph which should pass through origin. Reagents should be at room temperature $25 \pm 5°C$.

Method	Test	Blank
Hb diluting reagent	5.0 ml	5.0 ml
Fresh whole blood	0.02 ml	—

Mix well, allow to stand at room temperature for 3 minutes and measure optical density/transmittance of the test against blank at 540 nm.

Record the readings: The colour is stable for more than 24 hours in well stoppered tubes, kept in dark.

From the optical density reading of the test specimen determine the concentration of Hb in g/dl from the calibration curve.

If the optical density reading of test specimen is 0.385, then from the optical density reading of 0.385 draw a straight line parallel to the horizontal axis until it intersects the calibration curve. From this intersection draw a line parallel to the vertical axis down to horizontal axis. Alternatively if a single standard reading is taken the following calculation method may be used:

Calculation

$$Hb = \frac{O.D.\ of\ unknown}{O.D.\ of\ standard} \times \frac{Conc.\ of\ standard\ in\ mg/dl \times dilution\ factor}{1000}\ g/dl$$

$$Example\ \frac{0.385 \times 60 \times 251}{0.418 \times 1000} = 13.8\ g/dl$$

(2) Sahli's acid haematin method

Principle: Hb is converted into acid haematin by hydrochloric acid. The brown color of the compound is matched against a brown glass standard in a comparator.

Apparatus: Sahli-type haemoglobinometer consisting of the comparator with glass standards, a square Hb tube marked both in grams and percentage figures and Hb pipette marked at 20 cu mm, 0.1 N HCl and distilled water.

Technique:

1. Fill the Hb caliberated tube upto the mark 20 (not less) with 0.1 N HCl by means of a dropper.

2. Fill the Hb pipette exactly upto 20 cu mm mark by gentle controlled sucking; the pipette is held horizontally while taking the blood. If a slight excess is drawn in, it may be removed by touching the point of the pipette with the finger or gauge. If a great excess has been drawn in, inaccuracy will result, in this case the pipette must be cleaned, dried & refilled. Wipe off with gauge the blood on the outside of the pipette.

3. Empty the pipette into acid in the tube by keeping the point of the pipette to the bottom of the tube and gently blowing off the blood without causing bubbles. Rinse the pipette at least three times by drawing in and discharging the blood acid mixture.

4

Now withdraw the pipette half way up the tube and rinse the outside of pipette with a few drops of the acid.

4. Mix the acid haematin solution in the tube with the glass rod and allow the tube to stand for 10 minutes. In this interval at least 95 per cent of the colour of acid haematin is developed.

5. Now dilute the solution of acid haematin by adding distilled water, drop by drop, stirring the mixture all the time with glass rod. The comparator is held against good daylight and the addition of water continued till the colour of solution matches perfectly with that of the standards. Take the reading in grams per cent. The bottom of the meniscus is read.

Normal Range of Hb

Men	15.5 ± 2.5 g/dl
Women	14.0 ± 2.5 g/dl
Infants (full term cord blood)	16.5 ± 3.0 g/dl
Children 3 months	11.0 ± 1.5 g/dl
Children 3–6 years	12.0 ± 1.0 g/dl
Children 10–12 years	13.0 ± 1.5 g/dl

TOTAL RED BLOOD CELL COUNT (T.R.B.C)

Specimen: Erythrocyte count can be done on oxalated blood or on capillary blood directly collected into the pipette. In the former case, the sample, unless refrigerated must not be more than 6 hr old.

Apparatus

Red Cell pipette	
Diluting fluid: 40% formaldehyde	10 ml
Trisodium citrate (3% w/v)	990 ml
or	
Trisodium citrate	3.8 gms
Formalin	1 ml
Distilled water	99 ml
Neubauer's chamber with cover-slip.	

Technique

1. If oxalated blood is to be used, first mix it thoroughly by gentle shaking.

2. Fill the red cell pipette exactly upto 0.5 mark by holding the pipette almost horizontally. The pipette must be clean and dry.

3. Now draw in the diluting fluid upto the mark 101 (dilution 1 in 200). While filling the bulb the pipette should be gently rotated to obtain good mixing (Fig. 2).

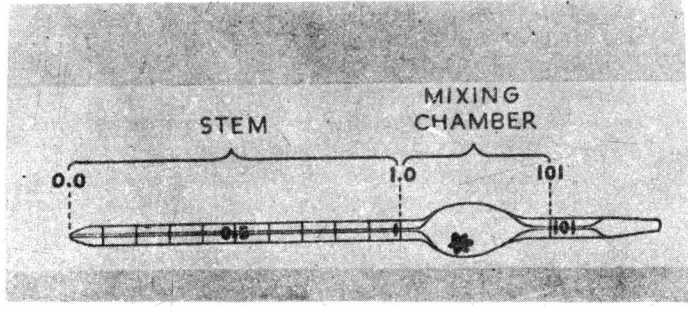

Fig. 2 R.B.C. pipette

4. The cover slip is placed over the Neubauer's chamber so as to cover both the ruled platforms evenly.

5. Now load the chamber. This is done in three steps:
   (a) Mix the contents of pipette for 3 minutes.
   (b) Expel 6 drops from the pipette to remove the fluid in the stem which has not been mixed with blood.
   (c) By holding the pipette at an angle of 45° and touching the space between the cover slip and the chamber by the point of the pipette, an appropriate drop of the mixture is allowed to run under the coverglass by capillary action; it must be sufficiently large to cover the whole ruled plateform yet not large enough to fill the moat. Also there must be no air bubbles.

6. Allow two minutes for setting of the cells and then count.

7. The count is done as follows:

In the erythrocytic count, the central double ruled square is used. Red cells lying in 80 very small squares have to be counted. These 80 small squares, comprise 5 medium sized squares, each of which is bound by a triple line (Fig. 3). It is recommended that the five medium sized squares chosen for counting cells should consist of four corners and one central; this is to secure an even distribution of cells. In counting, cells which touch the left hand lines or the upper lines of the square are taken to be within that square and those which touch the lower or right hand lines are omitted as outside the square.

To obtain accuracy at least 400 to 600 cells must be counted. If the count of the 80 small squares is less than this figure, more squares must be counted.

Calculation : The total area of the whole large central square is 1 sq mm. The smallest square has side of 1/20 mm so that its area is 1/400 sq mm and since the depth is 1/10 mm, its volume is 1/4000 cu mm. Total volume of 80 small squares is therefore 80/4,000 cumm = 1/50 cumm.

Dilution is 1 in 200

R.B.C. Count
= Dilution × 1/Voulme × Number of cells counted (N)
= 200 × 50 × N
= 10,000 × N cells/cumm.

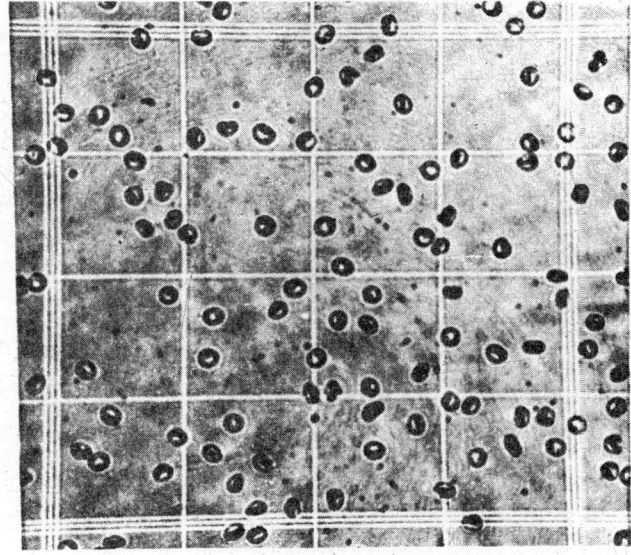

Fig. 3 Micro photograph showing R.B.C. in Neubauer Chamber

Sources of Error

1. Sampling error in collection of blood.
2. Equipment error in the pipette and haemocytometer.
3. Technical errors involved in the exercise from the filling of the pipette to the final count.
   Inherent or field errors of the distribution of cells in the counting chamber.

Normal Values

Men	$5.5 \pm 1.0 \times 10^{12}/l$
Women	$4.8 \pm 1.0 \times 10^{12}/l$
Infants (full term cord blood)	$5.0 \pm 1.0 \times 10^{12}/l$
Children 3 months	$4.0 \pm 1.0 \times 10^{12}/l$
Children 1 year	$4.4 \pm 0.8 \times 10^{12}/l$
Children, 3–6 years	$4.8 \pm 0.7 \times 10^{12}/l$
Children 10–12 years	$4.7 \pm 0.7 \times 10^{12}/l$

DETERMINATION OF PACKED RED CELL VOLUME (PCV) AND ABSOLUTE INDICES

Principle: An oxalated sample of the blood is centrifuged to pack red cells to the maximum. The volume of packed red cells is determined. The procedure is reliable because of its reproducibility.

Specimen: Though haematocrit determination (PCV) can be done on capillary blood (with the use of special haematocrit) venous blood is preferred. The blood must be oxalated with the special mixture of potassium and ammonium oxalate. The sample must be processed within two hours of collection.

Apparatus: The Wintrobe haematocrit tubes, pasteur pipettes and a centrifuge with a speed of 3000 r.p.m.

Procedure: The haematocrit tube must be clean and dry. Mix the oxalated sample of blood thoroughly by gently shaking for 3 minutes. With the pasteur pipette fill the haematocrit tube to the 10 mark. This is done by passing the pipette to the bottom of the haematocrit. There must be no air bubbles.

Fill a second haematocrit with either another sample of blood or with water. This tube is to counter balance the first one during centrifugation. Put the tubes in the centrifuge. Centrifuge at 3,000 r.p.m. for 30 minutes, preferably for 60 minutes. Take the reading of packed red cells. Recentrifuge for 5 minutes more at the same speed and take the reading again. There should be no difference between the two readings if the packing has been complete. If there is a difference, further centrifugation is indicated.

At the uppermost portion of packed red cells is seen a narrow dark band (due to reduced haemoglobin). The reading is made at the uppermost level of the band. Above the band will be seen a reddish grey layer of white cells. The volume of packed red cells read is for 10 ml. Multiply by 10 to get the value for 100. This value is the PCV. Normal range for adult males 43 to 54 per 100 ml of blood for adult females 37 to 47 per 100 ml of blood.

Calculation of MCV, MCH and MCHC (Absolute Indices):

$$\frac{MCV}{(\text{in cubic microns})} = \frac{PCV}{\text{RBCs in millions per cu mm}} \times 10$$

$$\frac{MCHC}{(\text{in per cent})} = \frac{\text{Hb in g per 100 ml}}{PCV} \times 100$$

$$\frac{MCH}{(\text{in picogms})} = \frac{\text{Hb in gm per 100 ml}}{\text{RBCs in millions per cu mm}} \times 10$$

CLINICAL USEFULNESS OF RED BLOOD CELL INDICES

Before electronic equipment became available less then 10 years ago, the RBC indices calculated after directly measuring the haemoglobin (Hb), the haematocrit (Hct) and the RBC count were:

$$MCV = \frac{Hct}{RBC} \qquad MCH = \frac{Hb}{RBC} \qquad MCHC = \frac{Hb}{Hct}$$

Now with the Coulter Counter type of automated equipment, a suspension of RBCs in a metered volume of electrolyte solution simply passes through a small orifice which is electrically charged. Since each RBC is a relative nonconductor, a change in the electrical charge occurs, which is then expressed as an RBC count. The magnitude of the charge change is proportional to the cell volume, and thus an MCV is derived as well. Finally, a haemoglobin is determined by an automated colorimetric method. Thus, only the Hb, MCV and RBC count are acutally measured, while the Hct, MCH, and MCHC are computed internallly using the above equations.

Normal Values for MCV, MCH, MCHC

The normal MCV in newborns is higher than at any other time of life, but beginning at a few months of age the MCV becomes lower than adult values. An MCV of 70, for example, may be normal for a 1 year old infant. This development change in MCV is paralleled by changes in the MCH. The MCHC is fairly constant throughout the life.

The Significance of the MCV

The MCV may be low, normal or high in various disorders, and specific diagnostic tests for anaemia should be based on clues provided by the MCV.

A. The Low MCV

Iron deficiency: The earliest changes in iron deficiency are a fall in bone marrow iron and a concomitant fall in serum ferritin. This is followed by a decrease in serum iron and rise in the quantity of RBC free erythrocyte porphyrin (FEP). The MCV then falls and finally the Hb drops. Currently, the MCV and the FEP are the most widely used screening tests for iron deficiency, but the serum ferritin may soon be both the screening and the diagnostic test.

Lead (Pb) poisoning: Microcytosis may be seen in lead poisoning but is not uniformly present, while a rise in FEP is almost invariably found. The FEP is now the standard screening test for Pb poisoning. The FEP tends to be much higher in Pb poisoning than in iron deficiency, although some overlap may exist.

Thalassemia minor: A low MCV is the hallmark of thalassemia minor, and the MCV may be used as a screening test of high sensitivity in the detection of beta thalassemia minor. In alpha thalassemia, the MCV on the average is slightly higher than in beta thalassemia. A Hb electrophoresis is best considered a confirmatory test for thalassemia.

A very simple calculation may be used to distinguish iron deficiency and lead poisoning from thalassemia minor based on the MCV and RBC count. The RBC count falls in iron deficiency and Pb poisoning but is normal in thalassemia minor. If the MCV is divided by the RBC count, a discriminate index is obtained where:

$$\frac{MCV}{RBC} < 12 = \text{Thalassemia minor}$$

$$\frac{MCV}{RBC} > 14 = \text{Iron deficiency or Pb poisoning}$$

Values between 12–14 are indiscriminate. Since these formulae are correct 95% of the time, a more rational selection of confirmatory tests is possible.

Miscellaneous: Other causes of microcytosis are much less common but include the anaemia of chronic disorders (this is usually normocytic, but 10 per cent are microcytic), severe protein malnutrition, sideroblastic anaemia, and copper deficiency.

B. Normocytic Anaemia

Anaemia with a normal MCV is usually caused by bone marrow failure, recent blood loss, or haemolysis.

C. The High MCV

Unlike in adults, macrocytosis in a child should not call B_{12} deficiency to mind first. The causes of a high MCV include:

1. Normal newborn: All normal newborns are macrocytic. In fact, an MCV of 94 or less should suggest a diagnosis of alpha thalassemia minor, the most common cause of microcytosis in newborns.

2. Reticulocytosis: Reticulocytes are very large and, when averaged with more mature RBCs, may produce a high MCV. A review of the peripheral blood smear will show that an elevated MCV is merely a reflection of young RBCs.

3. Down's syndrome: In Down's syndrome, the MCV averages 10 fl higher than normal.

4. Liver disease: This will deposit excessive lipids on the RBC, producing enlargement.

5. Hypothyroidism: A low T_4 commonly produces large speculated and targeted RBC.

6. Drugs: Any drug such as methotrexate which alters the DNA synthesis causes macrocytosis.

7. Folate deficiency

8. B_{12} deficiency: B_{12} and folate deficiency, in addition to producing macrocytosis, will cause hypersegmentation of neutrophils, distinguishing them from other causes of macrocytosis.

9. Miscellaneous: Other causes include preleukemic states and congenital pure RBC aplasia (Blackfan-Diamond syndrome).

Alterations of MCH and MCHC

Since the MCH falls as the Hb falls, relatively little information is obtained from the MCH itself. The same is somewhat true of a low MCHC, which adds nothing to what is already known from the MCV. A high MCHC is important to recognize, since it indicates that the haemoglobin content of the RBC is being very tightly packed. A high MCHC almost invariably means spherocytes are present and suggests such diagnosis as hereditary spherocytosis, ABO incompatibility, autoimmune haemolytic anaemia, and occasionally microangiopathic haemolytic anaemias.

Table 1

	MCV (fl)	MCH (pg)	MCHC
Normal adult	90 ± 10	31 ± 4	34 ± 3
Normal newborn	119 ± 9.0	36 ± 2	32 ± 2
Ages 10–17 mo	77 ± 7	26.1 ± 2.8	34.2 ± 1.6
18–48 mo	80 ± 6	27.0 ± 3.0	33.6 ± 1.4
4–7 yr	81 ± 5	27.6 ± 2.4	33.6 ± 1.6

ERYTHROCYTE SEDIMENTATION RATE (ESR)

If an anticoagulant is added to the blood and the specimen allowed to stand in a tube, red cells slowly sediment to the bottom of the tube leaving clear plasma as the supernatant. The rate of sedimentation estimated under standard conditions is known as the erythrocyte sedimentation rate (ESR). Sedimentation takes place in three stages:
1. Formation of rouleaux.
2. Sinking of rouleaux.
3. Packing of the rouleaux.

Influencing Factors

1. Difference in specific gravity between red cells and plasma.
2. The extent to which the red cells form roulex, which sediment more rapidly than single cells.
3. The ratio of red cells to plasma i.e. the PCV.
4. Plasma viscosity.
5. Verticality or otherwise of the sedimentation tube.
6. The bore of the tube.
7. Dilution, if any, of the blood.

Methods of Estimation

1. Wintrobe Method

Wintrobe Tube: Length — 110 mm
Diameter — 3.0 mm
Graduation of lower 100 mm from 0-100

Anticoagulant used: Double oxalate

Method: The tube is filled upto the 100 mm mark, allowed to stand in a vertical position at the room temperature, read the fall of red cells at the end of one hour (Fig. 4).

Advantage: Can be used for
1. Packed cell volume.
2. Buffy coat preparation.

2. Westergren Method

Westergren tube: Length — 300 mm
Diameter — 2.5 mm
Graduation in mm from 0 to 200

Anticoagulant used: 3.13% sodium citrate solution (0.106M) 0.5 ml of anticoagulant is used for 2 ml blood.

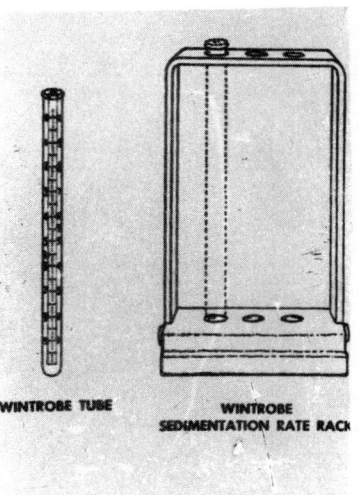

WINTROBE TUBE   WINTROBE SEDIMENTATION RATE RACK

Fig. 4 Wintrobe tube and Rack for E.S.R

Method: The mixture is drawn into a Westergren tube upto the zero mark and the tube set upright in a stand with a spring clip on top and rubber at bottom.

The level of the top of the red cell column is read at the end of 1 hour.

Precautions

1. The tubes must be scrupulously clean.
2. They must be filled properly without air bubbles.
3. They must be kept vertically.
4. Anaemia, if present will raise the ESR, irrespective of the primary condition.

Normal Values

Wintrobe Method: Men — 0 to 9 mm in 1st hour
Women — 0 to 20 mm in 1st hour
Westergren Method: Men — 0 to 5 mm in 1st hour
Women — 0 to 7 mm in 1st hour

Corrected ESR

The corrected ESR is needed to eliminate the influence of anaemia on sedimentation rate. the rate is then corrected according to the volume of cells by referring to chart for correction (Graph 1).

Find the horizontal line which represents the sedimentation in mm for 1st hour. Follow this across the chart until it intersects the vertical line which represents the blood cell volume per cent. Follow the nearest curved line until it intersects the heavy line at 42% per 100 ml, if the patient is female, or the line at 47% if the patient is male. Then, at the point of intersection, read the value on the horizontal line for the corrected sedimentation rate. The normal average sedimentation in one hour by this method is 9.6 mm for healthy female (0–20 mm) and 0–9 mm for healthy

Total Leucocyte Count (TLC)

Specimen: The leucocyte count may be done on oxalated blood or capillary blood. In the former case the sample must be examined within 6 hours of collection.

Graph 1

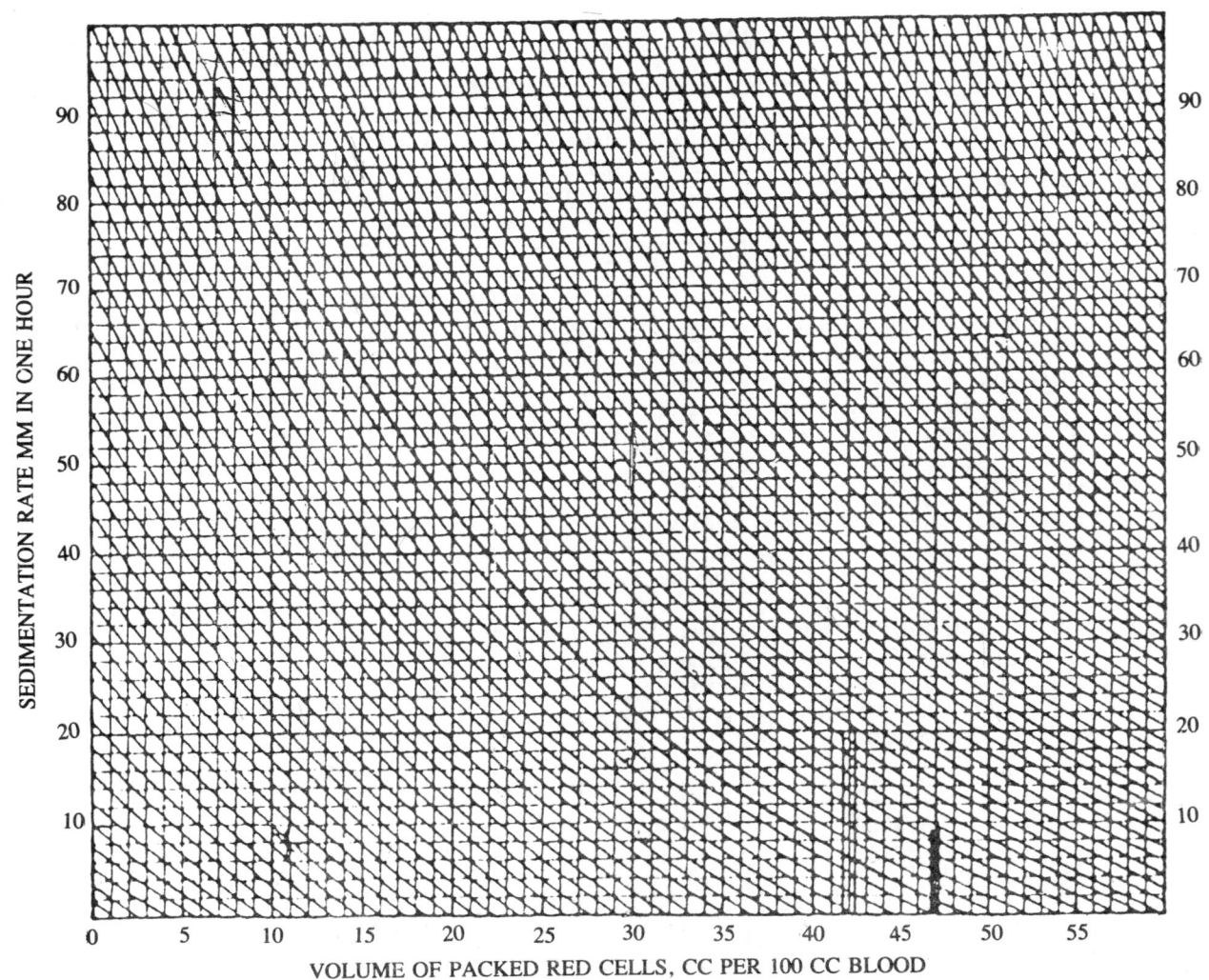

Apparatus

— A white cell pipette (white lead).
— Diluting fluid — 4% acetic acid with two drops of gention violet per litre.
— Neubauer's chamber with covership.
— Microscope.

Procedure

1. Draw blood in a clean dry pipette upto the mark 0.5 (Fig. 5) with all possible accuracy. The oxalated sample must be thoroughly mixed before use.
2. Wipe off the outside of the pipette with gauge.
3. Now draw the diluting fluid upto mark 11 (dilution 1 in 20). While drawing the fluid rotate the pipette.
4. Mix the contents of the pipette for 3 minutes.
5. Dispel the first 4 drops of the contents.
6. Adjust the Neubauer's chamber. It must be clean and dry. By holding the cover glass between the fingers at the edges, place

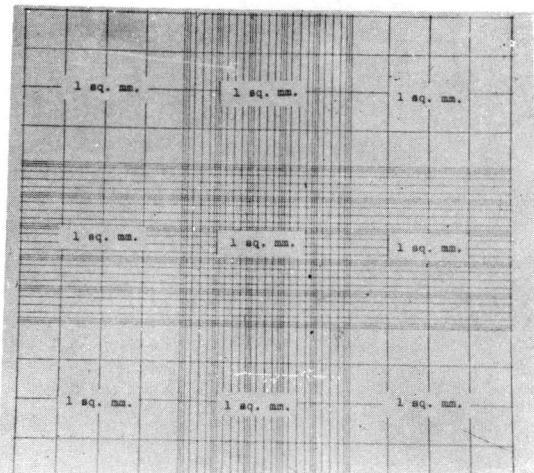

Fig. 6 Showing the ruled area of Neubauer Chamber

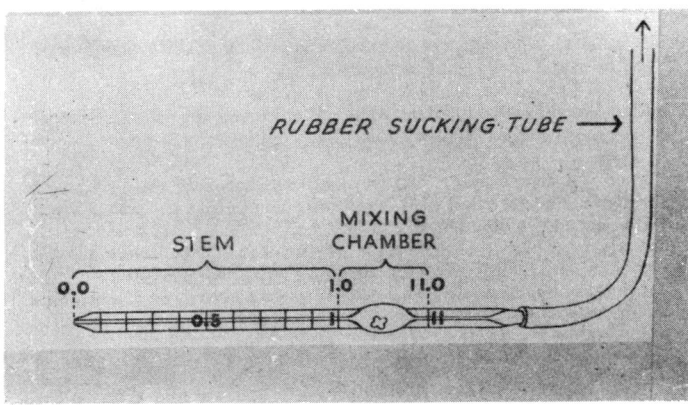

Fig. 5 White cell pipette with markings

it in such manner that both the ruled platforms are evenly covered by it. Load it with the mixture, by holding the pipette at angle of 45° and touching the space between the coverglass and the chamber by the point of the pipette, an appropriate drop of the mixture is allowed to run under the cover glass by capillary action. It must be sufficiently large to cover the whole ruled platform, yet not large enough to fill the moat. Also there must be no air bubbles.

7. Allow 2 minutes for setting of cells, then count.
8. The count is done as follows: The improved Neubauer chamber has two central platforms each of which is ruled. When the cover glass is in place there is a space of 0.1 mm depth over the ruled area. The surface of the ruled area is 3×3 mm (9 sq mm) (Fig. 6). Nine large squares can be recognised in the ruled area; the four corner squares are single ruled and the five central squares are double ruled. Each of the corner single ruled square is divided into 16 smaller squares (Fig. 7), the central double ruled square is divided into 400 very small squares. Each of the four large corner squres (with 16 small squares) has an area of 1 sq mm; each of the very small squares (400 in all) in the central square has an area of 1/400 sq mm. The central square is meant for the erythrocyte count; the four large corner squares are used for the leucocytic count. Fig. 8

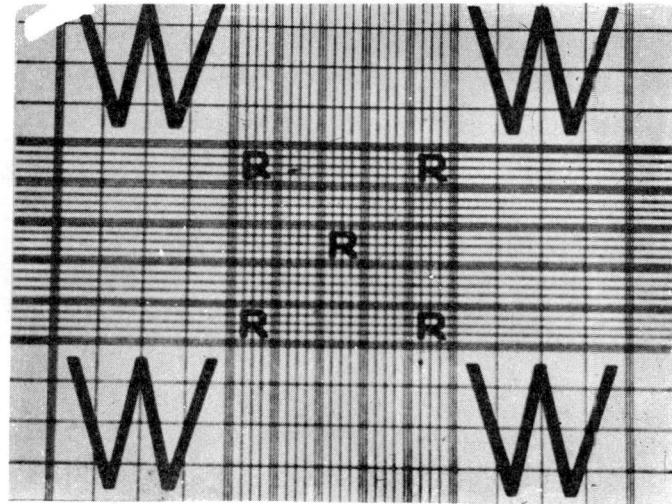

Fig. 7 Showing 'W' areas for white cell count

shows pattern of good and poor distribution of white blood cells and Fig. 9 shows procedure and score of counting. In counting, cells which touch the left hand lines or the upper lines of the square are taken to be within that square and those which touch the lower and right lines are omitted as outside the square. WBC. as viewed under low power magnification are shown in Fig. 10.

9. Calcualtion : The area of each large square is 1 sq mm, the depth of the chamber being 0.1 mm, the volume of the square is 0.1 cu mm.

Volume of four corner squares $= 0.1 \times 4 = 0.4$ cu mm

No. of cells in four corner squares $= N$
0.4 cu mm contains $= N$ cells.

$$1 \text{ cu mm contains} = \frac{N \times 20 \text{ (dilution factor)}}{0.4}$$

$$= N \times 50$$

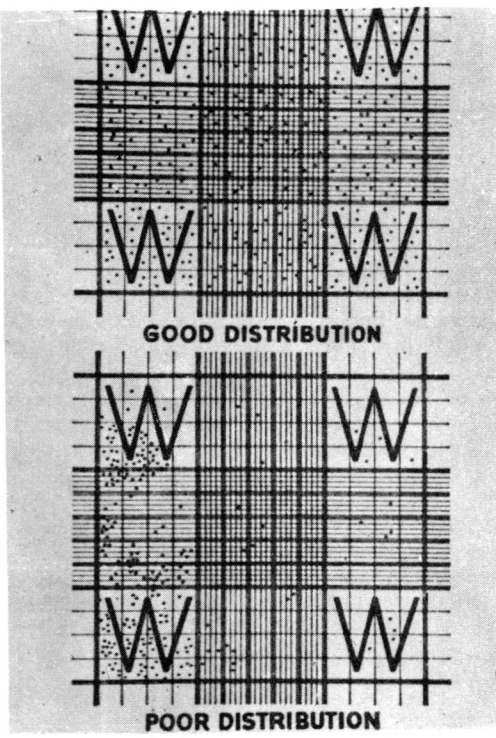

GOOD DISTRIBUTION

POOR DISTRIBUTION

Fig. 8 Showing pattern of good and poor distribution of W.B.C.

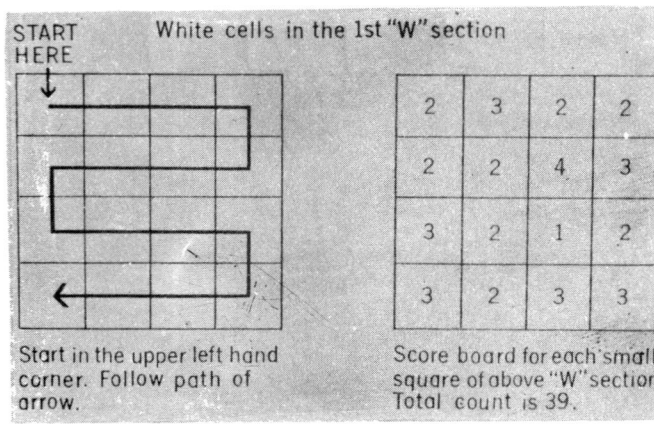

START HERE

White cells in the 1st "W" section

2	3	2	2
2	2	4	3
3	2	1	2
3	2	3	3

Start in the upper left hand corner. Follow path of arrow.

Score board for each small square of above "W" section Total count is 39.

Fig. Showing procedure and score of counting

Sources of Error

1. Sampling error in collection of blood.
2. Equipment error in the pipette and chamber.
3. Technical errors involved in the exercise from the filling of the pipette to the final count.
4. Inherent or field errors of the distribution of cells in the counting chamber. This can be minimised by counting large number of cells.

Range of T L C

Adults	$7.5 \pm 3.5 \times 10^3$/cu mm
Infants (full term 1st day)	$18 \pm 8 \times 10^3$/cu mm
Infants, 1 year	$12 \pm 6 \times 10^3$ cumm
Children 4–7 years	$10 \pm 5 \times 10^3$/cu mm
Children 8–12 years	$9 \pm 4.5 \times 10^3$/cu mm

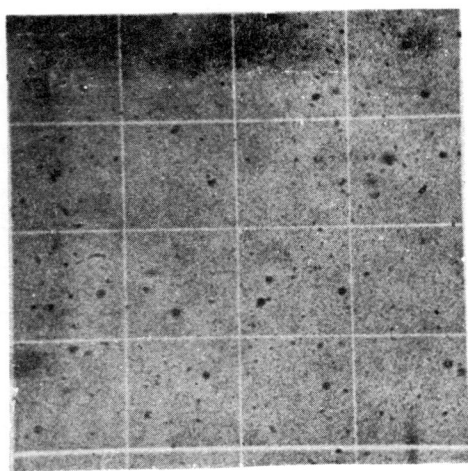

Fig. 10 W.B.C. as viewed under low power magnification ($\times 10$)

DIFFERENTIAL LEUCOCYTE COUNT (D.L.C.)

The slide should be chemically clean and wiped free from dust immediately before use.

The spreader

1. Should have a smooth edge.
2. Should be narrower in breadth than the slide on which film is to be made so that the edges of the film may be readily examined.
3. Should not be used for making more than six slides in succession without being cleaned.
4. Should be washed in running water and dried immediately after being used.

Preparation of Film

1. A small drop of blood is placed in the central line of a slide about 1–2 cm. from one end.
2. The spreader is placed at an angle of 45° to the slide and then moved back to make contact with the drop.
3. The drop should spread out quickly along the line of contact of the spreader with the slide (Fig. 11)
4. The moment this occurs the film should be spread by a rapid, smooth, forward movement of the spreader.
5. The drop should be of such size that the film is 3–4 cm in length

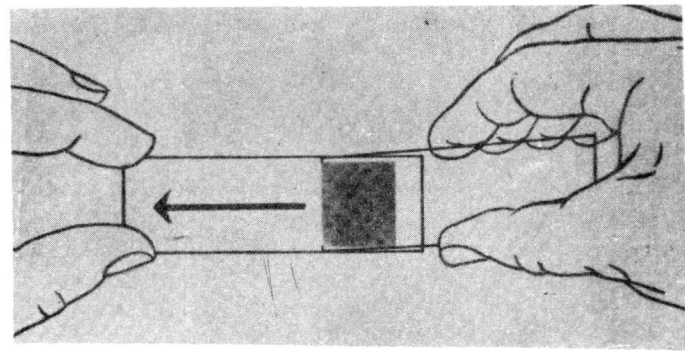

Fig. 11 Showing method of preparation of blood smear

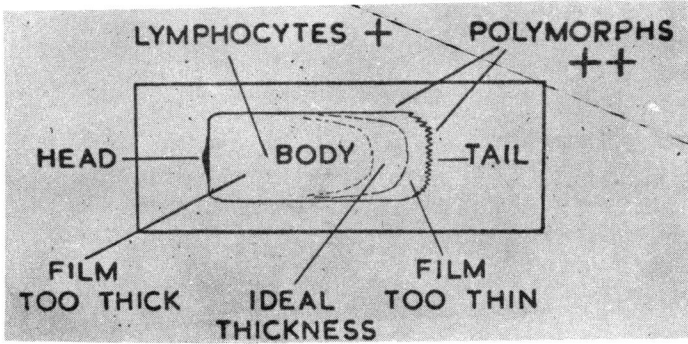

Fig. 12 Showing distribution of cells and parts of the smear

Qualities of a Good Film

1. Should not be too thin and the tail of the film should be smooth (Fig. 12).
2. There should be some overlap of the red cells, diminishing to separate near the tail.
3. The leucocytes in the body of the film should not be badly shrunken.

Procedure of Count

1. The cells should be counted using high power or oil immersion lens in a strip running the whole length of the film.
2. The lateral edges of the film are avoided.
3. The film should be inspected from the head to the tail.
4. If less than 100 cells are encountered in a single narrow strip, one or more additional strips should be examined until atleast 100 cells have been counted.
5. In patients with very high counts (as in leukemia) the cells should be counted in any well spread area where the cell types are easy to identify.

Sources of Error

If the film is made too thin or if a rough edged spreader is used many of the leucocytes, perhaps even 50% of them accumulate at the edges and in the tail. Moreover, a gross qualitative irregularity in distribution is the rule. Polymorphonuclear neutrophils and monocytes predominate at the margins and the tail and lymphocytes in the middle of the film. This separation probably depends upon differences in stickiness, size and specific gravity among the different classes of cells.

Giemsa Stain

Dissolve 3.75 gms powder stain in 375 ml methyl alcohol and then add 375 ml glycerol. Shake well. Keep in the incubator at 37°C for 4 days before use.

Phosphate Buffer *p*H 7.2
Solution A — 0.15 molar NaH_2PO_4, $2H_2O$ — 23.4 gms/litre
Solution B — 0.15 molar Na_2HPO_4 — 21.3 gms/litre
Mix solution A — 24.0 ml and solution B — 76.0 ml

Method of Staining

1. Air dried film is fixed in methanol for 2 minutes.
2. Pour Giemsa stain diluted 1:9 with buffer over the smear for 8–10 mintues.
3. Wash with buffer and dry.

Normal Differential Leucocyte Count (ADULTS)

Neutrophils	— 40–75%
Lymphocytes	— 20–45%
Monocytes	— 2–10%
Eosinophils	— 1–6%
Basophils	— 0–1%

Leishman Stain

0.15% in methyl alcohol.

Method of Staining

1. Pour enough stain on the smear to cover it fully.
2. Allow to act for 2 minutes.
3. Add twice the quantity of buffer to the stain.
4. Avoid overflow and suck the mixture in and out with the pipette to ensure thorough mixing. A scum will form on the smear.
5. Allow the diluted stain to act for 5 minutes.
6. Wash the smear.
7. Wipe to clean the back of the smear & allow it to dry and see.

When the white cell count rises above the normal values, it is referred to as leucocytosis.

When the white cell count drops below the normal values, it is referred to as leucopenia.

Some conditions where these abnormalities may be expected are listed in Table 2.

ABSOLUTE EOSINOPHIL COUNT

Eosinophil Diluting Fluid: (Dunger's solution)

Stock Solution

Eosin Yellow — 0.5 gm
Formaldehyde (40%) — 0.5 ml
Phenol (95%) (Aqueous) — 0.5 ml
Distilled water upto — 100 ml

Table 2. Conditions Accompanied by Abnormal White Cell Counts

High White Cell Count (leucocytosis)	Low White Cell Count (leucopenia)
appendicitis	measles
pneumonia	influenza
leukemia	brucellosis
tonsillitis	typhoid fever
meningitis	agranulocytosis
abscesses	infectious hepatitis
rheumatic fever	lupus erythematosus
diphtheria	cirrhosis of liver
smallpox	paratyphoid fever
chickenpox	protein therapy
peritonitis	radiation
erythroblastosis fetalis	myxedema
uremia	psittacosis
ulcers	sandfly fever
newborn	scrub typhus
pregnancy	dengue
menstruation	rheumatoid arthritis

Working Solution

6 ml of stock solution diluted with distilled water upto 100 ml.

Procedure: Suck blood upto 0.5 mark in a W B C pipette and dilute upto 11 mark with the diluting fluid. Gently rotate the pipette. Discard first 3 or 4 drops of fluid. Charge the neubauer counting chamber and allow it to stand for 3 minutes, so that the cells settle down.

Count all the eosinophils in the whole of the ruled area (i.e. 9 squares).

Calculation

ABSOLUTE EOSINOPHIL COUNT

$$= N \times 1/\text{Volume} \times \text{Dilution}$$

Volume $= \text{Length} \times \text{breadth} \times \text{depth}$
$$= 3 \times 3 \times .1 = 0.9 \text{ cumm}$$
$$= N \times \frac{1}{0.9} \times 20$$
$$= \frac{N \times 10 \times 20}{9} = \frac{N \times 200}{9}$$
$$= N \times 22.2/\text{cumm}$$

Normal value = (40–440 cells cumm.)

PLATELET COUNT

Direct Method

Specimen: Venous blood is collected by a clean puncture and delivered without frothing into a bottle or a tube containing the anti coagulant dipotassium EDTA. EDTA prevents the clumping of platelet or it may by collected by finger prick. Venous blood is preferred.

Procedure

1. Draw the blood into a clean dry R B C pipette upto the mark 0.5. The accuracy in filling the pipette has to be of high order.
2. Wipe off the outside of the pipette.
3. Draw the diluting fluid upto the mark 101.

   The diluting fluid (Rees-Ecker) has the following formula:

Sodium citrate	3.8 g
Brilliant cresyl blue	0.05 g
Neutral formalin	0.65 ml
Distilled water	100 ml

   Filter and centrifuge at 2.800 r.p.m. for 30 minutes. Stock the solution in a refrigerator in a well stoppered bottle and filter before use every time.

   Another good diluent is the formol citrate solution used for red cell count.
4. Shake the pipette for 5 mintues.
5. Discard the first 4 drops. Load the chamber; both the haemocytometer and the cover-slip must be scrupulously clean.
6. Allow the preparation to stand for 15 minutes in a moist chamber. An inverted petridish with a piece of wet filter paper in the top makes a good moist chamber.
7. Count under the high power with the light partially cut off. **Platelets are lilac-coloured. Count at least 300 platelets and** calculate by the formula.

$$\frac{\text{No. of platelets counted} \times 10 \times \text{dilution}}{\text{No. of 1 mm squares counted}} = \text{Platelets per cu mm}$$

Normal value — 1,50,000 to 4,00,000 cells/cu mm

RETICULOCYTE COUNT

Reticulocytes are young red cells which contain basophilic ribo-nucleoprotein but no nucleus. With Romanowsky stains they may show:—
1. Diffuse basophilia (Polychromasia)
2. Punctate basophilia
3. Filaments in the cells (Skein cells)

Basophilic ribo-nucleo-proteins (RNA) reacts with brilliant cresyl blue to form blue precipitate of granules or filaments. They take 1–2 days to ripe to mature RBC in spleen or peripheral blood. In smear they may be confused with:—
1. Papenheimer bodies which usually contain single dot like granular material & stain darker blue shade.
2. Heinz bodies stain lighter blue as compared to reticulocytes.

Staining Solution

Brilliant cresyl blue	1.0 gm
Sodium Carbonate (Anhydrous)	400 gm
Normal Saline	100 ml

First dissolve dye in Normal saline then add sodium carbonate. Mix and Filter the stain and keep at room temp

Procedure

Put 3–4 drops of staining solution in a small test tube. Add equal amount of oxalated or E D T A blood. Mix and keep in incubator at 37°C for 15–20 minutes. After that, gently mix the solution and prepare smears. If patient is anaemic, add more blood. If patients is polycythaemic, add less blood. Films are examined without fixing or counter staining, under oil imersion.

Calculation

Count 100 reticulocytes
For example — No. of reticulocyte in 150 fields = 100
Total No. of red cells in 150 fields = 3,000
Therefore, Reticulocyte % $= \frac{100 \times 100}{3000} = 3.3\%$

Normal Range

Adults and children	0.2 –2.0%
Newborn infants	2.0 – 6.0%

Decreased Reticulocyte Count

In aplastic anaemia and in conditions where the bone marrow is not producing red blood cells.

Increased Reticulocyte Count

In haemolytic anaemias, iron deficiency anaemias receiving iron therapy, thalassemia, sideroblastic anemias, and acute and chronic blood loss.

CHAPTER 2

NORMAL AND ABNORMAL HAEMOPOIESIS

NORMAL ERYTHROPOIESIS

In the adult normal erythropoiesis is described as "normoblastic". According to the monophyletic theory, the various cells concerned in normoblastic erythropiesis are the haemocytoblast, the pro-erythroblast, three types of normoblasts, the reticulocyte and the mature erythrocyte.

1. Haemocytoblast

A large cell, 18 to 24 microns in diameter, a large nucleus fills almost the whole cell; two or more nucleoli; cytoplasm agranular and stained dark blue. The cell is not readily identifiable, either by morphological or histochemical criteria.

2. Pro-erythroblast (Pro-normoblast):

Formed by differentiation from the haemocytoblast; measures 14 to 19 microns (2 to 3 times the mature erythrocyte); a large round nucleus fills three fourths of the cell; nuclear chromatin delicate with a reticulated pattern; nucleoli present; cytoplasm agranular and deep blue (non-haemoglobinised with a high content of ribonucleoprotein).

3. Early normoblast (basophilic normoblast type I):

Formed from the pro-erythroblast by division; measures 11 to 17 microns: nucleus large but without neucleoli; nuclear chromatin coarse and shows some lumps due to condensation; cytoplasm agrangular and blue (non-haemoglobinised).

4. Intermediate normoblast (polychromatophilic normoblast type II):

Formed by division from the early normoblast; measures 10 to 14 microns; nucleus smaller than that of the precursor and nuclear chromatin coarser with many lumps; cytoplasm bluish red (partial haemoglobinisation) (Fig. 13).

5. Late normoblast (Orthochromatic normoblast type III):

Formed by ripening of the intermediate normoblast; measures 7 to 10 microns (a little larger than the mature erythrocyte); nuclear chromatin very coarse, almost lumpy; cytoplasm red (fully haemoglobinised).

6. Reticulocyte

The smear has been stained supravitally by brilliant cresylblue. A non-nucleated cell of the size of a mature erythrocyte or a little larger, cytoplasm shows a network of reticulum stained blue (basophilic ribonucleoprotein).

7. Mature erythrocyte

Measure 7.2 microns in diameter, non-nucleated, biconcave disc, cytoplasm stained almost uniformly red with a faint central pallor.

ABNORMAL ERYTHROPOIESIS

1. Early megaloblast

A large cell, 3 to 4 times the size of a red cell; nucleus large, occupying three-fourths of the cytoplasm; nucleoli present; nuclear chromatin has a stippled appearance; cytoplasm blue (non-haemoglobinised). Note the resemblance to pro-erythroblast. The distinction made by the nuclear appearance).

2. Intermediate or polychromatic megaloblast

Smaller than the basophilic precursor; cytopasm purplish-red (haemoglobin has appeared).

3. Late or orthochromatic megaloblast

The cell is one and a half to two and a half times red cell; nucleus small and shrunken; clumps of chromatin but still a stippled appearance at places; no nucleoli; cytoplasm red (haemoglobinised).

4. Haemoglobinis megaloblast

The cytoplasm is red but otherwise it has all the features of an early megaloblast. Such a cell is considered very characterstic of Addisonian pernicious anaemia.

5. Macrocytes

The red cells have an increased diameter; the central pallor is absent.

ABNORMALITIES OF ERYTHROCYTES

Size: With some experience it is possible to say if the red cells are of normal size (normocytosis), diminished in size (microcytosis) or increased in size (macrocytosis). One judges the size by the diameter (normal average: 7.2 microns). In severe anaemia there is variation in the size of cells; this is anisocytosis. Megalocytes are large oval cells found in megaloblastic anaemias (Figs. 14 & 15).

Shape: Red cells with an irregular shape are called poikilocytes. The commonest irregularity is a pearshaped cell. Poikilocytosis, like anisocytosis, is a non-specific phenomenon found in all severe anaemias. In haemolytic anaemias the red cells are abnormally thick; they look like densely stained microcytes; the abnormality is known as microspherocytosis. Target cells are thin red cells with a relatively large diameter and resemble the concentric circles of a rifle target; they are seen in various anaemias, in obstructive jaundice and after splenectomy. Sickle-cells may be seen in stained smears; their presence, diagnostic of sickle-cell disease due to the abnormal haemoglobin S, is best demonstrated by special in-vitro technique. Burr cell with spiny periphery; they are seen in large number in uraemia. Schistocytes are red cell fragments found in many blood diseases with increased haemolysis (Fig. 16).

Colour: The intensity of the red colour of the erythrocyte in a stained smear is a rough indication of corpuscular haemoglobin concentration. In a hypochromic red cell the normal central pallor is increased. Hypochromasia indicates iron-deficiency.

Immature red cells: Immature red cells in the peripheral blood can only come from the marrow.

The correct significance of immature red cells in the peripheral blood can be best realised by studying their source, erythropoiesis in the marrow by means of marrow, biopsy. Abnormal erythropoiesis is called "Meagaloblastic" and is due to the deficiency of vitamin B_{12} or folic acid, or both.

Only common findings are referred to in what follows: Polychromasia (Polychromatophilia) is diffuse bluish-grey staining of the red cell. Basophilic stippling is the presence of multiple coarse granules in the red cell. Cells which show polychromatophilia and basophilic stippling are reticulocytes and their presence is indicative of active erythropoiesis, as in haemolytic anaemias; Pappenheimer bodies are small scanty basophilic granules in the red cell; unlike the granules of basophilic stippling, these bodies give a positive prussian blue reaction; they are siderophilic granules. Pappenheimer bodies are characteristically present after splenectomy. Cells with pappenheimer bodies or siderophil granules are known as siderocytes. Cabbot's rings are reddish purple rings or like the figure of eight. Howell-Jolly bodies are reddish blue nucleated fragments. Cabbot's rings and Howell-Jolly bodies are seen in severe anaemias and after splenectomy. They have no specific-significance (Fig. 17).

The nucleated red cell commonly encountered in the peripheral blood is the normoblast. An occasional normoblast is a normal finding in the newborn. A few normoblasts 2 to 5 per 100 leucocytes may be present in any severe anaemia. If present in large numbers, a haemolytic anaemia with an actively regenerating marrow is suspected. The presence of a megaloblast in the peripheral blood means that erythropoiesis must be megaloblastic and that the patient must be suffering from a megaloblastic anaemia.

NORMAL LEUCOPOIESIS

1. Cells of the myeloid or the granular series are produced normally only in the marrow.
2. Cells of the lymphoid series arise in the marrow to a small extent; their chief source is the lymphoid tissue of the body; lymph nodes and lymphoid tissue of the tonsils, the pharynx, the gastro-intestinal tract, the spleen and the thymus.
3. Cells of the monocytic series are probably derived from the reticulum cells of the marrow and the spleen. However, some consider myeloblasts and even lymphocytes as their ancestors.

a. Myeloid Series

1. **Myeloblast:** A large cell, measuring 11 to 18 microns (2 to 3 times the mature erythrocyte), nucleus round or oval, eccentric and with fine reticulated chromatin, 2 to 5 nucleoli, cytoplasm light blue, agranular, cytoplasm may show "Auer bodies" (red, rod-like structures) (Fig. 18).
2. **Promyelocyte:** Like the myeloblast nuclear chromatin coarser, nucleoli present, cytoplasm shows azurophilic granules.
3. **Myelocyte:** Measures 10 to 14 microns; nucleus round, oval, or kideny shaped with coarse chromatin, no nucleoli, cytoplasm contains coarse specific granules.

a. Neutrophil Myelocyte	: granules fine and pale pink.
b. Eosinophil Myelocyte	: granules large and deep pink.
c. Basophil Myelocyte	: granules large and deep purple, obscure the nucleus.

4. **Metamyelocyte** (neutrophil metamyelocyte or juvenile): Like the myelocyte, but the nucleus is deeply indented.
5. **Band Cell** (neutrophil stab cell): Size of the mature segmented cell; nucleus narrow, ribbon-like and bent on itself; chromatin condensed.
6. **Segmented Cell** (polymorphonuclear cell): Size 10 to 12 microns; nucleus shows lobes connected by filaments; cytoplasm contains granules.

a. Neutrophil segmented	: Cytoplasmic granules fine and pale pink violet (Fig 19).
b. Eosinophil segmented	: Cytoplasmic granules coarse and pink; nucleus like a spectacle (Bilobed) (Fig. 20).
c. Basophil segmented	: Cytoplasmic granules large, deep purple and obscure the nucleus.

b. Lymphoid Series

1. **Lymphoblast:** Measures 15 to 20 microns (2 to 3 times the mature erythrocyte); resembles the myeloblast very much; nucleus round or oval with reticulated chromatin but coarser compared to that of a myeloblast; there is a distinct nuclear membrane with condensation of chromatin on its inner surface; one to three clear-cut nucleoli; cytoplasm agranular, bluish, no Auer bodies (Fig. 21).
2. **Large lymphocyte:** Measures 10 to 14 microns; nucleus large, round or indented with pale-stained chromatin; cytoplasm abundant and pale blue; cytoplasm may show azure granules stained reddish blue.
3. **Small lymphocyte:** Equal in size to the mature erythrocyte or smaller; a round nucleus filling the cell; chromatin condensed and dark-stained; scanty pale blue cytoplasm containing azure granules.

c. Monocytic Series

1. **Monoblast:** A large cell 14 to 20 microns (2 to 3 times the mature erythrocyte); cell border may be irregular as if pseudopodia are present; nucleus round, oval or kidney-shaped and convoluted, chromatin fine and reticulated; nucleoli present, cytoplasm abundant, bluish grey; may show Auer bodies; no cytoplasmic granules.
2. **Monocyte:** of the same size as the precursor; nuclear chromatin coarser, nucleus round, oval, kidney-shaped, or convoluted, usually no nucleoli, cytoplasm abundant, greyish-blue "like frosted glass" and contains fine reddish-blue granules (Fig. 22).

ABNORMALITIES OF LEUCOCYTES

These mainly consist of the presence of immature leucocytes and of granulocytes with toxic granulations. Normally an occasional metamyelocytes or juvenile cells (about 1 per cent) are present. In pyogenic infections (with leucocytosis) their count goes up. A few myelocytes are common in the blood of infants and children. In adults a few myelocytes and an occasional myeloblast (without leucocytosis) may be found in severe anaemias and when the marrow is the seat of metastatic deposits of a carcinoma. However, in chronic myeloid leukaemia, the blood shows a large number of myelocytes (10 to 50 per cent) and fewer myeloblasts (2 to 5 per cent). In acute myeloid leukaemia, the myeloblast is the predominant cell in the blood (upto 90 per cent). In chronic lymphatic leukaemia, the predominant cell in the blood is the small lymphocyte, forming 85–99 per cent of leucocytes; lymphoblasts are rare. In acute lymphatic leukaemia, the lymphoblast is the predominant cell. In monocytic leukaemia, 50 to 90 per cent of leucocytes are

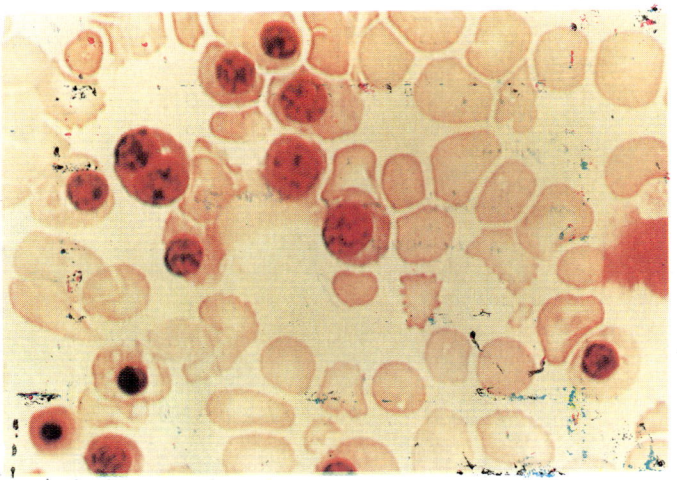

Fig. 13 Intermediate and late Normoblast

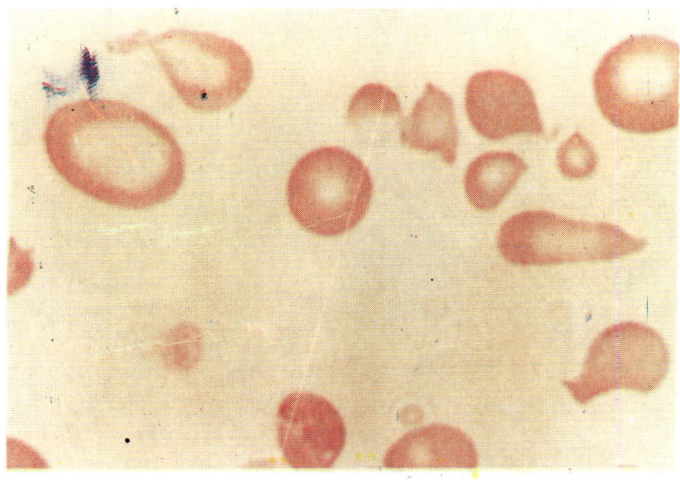

Fig. 15 Blood smear showing macrocytes

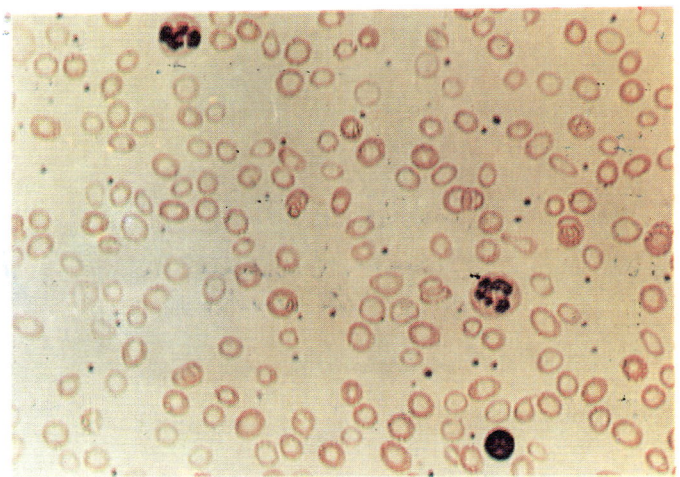

Fig. 14 Blood smear showing microcytes

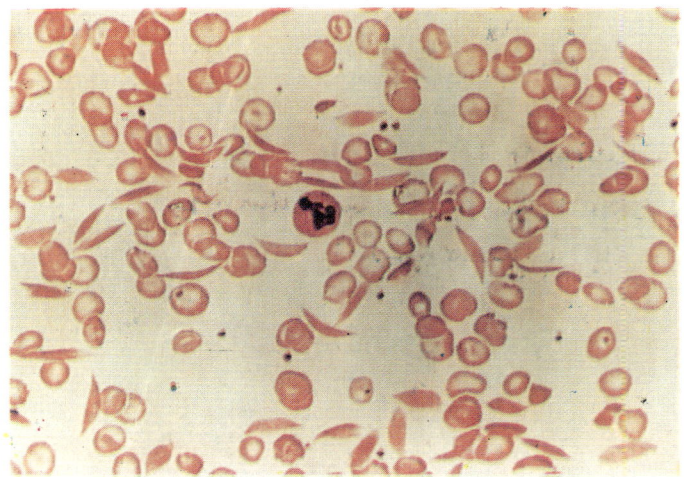

Fig. 16 Blood smear showing sickle cells

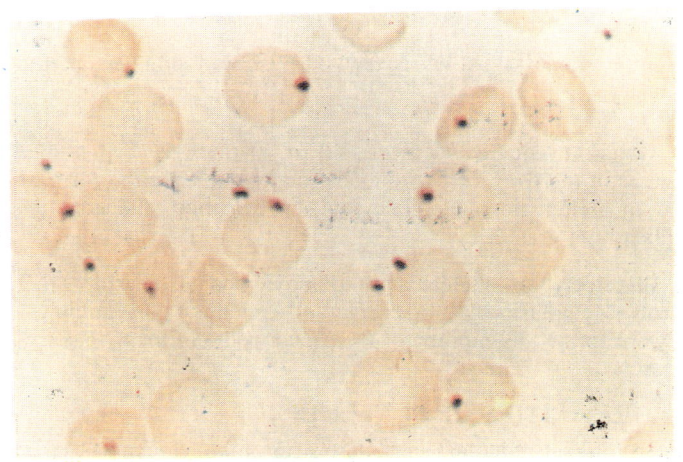

Fig. 17 Smear showing Howell-Jolly bodies

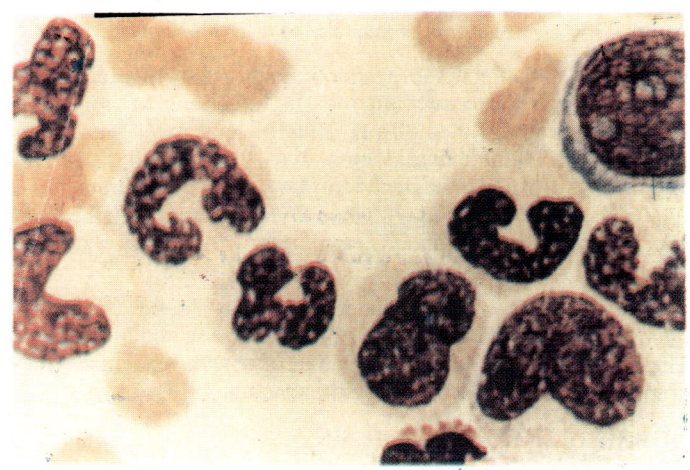

Fig. 18 Blood smear showing Myeloblast, Myelocyte,
Metamyelocyte and Band forms

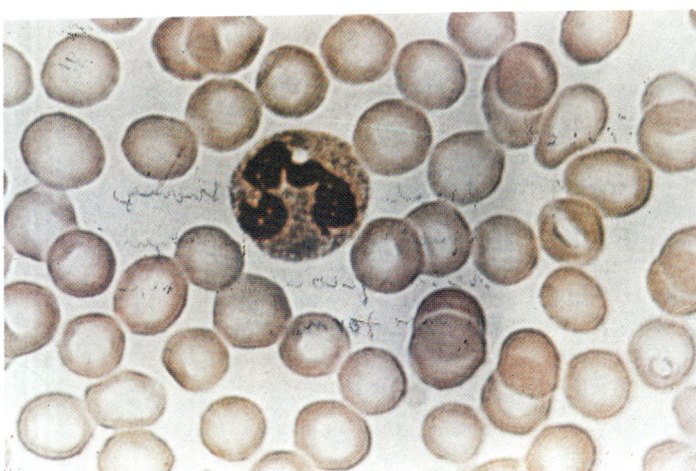

Fig. 19 Normal blood film showing polymorph

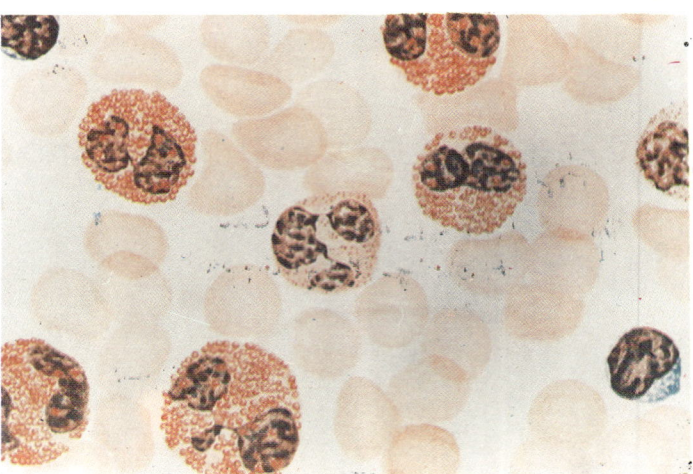

Fig. 20 Blood film showing Eosinophils

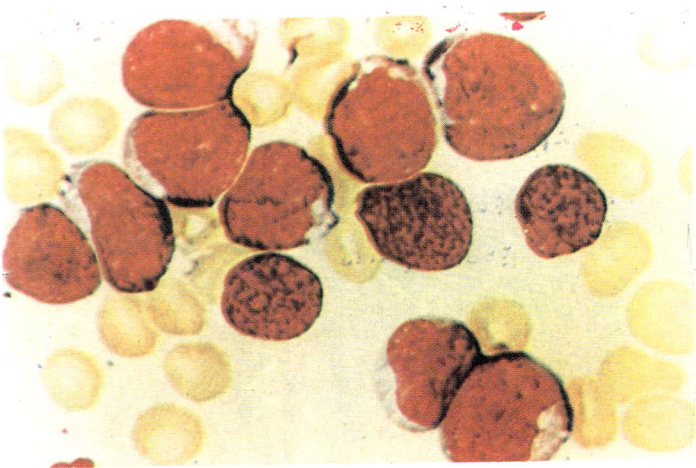

Fig. 21 Blood smear showing Lymphoblast

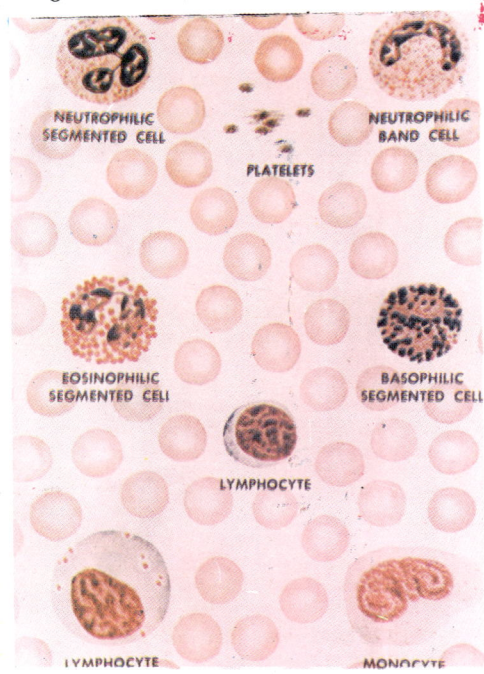

Fig. 22 Showing different types of leucocytes

monocytes and precursors (monoblasts), a few myelocytes and myeloblasts are also encountered. In Infectious Mononucleosis (Glandular lever), 40 to 80 per cents of leucocytes are ordinary lymphocytes, lymphocytoid monocytes "Abnormal cells". The last are primitive monocytes. Morphologically Infectious Mononucleosis can be confused with monocytic leukaemia; in the former the patient's serum contains agglutinins for sheep's red cells (Paul—Bunnel's test).

In severe acute infections, neutrophils may show vacuolation of the cytoplasm and their granules become coarse and blue-stained. These "toxic granules" are indicative of severe toxaemia. Heavy granulation is also seen in aplastic anaemias.

NORMAL THROMBOPOIESIS

1. **Megakaryoblast:** Measures 20 to 25 microns: nucleus single, oval or slightly indented; several nucleoli; cytoplasm scanty, blue and agranular.

2. **Promegakaryocyte:** Larger than the precursor; nucleus indented with coarser chromatin than that of the precursor; nucleoli

present; cytoplasm shows a few purplish red granules at the periphery.

3. **Megakarycocyte:** Measures 40 to 70 microns; cell border irregular in the form of pseudopods; many nuclei in the form of lobes in a ring; no nucleoli; cytoplasm pale blue and contains purplish-blue granules.

4. **Platelets:** Non-nucleated round or oval bodies; measure 2 to 3 microns; cytoplasm blue or purple and contains many granules. They are formed by nipping of the pseudopodia of the megakaryocytes.

ABNORMALITIES OF PLATLETS

A significant reduction of platelets (thrombocytopenia) can be judged in the smear. In essential thrombocytopenia, platelets may in addition show morphological abnormalities in the forms e.g. small size, giant forms or non-granularity of their cytoplasm. Abnormal variation in the size of platelets is a feature of myelosclerosis.

CHAPTER 3

ANAEMIA

ANAEMIA

Anaemia is a state in which the amount of haemoglobin or the number of red cells in the blood is below the normal limits. The red cell which is the carrier of haemoglobin has a limited life-span. To maintain haemoglobin and red cells within the normal limits new fully haemoglobinised red cells must be produced to replace the lost ones. Anaemia will, therefore ncessarily result (i) if the production of red cells is inadequate in quality or quantity, (2) if red cell destruction or blood loss exceeds the production, or (3) if these two factors combine. Anaemia is thus a symptom or sign of either of the two events mentioned above; it is not a disease. The objective behind investigating a case of anaemia is to unearth the underlying mechanism, to discover the cause of the imbalance between the production and the destruction of the red cell.

MECHANISM OF PRODUCTION OF ANAEMIA

The mechanism is three folds (1) diminished erythropoiesis (dyshaemopoietic anaemias), (2) blood loss (haemorrhagic anaemias); and (3) increased haemolysis (haemolytic anaemias). Diminshed erythropoiesis (dyshaemopoiesis) is either due to nutritional deficiency or due to marrow failure. Nutritional factors essential for erythropoiesis are: iron, traces of copper, cobalt, vitamin B complex (vitamin B 12, folic acid, pyridoxine, riboflavin and nicotinic acid), vitamin C, first class proteins, or possibly some internal secretions (thyroid, pituitary, sex hormones) and pigments (bile pigments and chlorophyll). The deficiency of these factors may be dietetic or due to defective absorption, or due to increased demands (pregnancy or period of growth). Dietetic defiency is a common cause of nutritional anaemias in our country. Failure of marrow (resulting in aplastic or hypoplastic anaemias) may be primary (idiopathic) or due to extraneous toxic factors (chemicals, drugs and irradiations). Blood loss may be acute or chronic and brought about by trauma or disease.

Table 3 *Classification of Anaemia Based on Pathophysiologic Factors*

Anaemia due to blood loss
Acute blood loss (external and internal bleeding)
Chronic blood loss (gastrointestinal, reproductive and urinary tract)
Fetal and perinatal blood loss.
Anaemia due to excessive destruction of red cells
Hereditary (elliptocytosis, spherocytosis, enzyme deficiencies, haemoglobinopathies)
Acquired (isoantibodies, autoantibodies, drug or chemically induced, mechanical and traumatic, infections, hypersplenism, paroxysmal nocturnal haemoglobinuria)
Anaemia due to decreased production of red cells
Nutritional deficiencies (inadequate nutritional intake; Fe, vitamin B_{12}, folate deficiency; defective absorption)
Bone marrow failure (endocrine, idiopathic, myelophthisic, toxic)

Increased haemolysis may be due to hereditary intracorpusular defects (spherocytosis, sickling) reducing the life-span of the red cell, or may be acquired and due to the action of haemolytic agents (physical, chemical, bacterial and antibodies)

In the aetiological diagnosis of anaemia the following points are important; the family history regarding anaemia, jaundice and bleeding in other members of the family; the personal history regarding dietary habits, occupation (contact with chemicals), drugs and chronic bleeding from any site; the physical examination (to detect lymphadenopathy, hepatosplenomegaly, and evidence of deficiency states); ancillary examinations like roentgenography and laboratory investigations.

Moderate anaemia may not be detectable by the physical examination. Two laboratory screening Procedures are available to decide the issue (1) estimation of haemoglobin and (2) haematocrit determination. In an adult haemoglobin below 12 gm per 100 ml. or P.C.V. below 37 per 100 ml indicates the presence of anaemia. If both haemoglobin estimation and determination of P.C V. are carried out, they are a check against one another.

The basic study consists of the cytological examination of the blood; this includes the determination of haemoglobin, the enumeration of red cells and leucocytes (with the reticulocyte count and platelet count in special cases), the differential count and the examination of the stained smear. The levels of haemoglobin and red cells will tell about the severity of the anaemic state and the examination of the smear will give information about the size of the red cell, its haemoglobin concentration and the presence of abnormal red cells. To know the morphologic type of anaemia with exactitude the first step is haematocrit determination which gives the corpuscular volume of the packed cell (P.C.V.) per 100 ml. of the blood. From P.C.V., haemoglobin in g per 100 ml and red cell per c mm, two values most essential for the morphologic typing of anaemias can be calculated. These are the mean corpuscular volume (M.C.V.) and the mean corpuscular haemoglobin concentration (M.C.H.C.)

The M.C.V. and the M.C.H.C. are absolute values based on actual figures obtained in a given patient and do not involve correlation with arbitrarily fixed normals as in the case of "indices" like the color index. The M.C.V. is sensitive indicator of the size of the red cell, except in case of spherocytosis where the diameter and the volume of the red cells do not preserve their normal relationship. The M.C.H.C. is a sensitive indicator of the haemoglobin saturation of the red cells with reference to its volume. A lowered M.C.H.C. — hypochromia means red cells are unsaturated and, therefore, is an indication for iron therapy.

An increase in the M.C.H.C. so called hyperchromia is a physiological impossibility. The following table shows the morphologic classification of anaemias on the basis of the M.C.V. and the M.C.H.C.

Table 4 *Anaemias: Common Morphologic Types And Their Causes*

Types of Anaemia	M.C.V. (fl) C. microns	M.C.H.C. percentage	Common Cause
1. Macrocytic normochromic	more than 94	more than 30	Deficiency of vitamin B12 or of folic acid; some times aplastic and haemolytic anaemia.
2. Macrocytic hypochromic	'More than' 94	'Less than' 30	Deficiency of Vitamin B12 or of folic acid plus iron.
3. Normocytic normochromic	Between 78–94	'Between' 30–33	'Haemorrhagic anaemias haemolytic Anaemias; hypolastic and aplastic Anaemias.
4. Microcytic normochromic	'Below' 78	'Between' 30–33	Anaemia due to infections.
5. Microcytic hypochromic	below 78	below 30	Deficiency or lack of iron.

IRON DEFICIENCY ANAEMIA

Characteristically the anaemia is microcytic (M.C.V. <74 c. microns) and hypochromic (M.C.H.C. <30 per cent). Proportionately haemoglobin is reduced much more than the red cell count. The smear of the peripheral blood shows red cells that are smaller than normal and poorly filled with haemoglobin so that the normal central pallor is exaggerated. In severe cases a few normoblasts may be present. The reticulocyte count is low. The leucocytes and platelets are reduced. The marrow shows normoblastic hyperplasia and the nucleated red cells show depletion of siderotic granules. The plasma iron is below 100μg./100 ml; in advanced cases it is below 35 μg. There is a specific orderly response to iron therapy. The common causes of iron-lack anaemia are: (1) increased demands for iron (period of rapid-growth, pregnancy) and (2) iron loss exeeding absorptin (chronic blood loss and malabsorption). In every case of iron-lack anaemia a diligent search must be made for the cause of blood loss which may vary from an innocent one like hookworm infection to a serious one like an ulcerated malignant growth; the prognosis depends upon removal of the ultimate cause of anaemia or blood loss (Fig. 14).

MEGALOBLASTIC ANAEMIA

Megaloblastic anaemias are of many different kinds, but all of them are ultimately due to deficiency of Vitamin B12 or of folic acid, or of both. The two large groups are: (1) hereditary constitutional megaloblastic anaemia (Addisonian pernicious anaemia) and (2) a symptomatic megaloblastic anaemia. The former is due to the absence of the intrinsic factor in the gastric juice a constitutional defect causing defective absorption of Vitamin B12. The anaemia is macrocytic (M.C.V. >100) and normochromic (M.C.H.C. normal). The leucocytes and platelets are reduced; the nuclei of neutrophils are hypersegmented (6 to 8 lobes). The marrow shows megaloblastic erythropoiesis and giant stab forms juveniles, and promyelocytes. The van den Bergh reaction on the serum is indirectly positive, the serum vitamin B12 is reduced below 100 μg. ml. and the serum iron is normal. Gastric analysis shows histamine fast achlorhydria. Hereditary constitutional megaloblastic anaemias react to treatment by liver extract, vitamin B12 and folic acid. The last drug, however, precipitates the complication of subacute combined degeneration of the cord and is, therefore, not used. The treatment has to be life long, since the defect is constitutional. Among the broad group of symptomatic megaloblastic anaemias the commoner subvarieties are as follows:—

(a) nutritional megaloblastic anaemia is due to dietetic deficiency of Vitamin B12 or folic acid; it may be seen in infants, **adult. males, non-pregnant females and pregnant females** (so called prenicious anaemias of pregnancy).

(b) **due to the malabsorption syndrome; in tropical sprue** idiopathic steatorrhoea, ceoliac disease, regional ileitis and patients with gastrectomy & with intestinal obstruction.

(c) **due to the fish tapeworm diphyllobothrium latum which** utilizes vitamin B12 in the bowel and deprives the body of the element.

(d) due to anti convulsant drugs, folic acid antagonists, and deficiency of ascorbicaacid: in these conditions the inadequate utilization of folic acid causes megaloblastic anaemia.

These symptomatic anaemias show the following differences from the hereditary constitutional type. The anaemia may not be macrocytic and it may be hypochromic. In peripheral blood, the presence of hypersegmented neutrophils and megaloblasts are the only diagnostic features. The marrow picture is indentical. The van den Bergh reaction may be negative. Either vitamin B12 or folic acid of the serum, or both may be low; the serum iron may be low. Histamine-fast achlorhydria may not be present. Special tests are required to demonstrate specific defects like malabsorption, steatorrhoea or the presence of tapeworm. Once the defect is removed the anaemia is cured and life-long maintenance therapy is not required.

HAEMOLYTIC ANAEMIA

Haemolytic anaemias are due to an accelerated destruction of erythrocytes. The reduced life span of erythrocytes (normally 120 days) leads to increased rate of erythropoiesis, with an increase in the number of reticulocytes. If the rate of erythrocyte destruction is only moderately accelerated, anaemia will not develop because the bone marrow can compensate for the disorder (so called compensated haemolysis). If, however, the destruction takes place at a high rate, anaemia with increased serum bilirubin and serum iron values will develop.

Causes

a) Distubrances of cellular origin	— Congenital spherocytosis — Congenital ovalocytosis — Sickle cell anaemia — Thalassemia — Haemoglobin C and other haemoglobinopathies. — Paroxysmal nocturnal hemoglobinuria — Enzymopenic anaemias due to a defect in the anaerobic erythrocytic glycolysis.
b) Disturbances of extracellular origin	— Due to infectious agents (Plasmodium malariae) — Due to chemical agents (lead, benzene, phenacetin containing drugs, etc.)

— Autoimmune haemolytic anaemias
— Paroxysmal cold haemoglobinuria
— March haemoglobinuria.

c) Disturbances of cellular and extracellular origin
— Disturbances in the aerobic erythrocytic glycolysis and effects of drugs (e.g. glucose-6-phosphate dehydrogenase deficiency)
— Haemoglobin Zurich and other drug-sensitive haemoglobinopathies.

With the exception of paroxysmal nocturnal haemoglobinuria, the anaemias with a cellular disturbance are all congenital and hereditary. In the forms due to extracellular causes an agent foreign to the body (infections, chemical, etc.) affects the viability of the erythrocytes. In the anaemias due to a combined cellular and extracellular disturbances, agents foreign to the body affect the viability of the erythrocytes only if the latter already show a hereditary anomaly which in itself is of no significance.

HAEMOLYTIC ANAEMIA OF CELLULAR ORIGIN

Congenital spherocytosis

This anaemia, inherited as a dominant autosomal trait, is characterized by small round cells that do not show a central pale area. In the blood smear only a certain number of erythrocytes posses this form. In addition, there is some polychromasia indicating reticulocytosis. The spherocytes are characterized by increased osmotic fragility. They are preferentially destroyed in the spleen, this being the cause of splenomegaly. Splencectomy cures the anaemia: the spherocytes persist and are even more numerous than before, because they no longer undergo an accelerated destruction in the spleen.

Congenital Ovalocytosis

Congenital ovalocytosis can be present with or without haemolysis. The reason for this difference is not known. In both diseases the blood picture is characterized by the presence of a great number of oval erythrocytes. The haemolytic form is usually accompanied by anaemia, reticulocytosis and erythropoietic bone marrow hyperplasia. In this form splenectomy will lead to recovery (Fig. 23).

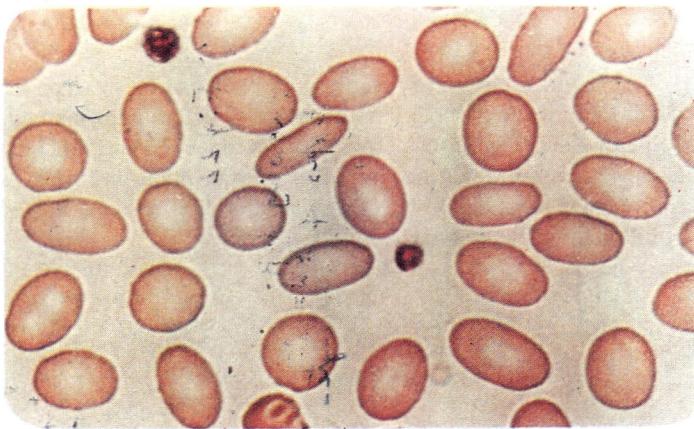

Fig. 23 Blood smear showing ovalocytes

Table 5. *Hereditary Haemolytic Disorders*

Red cell membrane disorders
Altered phospholipid concentration
Hereditary elliptocytosis
Hereditary spherocytosis
Hereditary stomatocytosis
Enzyme abnormalities
Defect in Embden-Meyerhof pathway (pyruvate kinase deficiency: rarely deficiencies of triose isomerase, glucose phosphate isomerase, 2, 3-diphosphoglycerate mutase, glyceraldehyde-3-phosphate dehydrogenase, hexokinase, phosphyglycerate kinase, and phosphofructokinase)
Defect in pentose phosphate pathway (deficiency of glucose-6-phosphate dehydrogenase, 6-phosphogluconate dehydrogenase)
Deficiency of glutathione reductase and peroxidase or ATPase
Haemoglobin or haemoglobin synthesis abnormalities
Erythropoietic porphyria
Haemoglobinopathies (sickling haemoglobins, hemoglobin C)
Thalassemia

Table 6. *Immune Haemolytic Anaemia with Demonstrable Antibodies and acquired Red Cell defects*

Acquired red cell defects
Paroxysmal nocturnal haemoglobinuria
Nutritional deficiencies (vitamin B_{12}, folic acid, iron)
Haemolytic disorders and isoantibodies
Erythroblastois fetalis (ABO, Rh)
Most transfusion reactions
Acquired autoimmune haemolytic disease
Warm-reactive antibodies
Idiopathic
Secondary to lymphoma, lupus erythematosus, infectious monocucleosis
Cold-reactive antibodies
Cold heamagglutinin disease
Secondary to pneumonia, lymphoma, infectious mononucleosis
Paroxysmal cold haemoglobinuria
Drug-dependent antibodies

Table 7 *Haemolytic Disorders not Associated with Demonstrable Antibodies*

Haemolytic disorders caused by chemicals (heavy metals, arsine, naphthalene, phenylhydrazine, oxidant and surface-active compounds, hypotonic solutions)
Haemolytic disorders caused by infectious agents (bacterial toxins, haemolysins, parasites)
Haemolytic disorders caused by physical agents (thermal injury, hyperoxemia)
Haemolytic disorders caused by unknown mechanisms (infections, liver disease, malignancy, renal disease)
Microangiopathic haemolytic anaemia (associated with cardiac valve prosthesis, carcinomatosis, eclampsia, haemolytic uremia syndrome, malignant hypertension, thrombotic thrombocytopenic purpura)

Haemolytic Anaemias of Extracellular Origin

Plasmodia directly infest the erythrocytes and lead to their destruction in the reticuloendothelial system.

Industrial poisons and drugs, lead poisoning is characterized by erythrocytes with basophilic stippling. Phenacetin containing drugs, occasionally also sulfonamides, cause an inclusion anaemia if taken in large amounts. The Heinz inclusion bodies consist of denatured methemoglobin and can only be demonstrated as coarse blue dots by means of brilliant cresyl blue supravital staining. The methemoglobin has lost the ability to transport oxygen because the divalent Hb Fe^{++} has been oxidized to the trivalent Fe^{+++} by the drugs.

Autoimmune haemolytic anaemias

On rare occasions the human body forms antibodies against its own erythrocytes. The cells carrying such antibodies can be detected by the direct Coombs' test. They are destroyed at an accelerated rate in the reticulo endothelial system. In the peripheral blood such cells can appear as spherocytes. The number of reticulocytes is always increased. Accordingly one finds an increased number of polychromatic erythrocytes in the peripheral blood.

Glucose-6-phosphate dehydrogenase deficiency (G-6-PD deficiency):

This most frequent defect of erythrocytic aerobic glycolysis preferentially affects individuals of the black race and of certain areas of Southeast Asia. Haemolytic anaemia will develop only if the carriers of this defect take drugs possessing oxidizing activity (antimalaria drugs, sulfonamides, phenylbutazone, etc.). The favism observed in Sardinia is due to the same biochemical disorder, the ingestion of fava beans triggering the haemolysis. The haemolytic crisis is confined to the period of drug-intake. After discontinuation of the triggering agent, the blood picture recovers spontaneously.

Haemoglobin Zurich

This is the first haemoglobinopathy shown to manifest itself as an acute intravascular haemolysis only after the intake of certain drugs (e.g. sulfonamide). During acute haemolysis a great number of strikingly large inclusion bodies appear. Remission is spontaneous; the haemolytic crisis, however, are usually so severe that they have to be treated with blood transfusion.

Paroxysmal nocturnal haemoglobinuria (PNH)

This uncommon hemolytic anaemia is the only anaemia due to an intrinisic cell defect which is not hereditary. It is characterized by intravascular haemolysis with hemoglobinuria occurring predominantly at night. The PNH erythrocytes show decreased resistance to acid and heat. In addition they haemolyse very easily in a hyperosmotic medium. These properties are used in the performance of the following diagnostic tests: Ham's acid serum test, the Maier-Hegglin heat resistance test and the sucrose haemolysis test. The anaemia is usually accompanied by leukopenia (neutropenia) and thrombocytopenia. In severe cases treatment is limited to the administration of erythrocyte concentrates.

OSMOTIC FRAGILITY TEST

Normal red cells, when placed in hypotonic salt solutions, absorb fluid, thus causing the volume to increase and the shape to change from that of biconcave discs to spherical forms. Further expansion of volume leads to cell rupture or hemolysis. Cells which are thicker than normal or spherical canot expand as much as can normal cells without placing their capsule under tension and therefore they hemolyze more readily in low salt concentrations than do normal cells. On the other hand, cells which are thin (leptocytes), sickled cells or cells with surface folds (target cells) are capable of a greater than normal percentile expansion of volume before reaching the spherical shape. These thin cells

therefore do not hemolyze in hypotonic salt solutions as readily as do normal cells.

For testing the osmotic fragility of erythrocytes, blood is placed in a series of tubes containing descending concentrations of sodium chloride. The degree of haemolysis or the point of beginning and complete hemolysis is noted. Control tests are always needed for there are many variables such as the criteria used in evaluating hemolysis, the accuracy of measurements of the salt concentrations, the chemical purity of the salt, cleanliness of glassware, the amount of blood in relation to the anticoagulant, the final pH, any contamination, and the time elapsed between the drawing of blood and the reading of the test.

Methods

Qualitative

A stock solution of sodium chloride is prepared by dissolving 1 gm of C.P. sodium chloride, which has been dried in a desiccator, in 100 ml of distilled water. By using varying amounts of this 1 per cent salt solution and making up to 10 ml, with distilled water, the desired ranges of salt concentration are prepared. Thus, if a 0.64 per cent solution is desired, 6.4 ml of stock solution are mixed with 3.6 ml of water; for a 0.60 per cent solution, 6.0 ml of stock solution plus 4.0 ml of water; etc.

The usual range is provided by making up a duplicate series of 10 tubes, each set having concentrations 0.64 to 0.28 per cent of intervals of 0.04 per cent. It is important to mix water and saline by inversion of the tube.

After venous blood is collected, 1 drop of blood is added to each tube. If the patient is anemic, 2 drops are preferred. The blood first may be mixed with EDTA and 0.1 ml or 1 drop from a 1 ml pipette added to each tube. The blood from the control and the patient must be handled in exactly the same way. After thoroughly mixing, the tubes are allowed to stand for several hours, preferably in a refrigerator, until the red cells settle. If more rapid reading is desired, the tubes may be centrifuged.

The point of beginning hemolysis in each series is noted by looking for the tube with the highest concentration in which the pink tinting of the supernatant fluid is detectable. A bright light, a white background, and comparison with other tubes help in determining this end point.

The point of complete hemolysis is indicated by the tube in which there are no red cells left intact. Aids is determining this end point are a slight agitation of the sediment to see if whorls of cells come up from the bottom, or the reading of point through the solutions as a means of detecting turbidity. The solution at the point of complete hemolysis is clear.

Example of report :

	Beginning hemolysis	Complete hemolysis
Patient	0.48% NaCl	0.36% NaCl
Control	0.44% NaCl	0.32% NaCl

A difference of more than one tube is significant.

Quantitative

Principle

Blood in known quantities is added to measured amounts of varying concentrations of sodium chloride buffered to pH 7.4 with sodium phosphates. The degree of hemolysis in each mixture is measured photoelectrically. A stock solution of buffered sodium chloride, which is osmotically equivalent to 10 per cent NaCl, is made by dissolving NaCl 180.0 gm, Na_2HPO_4 27.31 gm and NaH_2PO_4. $2H_2O$ 4.86 gm in approximately 1,000 ml of distilled water, after which the solution is made up to a volume of 2,000 ml of distilled water. This stock solution will keep for months if stored in a stoppered bottle. In preparing a series of hypotonic solutions, a working 1 per cent solution is prepared, from which a series of final solutions are prepared which are equivalent to 0.85, 0.75, 0.65, 0.60, 0.55, 0.50, 0.45, 0.40, 0.35, 0.30, 0.20, 0.10 and 0.00 per cent NaCl. These final dilute solutions will keep in the refrigerator for several weeks. They should be discarded if they become cloudy owing to growth of molds.

Equipment

1. Test tube rack containing two series of 13 matched colorimeter tubes which are chemically clean and which have been rinsed with distilled water and dried.
2. Calibrated serological pipettes, 10 ml.
3. Sahli pipettes, 20 cu mm.
4. Photoelectric colorimeter, green filter 510 mμ.

Procedure

Five milliliters of buffered salt solution equivalent to 0.85 per cent NaCl are placed in the first test tube of the front row of tubes and a similar amount in the first test tube of the back row. Next 5 ml of the 0.75 per cent solution are placed in the third pair of tubes, and so forth. Distilled water (5 ml) is placed in the last pair of tubes.

Five milliliters blood are collected from the patient and the control at approximately the same period of time. The venous blood may be heparinized or defibrinated. For defibrination place 5 ml blood in a 60 ml Erlenmeyer flask containing one glass bead (size 3 to 1 mm) for each milliliter of blood. The flask should be gently rotated for 5 minutes or until the fibrin collects around the beads.

Using a Sahli pipette, 20 cu mm of blood to be tested are placed in each of the buffered salt solutions in the front series of tubes. After each addition of blood to the respective hypotonic saline solution, the pipette should be rinsed several times and the residual contents blown out forcefully. There is no need of thoroughly drying the pipette each time or using a separate pipette for each specimen. Twenty cubic millimeters of heparinized or defibrinated blood from the normal control patient are now added to each of the 13 tubes in the back control row of tubes. The blood and saline is mixed and allowed to stand at room temperature for 30 minutes, after which the tubes are centrifuged for 5 minutes at approximately 900 × g. Following this the tubes are in turn placed in a photoelectric colorimeter and the optical density is determined. The supernatant fluid in the 0.85 per cent NaCl tubes serves as a "blank" and the supernatant fluid in the distilled water tube (0.00 per cent NaCl) serves as the tube of reference for complete or 100 per cent hemolysis. The degree of hemolysis as revealed by the scale reading of the dial is noted for each of the tubes. The degree of hemolysis in each tube is expressed in terms of percentage of the scale reading of the completely hemolyzed reference tube. The plotting on graph paper of the per cent of hemolysis of the patient and the control against the varying concentrations of buffered saline is recommended.

The test can be made more sensitive by allowing the blood to remain in contact with the hypotonic salt solutions for 24 hours at 37°C.

Because the quantitative test using multiple tubes is so time consuming, one may perform a screening test by determining the per cent of hemolysis in the 0.50 per cent tube.

Interpretation

In normal individuals a sigmoid type of curve is obtained in which there is 50 per cent hemolysis in the 0.50 to 0.40 per cent NaCl range.

Clinical applications

When normal blood is mixed with descending concentrations of hypotonic salt solution, some of the red cells undergo hemolysis within the range of 0.48 to 0.40 per cent NaCl (average 0.44 per cent) and there is complete hemolysis between 0.40 and 0.32 per cent NaCl (average 0.34 per cent).

In hereditary spherocytic anemia, and in certain patients with acquired hemolytic jaundice, there is partial hemolysis in concentration above the control and often above 0.50 per cent NaCl. In thalassemia, sicklemia and obstructive (regurgitant) jaundice, hemolysis occurs at levels lower than the control and there is often a greater spread than normal between the tubes in which there is beginning hemolysis and complete hemolysis. In sicklemia and thalassemia, and perhaps in other conditions, it is thought that the red cells are not only thinner than normal, and therefore can expand to a greater extent before hemolysis occurs, but that these cells act as poor osmometers and do not imbibe fluids as readily as do normal cells.

The fragility test is a fairly time-consuming procedure which is not indicated unless hemolytic jaundice is suspected.

Indications for ordering the test and unexplained jaundice of a hemolytic type, abnormal red cell regeneration and splenomegaly. The test is not needed in the diagnosis of sickle cell anemia or in obstructive jaundice. In the majority of cases of anemia in which there is neither evidence of abnormal blood destruction, nor compensatory regenerative signs, the test should not be ordered, for it will be of no value and will add pain, expense and unnecessary labour.

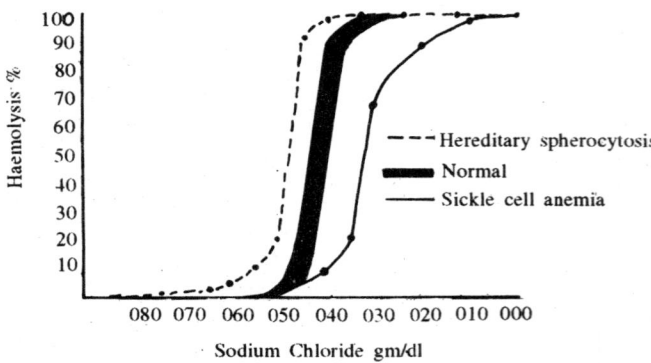

Fig. 23A. Quantitative osmotic fragility test. Range of normal variation indicated by stippled area.

CHAPTER 4
HAEMOGLOBINOPATHIES

NORMAL AND ABNORMAL HAEMOGLOBINS

Normal haemoglobin consists of a haeme-component and a globin component which is a glycoprotein. Haemoglobinopathies are disorders of the globin component of haemoglobin. These globin components are coded for by 5 different alleles namely alpha (α); beta (β) gama (γ); delta (δ) epsilon (ϵ).

Each globin component consists of a pair of chains as: $\alpha\alpha$ ($\alpha2$); $\beta\beta$ ($\beta2$); $\gamma\gamma$ ($\gamma2$); $\delta\delta$ ($\delta2$); $\epsilon\epsilon$ ($\epsilon2$).

Various normal haemoglobins include.
1. Normal adult haemoglobin (HbA)$\alpha2$ $\beta2$ — 95–98% of adult haemoglobin.
2. Fetal haemoglobin (HbF) $\alpha2$ $\gamma2$ — 70–90% of fetal haemoglobin at birth.
3. HB A-2 — $\alpha2\delta2$ — 2–3% of normal adult haemoglobin.
4. $\alpha2$ $\epsilon2$ — Gower II (Present at 6–8 wk of I.U. Life).
5. $\epsilon4$ — Gower I.

Abnormal Haemoglobins may be due to

1. Qualitative defects — result in Hb C, D, E, H, S eg. Sickle cell anaemia (Structural).
2. Quantitative defects-result in normally increased or decreased production of globin chains eg. Thalassemias.
3. Mixed defects. Sickle thalassemias.

HEMOGLOBINS

NORMAL	ABNORMAL
A,F,A2	S,C,D,E,G,H, I,J,K,L,O,P,Q

Sickle cell anaemia

The sickle cell anaemia is the first haemoglobinopathy whose basic defect was explained biochemically. The abnormal haemoglobin S is characterized by the substitution of a single amino acid in the β-chain of globin (glutamine in position 6 is substituted by valine).

The sickle cells are rarely visible in fresh blood smears. The transformation of round erythrocytes into sickle cells takes place in an oxygen poor medium or by lowering of pH. The sickling of cells in the blood vessels leads to an increase in viscosity until total occlusion of the capillaries has taken place by rigid sickle cells hooked into each other. The symptoms of homozygous patients with sickle cell anaemia are characterized by multiple recurring microinfarcts in various organs (brain, heart, joints, kidneys, etc). Heterozygous sickle cell carriers are almost free of symptoms.

The treatment of sickle cell anaemia is limited to blood transfusion.

Thalassemia (Mediterranean Anaemia)

The anaemia, which frequently affects inhabitants of Mediterrnean countries, is being increasingly encounter in northern Europe with the influx of labor from southern countries. The homozygous form is designated thalassemia major the heterozygous thalassemia minor.

Thalassemia major is a severe anaemia with considerable enlargement of liver and spleen, already manifesting itself in early childhood. The peripheral blood shows pronounced anisocytosis with hypochromic erythrocytes and a clear tendency to microcytosis. Apart from microcytes one encounters poikilocytes, target cells & erythrocytes with basophilic stippling. The appearance of erythroblasts in the peripheral blood is a characteristic finding. In most cases treatment is limited to blood transfusions. Despite this, life expectancy does not extend beyond childhood or adolescence.

Thalassemia minor usually follows an asymptomatic course. In most cases diagnosis is made accidentally or on checking family members of known thalassemia cases. In the blood smears one finds purely erythrocytic changes which are less marked than in thalassemia major (hypochromasia, microcytes, target cells and basophilic stippling) (Table 10); there are no erythroblasts in the peripheral blood. Characterstic is, at first glance, the paradoxical discrepancy of hypochromic blood picture with increased serum iron. This finding can be explained by a defect in haemoglobin synthesis (hypochromic erythrocytes) and by an increased rate of erythrocyte destruction (increased serum iron). Thalassemia minor requires no treatment.

To diagnose thalassemia the abnormal proportion of the three physiological haemoglobins is used (normal values in the adult: Hb $A_1 \geqslant 96\%$ Hb $A_2 < 3\%$, Hb F Fetal Hb $\leqslant 0.75\%$. In thalassemia major Hb A_2 and Hb F are increased and in thalassemia minor only Hb A_2.

Table 10. *Blood Cells in Thalassemia Major, Thalassemia Minor, and Iron Deficiency Anaemia*

	Thala-ssemia major	Thala-ssemia minor	Iron deficiency anaemia
Peripheral blood			
Anisocytosis	2–4 +	1–2 +	1–2 +
Hypochromic Microcytosis	2–4 +	1–3 +	2–4 +
Poikilocytosis	2–4 +	1–2 +	0–1 +
Polychromasia/ basophilic stippling	2–3 +	1–2 +	No
Target cells	3–4 +	2–3 +	0–1 +
Howell-Jolly bodies	Occasional	No	No
Normoblasts	Occasional	Seldom	Seldom
Reticulocytes	Significantly increased	Moderately increased	Decreased to normal
Platelets	Normal to increased	Normal	Normal increased or decreased
White blood cells	Normal to increased	Normal	Normal to decreased
Bone marrow			
Erythroid hyperplasia	3–4 +	Normal to 2 +	3–4 +
Haemosiderin	3–4 +	Normal to 2 +	Absent

Various Laboratory tests for detection of haemolytic disorders are shown in Table 11.

Table 11. *Laboratory Tests used in the Differentiation of Haemolytic Disorders*

Tests for evidence of haemolysis, increased haemoglobin metabolism and excretion of haemoglobin breakdown products
C_{Hb}, reticulocyte count, red cell morphology
Serum bilirubin, urinary and fecal urobilinogen
Plasma haemoglobin, haptoglobin, and haemopexin
Haemosiderin in urinary sediment (mechanical red cell injury, paraoxysmal nocturnal haemoglobinuria — PNH — thalassemia)

Tests for red cell resistance and survival
Osmotic fragility, fragility after incubation at 37°C
Red cell survival studies (^{51}Cr)

Test for red cell enzyme deficiency
G6PD deficiency, other pentose phosphate pathway defects
Pyruvate kinase
Other enzyme assays

Tests for haemoglobinopathies and thalassemia

Acidified serum test (Ham's test) for PNH

Tests for the presence of antibodies
Direct and indirect antiglobulin (Coombs) test
Blood group determination (ABO, Rh, others)
Testing serum for free antibodies (20°C, 37°C)
Determination of antibody immunoglobulin class (IgG, IgM)
Testing with cells preincubated with suspected drugs.
Complement activity determination
Determination of other serologic abnormalities.

INVESTIGATION OF THE HAEMOGLOBINOPATHIES

Collection of Blood and Preparation of Haemolysates

Blood can be collected into any anticoagulant, but if the samples have to be transported, ACD is the most suitable.

For routine analysis wash the red cells three times in 9.0 g/l NaCl (saline) and then lyse them by adding to the packed cells 2 volumes of water and 1 volume of toluene or carbon tetrachloride (CCl$_4$). Both of these solutions are toxic and should be used with care. Mouth pipetting must be avoided. After shaking in a mechanical agitator, centrifuge the mixture at 3000 rpm (1200 g) for 30 min and pipette off the clear Hb solution. Preferably, however, since organic solvents precipitate unstable Hbs and free globin chains, better results are obtained by lysing the cells in 2 volumes of water (without toluene) and centrifuging at 20,000 rpm (18000 g) at 4°C for 20 min.

In a routine laboratory, if many samples are to be analysed, a practical rapid alternative is to lyse the once-washed packed cells with a few drops of a solution containing 20 g/l saponin plus 10 g/l KCN. However, this type of haemolysate does not keep for more than 1–2 days at 4°C at room temperature, as it tends to gel.

Storing specimens prepared by either procedure at −20°C is satisfactory only for a few weeks, but lysates can be stored indefinitely in liquid nitrogen.

When it is suspected that a patient is suffering from a haemoglobinopathy, the clinical history and ethnic group, family history, the physical findings and the blood picture provide important information. However, for a definitive diagnosis, an abnormal Hb and/or the laboratory features of thalasaemia have to be demonstrated.

The International Committee for Standardization in Haematology (ICSH) Expert Panel on Abnormal Haemoglobins and Thalas-saemia have proposed a recommended procedure for the identification of haemoglobinopathies. The proposals have been incorporated in the recommendations in this chapter.

The laboratory investigations should be carried out in several stages:

1. **Preliminary tests**
   a. Blood count and film.
   b. Zone electrophoresis of Hb at an alkaline *p*H on cellulose acetate.
   c. Tests for sickling and/or solubility.
   d. Quantitation of Hb A$_2$.
   e. Quantitative and qualitative distribution of Hb F.

2. **Identification of abnormal haemoglobins**

   If indicated, further electrophoresis techniques to identify abnormal Hbs:

Preliminary Tests

Blood count and film

A full blood count, including red-cell count, haemoglobin level, mean cell volume and mean cell haemoglobin, provide valuable information in the diagnosis of both α and β thalassemias, whilst examination of blood films may show characteristic red-cell changes, e.g. target cells and Hb C and sickle cells with Hb S.

Cellulose acetate electrophoresis at alkaline *p*H

For routine work, the best method for separating abnormal Hbs is by electrophoresis on cellulose acetate membrane. This method is simple and generally satisfactory for distinguishing the common types of Hb. Various buffers can be used for Hb electrophoresis at an alkaline *p*H, with a continuous or discontinuous system.

Continuous buffer system

Tris-EDTA-borate, *p*H 8.9. Tris-(hydroxymethyl)-aminomethane 14.4 g; EDTA (disodium salt) 1.5 g; boric acid 0.9 g; water to 1 litre.

Discontinuous buffer system

Tris-EDTA-borate, *p*H 9.1 (anode chamber). Tris-(hydroxymethyl)-aminomethane 25.1 g; EDTA (disodium salt) 2.5 g; boric acid 1.9 g; water to 1 litre.

Barbitone, *p*H 8.6 (cathode chamber). Sodium diethylbarbiturate 25.75 g; barbitone (diethyl barbituric acid) 4.6 g; thiomersal (preservative) 0.25 g; water to 5 litre.

Method

Soak cellulose acetate membrane strips in the buffer used (a mixture of equal volumes of the two buffers in the discontinuous system) and, after blotting, place them across the bridges of the electrophoresis tank. Secure the strips using wicks of Whatman No. 1 filter paper, soaked in buffer.

Apply the haemolysate near to the cathode bridge. A variety of applicators are available commercially, or a fine pen or fine capillary tube may be used.

Then carry out electrophoresis at 200-300 V (approximately 1 mA/cm width of strip). Separation should be complete within 30 min. Then stain the strips for c 2 min in 0.2% ponceau S in 3% trichloracetic acid. Remove excess stain with 7% acetic acid, made up in tap water.

The relative electrophoretic mobility of some Hbs at pH 8.9 are shown in Chart 1.

Control preparation

It is advisable to electrophorese a known control sample with each electrophoresis.

The following method is recommended for preparing a control haemolysate containing Hbs A, F, S and C:
1. Obtain the following fresh blood samples (in any anticoagulant): AC; SS; F (cord blood).
2. Wash the cells three times with saline. Lyse the cells with a half volume of water and add 1 volume of CCl_4. Mix vigorously and then centrifuge for 10 min at 3000 rpm (1200 g).
3. Add a few drops of 0.3 mol/1 KCN (2g/dl) to the haemolysate to stabilize the Hb as cyanmethaemoglobin (HiCN).
4. Adjust the Hb concentrations of the haemolysates with water to within 20 g/l;
5. Mix equal volumes of the three haemolysates.
6. Check the mixture by electrophoresis.
7. Dispense in 0.5 ml volumes. If stored at 4°C they should be stable for several weeks; however, if stored in liquid nitrogen they should be stable for several months.

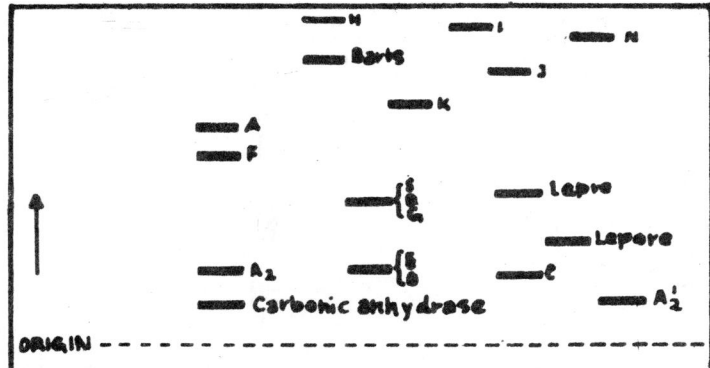

Chart 1:

TESTS FOR HB S

Tests to detect the presence of Hb S depend on the decreased solubility of the abanormal Hb at low oxygen tensions.

Sickling in whole blood

The sickling phenomenon may be simply demonstrated in a thin wet film of blood sealed between slide and cover-glass by means of a petroleum jelly-paraffin wax mixture. Sickling develops in the various types of sickle-cell disease and also in Hb S trait. In homozygous Hb S disease (or Hb SC disease or Hb `S/β-thalassaemia) marked sickling is usually visible after incubation for 1h or less at·37°C and filamentous forms are conspicuous. In Hb S trait the process is slower and the changes are less severe and incubation for as long as 12 h may be necessary for the changes to develop. They can, however, be hastened by the addition of reducing agents to the blood, e.g. sodium dithionite.

Method using reducing agent

Reagents

(A) Sodium dithionite ($Na_2S_2O_4$), 0.114 mol/l: 19.85 g/l. Prepare freshly just before use.

(B) Disodium hydrogen phosphate (Na_2HPO_4), 0.114 mol/1 16.2 g/l. For use, mix 2 volumes of A with 3 volumes of B to obtain a final pH of 6.8.

Add 5 drops of the freshly prepared reagent to 1 drop of anti-coagulated blood on a slide. Cover immediately with a cover-glass and seal with petroleum jelly-paraffin wax mixture. Sickling takes place almost immediately in Hb S disease and should be obvious in Hb S trait within 1 h.

Qualitative solubility test

Hb solubility tests provide a rapid method for the detection of Hb S. They are particularly useful for tentatively discriminating between Hb S homozygotes and Hb S with Hb A or an abnormal Hb or thalassaemia. It is, however, inadvisable to give an opinion on the exact genotype of the patient (e.g. Hb AS, SS or SC) without confirmation by electrophoresis.

ESTIMATION OF HB A_2

The International Committee for Standardization in Haematology has made recommendations for two methods suitable for Hb A_2 estimation. The first uses separation of Hb A_2 by electrophoresis on cellulose acetate membrane, based on the method of Marengo-Rowe. The second method is the microcolumn technique of Efremov et al. The microcolumn method is simpler and more precise, but the electrophoretic method provides a useful screen for the presence of some abnormal Hbs; it is more suitable for the laboratory performing tests only intermitently.

Electrophoresis

Reagent

Buffer, 0.13 mol/1 tris-EDTA-borate, pH 9.1. Tris-(hydroxymethyl)-aminomethane 82.5 g; EDTA (disodium salt) 7.8 g; boric acid 4.6 g; water to 5 litre.

Method

Soak two cellulose acetate strips per sample in buffer and blot. Place the strips across the bridges of the tank. Secure with buffer-soaked filter paper wicks.

Apply approximately 10μl of a haemolysate (approximately 10 g/dl) between the cathode bridge and mid-point of the strip, leaving not less than a 0.5 cm gap at each side of the strip. A glass capillary tube is a suitable applicator. Apply 200 V until there is a clear separation, which normally takes place within 60–100 min. Then cut out the Hb A and Hb A_2 zones and elute them in 20 ml and 4 ml, respectively, of buffer, for a minimum of 30 min. Set up a normal control with each batch of samples.

Read the absorbance (A) at 413 nm and determine the percentage of Hb A_2 by the equation below. Treat a Hb-free piece of cellulose acetate similarly, and use as a blank.

Calculation

$$\% \text{ Hb } A_2 = \frac{A^{413}HbA_2}{(A^{413}HbA \times 5) + A^{413}HbA_2} \times 100$$

Normal range 1.8–3.5%.

ESTIMATION OF HB F

Hb F may be estimated by several methods, all of which are based on its resistance to denaturation at alkaline pH.

For small amount of Hb F the method of Betke et al. is most

reliable, whilst for levels of over 50%, and in cord blood, the method of Jonxis and Visser is preferable

Method of Jonxis and Visser

Add 0.1 ml of blood or haemolysate (approximately 100 g/l) to 10 ml of water; then add 2 drops of 10% NH_4OH solution. Measure the absorbance at 576 nm (A_B) Then add 0.1 ml of the same blood or lysate to 10 ml of 0.06 mol/1 NaOH; add 2 drops of 10% NH_4OH solution at room temperature. Mix thoroughly and measure the absorbance every min for 15 min at 37°C for 15 min, cool to room temperature and measure the absorbance (A_E). The ratio $A_B{:}A_E$ should be constant.

Calculate the percentage of undenatured Hb at each minute:

$$\frac{A_T^{576} - A_E^{576}}{A_B^{576} - A_E^{576}} \times 100.$$

Then plot the percentage on the logarithmic scale of semi-logarithmic paper, against time. This should produce a straight line from which the original amount of Hb F, i.e. that at zero time, can be found by extrapolation.

Quantitative Alkali Denaturation Method for estimation of fetal haemoglobin

1. Take 9.5 ml of Drabkin's solution in a test tube, add 0.5 ml of haemolysate. Cyanmethaemoglobin (HiCN) is formed. Mix well.
2. Transfer 2.8 ml of HiCN solution in a tube and keep at 20°C. To this add 0.2 ml of 1.2N NaOH solution. Mix rapidly, incubate for 2 minutes at 20°C. Mix again and let stand for 5–10 minutes. Filter through Whatman filter paper number 3.
3. Prepare the total hemoglobin by adding 0.4 ml of the original HiCN solution to 6.5 ml of distilled water.
4. Using Drabkin's solution as blank at 540 nm read the total haemoglobin and filtrate.
5. The optical density should fall between 0.05 and 0.5. If it is beyond 0.5 dilute the haemolysate with distilled water and repeat the said procedure.
6. Calculate as

Haemoglobin F percentage or HbF
$$= \frac{\text{O.D of filtrate}}{\text{O.D of total haemoglobin}} \times \frac{100}{10}$$

Significance

In infants aged 1 yr the level of HbF should not be more than 1%. The normal range for adults is 0.5–0.8%.

Increased levels are found in many disorders, notably in β-thalassaemia trait and sickle-cell disease. But any haematological condition, congenital or acquired, may be associated with a slight increase.

HbF and HbS concentration of various haemoglobinopathies are summarised in Table 12.

Table 12 *HbF and HbS concentration as percentage of total Hb concentration in various disorders is given below:—*

Disorder	HbF%	HbS
Normal	<1% (in adults)	not present
Sickle cell trait (AS)	normal	30–40%
Sickle cell anaemia (SS)	1–20%	75–95%
HbS β thalassemia		
[Sβ⁺(some β chains present)]	2–10%	60–85%
[Sβ° (no β chains present)]	5–30%	76–90%
HbS-C (SC)	1–5%	50–55%
HbS-D (SD)	1–5%	95% (S + D)
β Thalassemia major	10–98%	—
α Thalassemia	reduced	—

CHAPTER 5

BONE MARROW SMEARS

SIGNIFICANCE OF BONE MARROW SMEARS AND INDICATIONS

The red cells, white cells, and platelets are manufactured in the bone marrow. If the manufacturing process is abnormal, it may indicate disease. The manufacturing process may be studied by obtaining a smear of the bone marrow and evaluating the cells.

The normal values for bone marrow smears are given in Table 13.

What is the M:E ratio? The M:E stands for myeloid-erythroid. Thus, the M:E ratio is the myeloid erythroid ratio. It is the ratio of white cells to nucleated red cells.

For example, if a bone marrow smear shows 80% white cells and 20% nucleated red cells, the M:E ratio is 4:1.

The M:E ratio is often referred to as the WBC:Nucleated RBC ratio.

The average M:E ratio is 4:1, with a normal range of 6:1 to 2:1.

An increased M:E ratio (7:1 or more) may be found in infections, granulocytic leukemia, leukemoid reactions, and a decrease in the number of nucleated red cells.

A decreased M:E ratio (1:1 or less) may be encountered in either a decrease in the production of white cells or an increase in the production of red cells.

Bone marrow smears are of particular interest to the physician in the following diseases: aplastic anaemia; pernicious anaemia, leukemia, purpura haemorrhagica, agranulocytosis, and multiple myeloma (Table 14).

INDICATIONS FOR BONE MARROW ASPIRATION

Absolute indications:
— Megaloblastic macrocytic anaemia.
— Aleukemic or subleukemic leukemia.

Diagnosiic importance
— Multiple myeloma.
— Aplastic anaemia.
— Gaucher's disease.

Confirmatory importance
— Leukemias of all types.
— Haemolytic anemia.
— Idiopathic thrombocytopenic purpura..
— Idiopathic granulocytopenia.
— Leishmaniasis.
— Disseminated lupus erythematosus
— Metastatic diseases.
— Myeloproliferative disorders.
— Lipid storage.
— Sideroblastic anaemia.
— Iron deficiency anaemia.
— Lymphoma (staging).

PREPARATION AND STAINING OF BONE MARROW SMEARS

1. Place a small amount of bone marrow on a glass slide.

2. Make a bone marrow smear in the same manner that you would make a blood smear.
3. Make about 5 more bone marrow smears.
4. Make a finger puncture on the patient.
5. Make two blood smears for a differential white cell count.
6. Write the patient's name and date on both the bone marrow smears and blood smears.
7. Allow the bone marrow smears and the blood smears to dry. (It takes about 20 minutes for bone marrow smears to dry).
8. Then stain both the marrow smears and blood smears with **Giemsa stain** and buffer solution.
9. After staining the bone marrow smears and blood smears, allow them to dry. (It requires about 10 minutes.)
10. Make the study of bone marrow cells which is given below.

THE PROCEDURE GIVEN BELOW IS RECOMMENDED FOR STUDYING THE MARROW FILMS:

1. Naked eye inspection of the slides to select the smear-containing particles.
2. With 10x objective survey the particles whether they are normoplastic, hypoplastic or hyperplastic.
3. Select a cellular area (usually in the tail portion of the film around particles), study the cytologic details by high power-40x and oil immersion-100x objectives.

Note the under-mentioned points

Cellularity: Normo/hypo/hyper plastic marrow particles. Cellularity is better defined by studying histoglogic sections of aspirated particles, though crude estimates can be given on films. The normal cellularity of the marrow varies with age being more in infants and least in elderly individuals.

Next look for *reaction of erythropolesis,* whether it's normoblastic, megaloblastic or micro-normoblastic. Look for maturity of leukopoietic cells. The M:E ratio is based on a count of 500 to 1000 marrow cells. In the normal adult the reaction is normoblastic, leukopoietic maturity is normal and **M:E ratio** is about 3 or 4:1. The M:E ratio at birth is 1.85:1, during the first two weeks it reaches its peak of 11:1. It then gradually drops to the (years 1 to 20) average of 3:1.

Table. 13 *Cell distribution in Bone marrow and peripheral blood*

Types of cells	Marrow%		Peripheral blood%	
	Average	Range	Average	Range
Myeloblasts	2.5	0.5–5	0	
Promyelocytes	6	1–8	0	
Myelocytes	15	8–20	0	
Neutrophilic	12	5–19	0	

Cell type	Value	Range		
Eosinophilic	1.5	0.5–3.0	0	
Basophilic	0.3	0.0–0.3	0	
Metamyelocytes	29	14–36	0	
Neutrophilic	26.4	13–32.0	0	
Eosinophilic	2.0	0.5–3.0	0	
Basophilic	0.3	0.0–0.3	0	
Segmented granulocytes	32	17–43		
Neutrophils	27	15–35	60	50–70
Eosinophils	4	1–7	2	1–4
Basophils	1	0.5–1.5	0	0–1
Monocytes	2	0.4–4.0	5	2–10
Lymphocytes	13	5–20	30	20–40
Pronormoblasts	0.6	0.2–4	0	
Early normoblast	2.4	1.5–5.8	0	
Intermediate normoblast	10.6	5.0–20.0	0	
Late normoblast	6.6	3.0–20.0	0	
Megaloblasts	0.2	0–0.5	0	
Megakaryocytes	0.4	0.04–2.0	0	
Reticulum cells	1.0	0.2–3.0	0	
Plasma cells	0.6	0–2.0	0	
M:E Ratio	3–4 : 1			

Table 14 *The More significant Bone marrow abnormalities in various diseases*

Disease	Abnormality	Normal Values
Aplastic anaemia	hypoplastic (**defective and incomplete development of cells**)	normoplastic
Iron deficiency anaemia	hyperplastic (overactive): increase in nucleated red cells (30–60%)	normoplastic 8–30%
Pernicious anaemia	increase in nucleated red cells (30–50%): presence of "pernicious anemia type" nucleated red cells	8–30% 8–30%
Hereditary spherocytic anaemia	increase in nucleated red cells (30–60%)	8–30%
Sickle cell anaemia	increase in nucleated red cells (40–70%)	8–30%
Thalassemia major	increase in nucleated red cells (30–60%)	8–30%
Acute granulocytic leukemia	increase in myeloblasts (15–50%)	0–5%
Chronic granulocytic leukemia	increase in myeloblasts (5–15%) increase in myelocytes and metamyelocytes	0.5%
Acute lymphocytic leukemia	increase in lymphoblasts (15–75%)	0%
Chronic lymphocytic leukemia	increase in lymphocytes (30–90%)	5–15%
Monocytic leukemia	increase in monocytes (20–60%)	0–5%
Plasmacytic leukemia	increase in plasmacytes (15–75%)	0–1%
Purpura hemorrhagica (idiopathic thrombocytopenic purpura)	number of megakaryocytes **is normal or increased;** **platelet formation** is decreased	0–3%
Polycythemia vera	hyperplastic; percentage of white cells, red cells, and platelets is normal	normoplastic
Agranulocytosis	granulocytes are decreased during height of disease but increased during recovery: percentage of nucleated red cells is normal: percentage of megakaryocytes is normal	8–30% 0–3%
Infectious mononucleosis	increase in lymphocytes (15–35%)	5–15%
Multiple mycloma	10–90%	0%
Hodgkin's disease	presence of Sternberg-Reed cells	0%
Gaucher's disease	presence of Gaucher's cells	0%

CHAPTER 6

LEUKEMIAS AND MYELODYSPLASTIC SYNDROMES (M.D.S.)

LEUKEMIAS

Leukemia is a morbid condition characterised by wide spread hyperplasia of leucopoitic tissue, either myeloid or lymphatic, which is usually associated with qualitative and quantitative changes in the white cells of the circulating blood.

Exposure to ionizing radiation increases the incidence of leukemia in animals, and in man exposure to doses of 100r or over carries a definite risk of leukemia.

Leukemias are classified as
1. Myeloid Leukemia (Acute and chronic)
2. Lymphatic Leukemia (Acute and chronic)
3. Monocytic Leukemia (Acute, sub acute)
4. Atypical Leukemias:
   (a) Aleukemic leukemia
   (b) Chloroma
   (c) Plasma cells leukemia
   (d) Eosinophilic, Basophilic, mast cell leukemias
   (e) Megakaryocytic leukemia etc.

ACUTE LEUKEMIAS

Two main forms of acute leukemias are recognised: myeloid (AML), more frequent in adults (more than 20 years), and lymphoblastic (ALL), predominantly in children (<15 years) (Fig. 24 & Fig. 25).

AML: 6 types of AML (FAB classification) can be identified by morphology with help of cytochemistry. The main features of each type M_1 to M_6 are summarized in the Table. 15.

Table 15 *(FAB) French American British Classification*

Types	Main Features
M_1 (Myeloblastic)	* Blasts with few or no granules (90%) * Auer rods +
M_2 (Myeloblastic)	* Blasts (30%) * Maturation beyond promyelocytes * Abnormal neutrophils
M_3 (Promyelocytic)	* Hypergranular promyelocytes * Faggets * Bilobed nuclei * Hypogranular variant
M_4 (Myelo Monocytic)	* Blasts (30%) * Evidence of granulocytic and monocytic differentiation
M_5 (Monocytic)	(a) Monoblasts (b) Monoblasts, promonocytes & monocytes (a) & (b) 80% monocytic cells
M_6 Erythro Leukemia	* Over 50% of erythroid cells, often bizarre, Myeloblasts with Auer rods

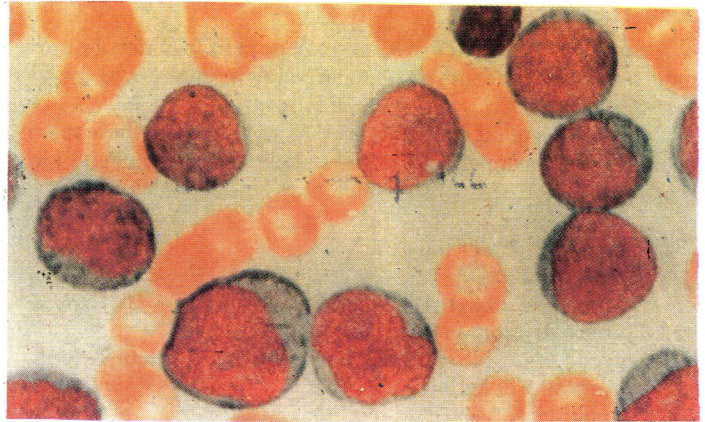

Fig. 24 Blood film of A.M.L.

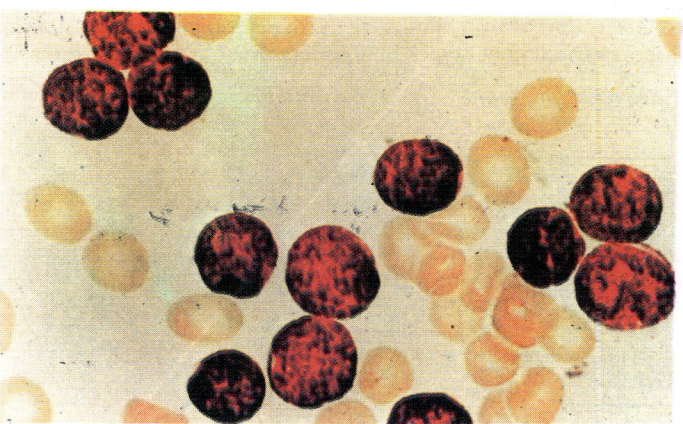

Fig. 25 Blood film of A.L.L.

CYTOCHEMISTRY OF AML

Certain cytochemical reactions are essential in distinguishing AML from undifferentiated forms of ALL (e.g. L_2). This is particularly so in cases where the cells are immature, e.g. in M_1 (myeloblastic leukemia poorly differentiated). The peroxidase, Sudan Black B and chloracetate estrase reactions reveal granulocytic differentiation in M_1, M_2, M_3 and M_4 types of AML. Whilst the non specific esterases (nephthol acetate (NASDA) and alpha-nephthol acetate esterase (ANAE) ± sodium fluoride (NaF), and the acid phosphatase and lysozyme reactions, demonstrate monocytic differentiation. Non specific esterase reactions are usually weak or negative in M_3. In erythroleukemia (M_6) the PAS (Periodic Acid Schiff) reaction may be strongly positive.

Cytochemical reactions are usually done to detect the deficiency of enzyme contents of mature neutrophils in AML, particularly in M_2 and M_6. The NAP (neutrophil alkaline phosphatase), score is often low in M_2 (myeloblastic leukemia with maturation). The peroxidase, Sudan Black B and chloroacetate reactions may also be negative in variable proportions of neutrophils in AML, more frequently in M_2 and M_6. The NAP scores are usually normal and high in ALL and M_5.

In acute megakaryoblastic leukemia, the blast cells appear undifferentiated, and may resemble lymphoblasts. The cytochemical profile of these cells is similar to that of megakaryocytes i.e. positive reactions with PAS, acid phosphatase and ANAE (NaF-sensitive as in monocyte). The cytochemical classification of some leukemias is possible by use of 7 different tests.
1. Nephthol AS-D chloroacetate esterase (NASDCA) activity.
2. Alpha-nephthyl acetate esterase (NA).
3. Alpha nephthyl butyrate esterase (NB) activity.
4. Myeloperoxidase (M.P.) activity.
5. Sudan Black B (SB) reaction.
6. Acid phosphatase (AP) activity.
7. Periodic Acid Schiff (PAS) stain.

The characteristics and interpretations are shown in microphotograph (Fig. 26 to Fig. 32).

ACUTE LYMPHOCYTIC LEUKEMIA (A.L.L.)

Three morphological types have been described by the FAB group: L_1, L_2, and L_3. The differences in age incidence (L_1 is more common in children and L_2 more frequent in adults), the strong correlation of L_3 with B-ALL (with monoclonal membrane immunoglobulins) and the difference in prognosis between L_1 and L_2 (worse in L_2) within similar age groups together suggest that the three morphological types may reflect true biological differences.

Table 16. *Cytochemistry and the immunological classification of ALL.*

Method	Common-ALL	Null-ALL	T-ALL	B-ALL
Morphology	L1-L2	L1-L2	L1-L2	L3
PAS	+ or + + coarse granules	– or + +	– or +	–
Acid phosphatase	– or +	– or + +	+ + or + + +	–
ANAE	–	– or +	+ or + +	–
Peroxidase	–	–	–	–
Sudan black B	–	–	–	–
Lysozyme	–	–	–	–

L_1 lymphoblasts tend to be small and to have scanty cytoplasm; the nucleo-cytoplasmic (N:C) ratio is high in the majority and they have a small and not easily visible nucleolus; the nuclear membrane is often regular. L_2 lymphoblasts, in contrast to L1, are larger, have more abundant cytoplasm (low N:C ratio) and have one or more prominent nucleoli; the nuclear outline is irregular in over 25% of cells. The differences between L_1 and L_2 can be more easily resolved in borderline cases by the simple scoring system proposed by the FAB group. L_3 (or Burkitt type) cells, because of their resemblance to cells of the endemic African lymphoma are uniformly large, have finely stippled nuclear chromatin and, characteristically, a deep basophilic cytoplasm often associated with prominent vaculolation.

Three cytochemical tests are useful in the study of ALL; the PAS, acid phosphatase and ANAE reactions. They do not correlate with the L_1, L_2 or L_3 morphological types but they do show a relationship to the immunological subtypes of ALL.

In cases in which the cells are undifferentiated (usually L_2 blast cells in adult patients), it is important to exclude AML (usually M_1 and M_5a). For this, the peroxidase, Sudan Black B and NASDA reactions should be shown to be negative. ANAE can show in ALL a granular reaction, but this is not the strong diffuse pattern (NaF-senstive) seen in M_5. The PAS reaction is often postive in ALL — at least, in a proportion of blasts, as shown by coarse granules or blocks of positively-reacting material (usually glycogen). This pattern of reaction, particularly with a negative background, is rarely seen in AML; it is more typical of the common form of childhood ALL which can be defined by immunological tests for the ALL antigen described as non-B, non-T ALL (negative B and T markers) or common-ALL.

In T-ALL (positive T-cell markers), the PAS reaction is negative in two-thirds of cases; in B-ALL it is negative in the majority. The differences shown by the PAS reaction probably reflect the different proliferation kinetics of the immunologically-defined subtypes of ALL. For example, in B-ALL (PAS-negative) a greater number of cells are in cycle; this is also reflected in the numerous mitotic figures seen in bone marrow with L_3 morphology. The acid phosphatase test gives a consistently localized positive reaction in T-ALL and pre-T-ALL blast cells.

CHRONIC LEUKAEMIAS

Definition

Primary malignancies of haemopoietic cells in which the clinical course is measured in months and years in contrast to the acute leukaemias.

Many of the malignant cells are differentiated and these relatively mature cells appear in large numbers in the peripheral blood, giving rise to leucocytosis which may be very marked.

Classification

I. Myeloid origin
1. Chronic granulocytic (synonymous myeloid) — CGL or CML.
2. Chronic myelomonocytic (CMML).
3. Chronic erythroleukaemia (Di Gughelmo's syndrome).

II. Lymphoid origin
1. Chronic lymphocytic (B-cell or T-cell).
2. Prolymphocytic (B-cell or T-cell).
3. Hairy cell (leukaemic reticuloendotheliosis).

THE CYTOCHEMICAL CLASSIFICATION OF SOME LEUKEMIAS IS POSSIBLE BY USE OF 7 DIFFERENT TESTS.

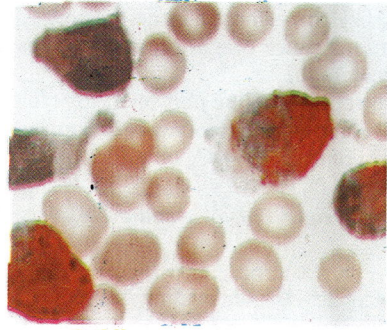

Fig. 26

NAPHTHOL AS-D CHLOROACETATE ESTERASE [NASDCA] activity is exhibited by cells of granulocytic lineage. NASDCA activity appears at differentiated myeloblast/progranulocytic stage of cellular development.

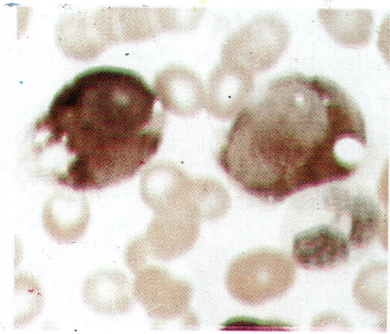

Fig. 27

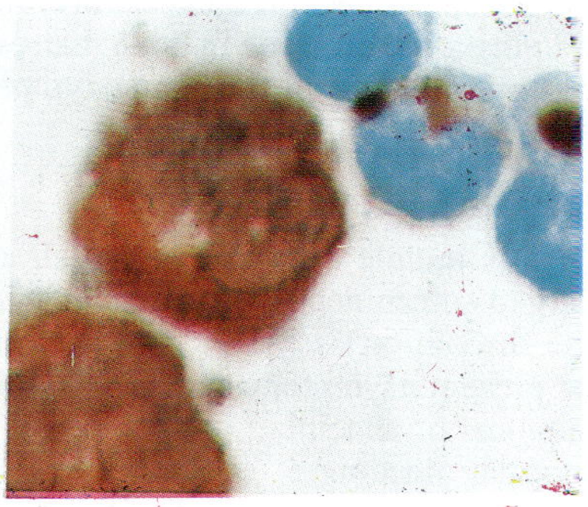

Fig. 28

α-NAPHTHYL ACETATE ESTERASE [NA] AND α-NAPHTHYL BUTYRATE ESTERASE [NB] activities are used to recognize cells of monocytic origin. At pH 7.6, NA is seen almost exclusively in monocytes and histiocytes, with occasional granules in polymorphonuclear leukocytes and lymphocytes. At this pH, megakaryocytes and erythroblasts exhibit intense NA activity. Sodium fluoride inhibits monocyte enzymes and is used to distinguish monocyte activity from other esterase activity.

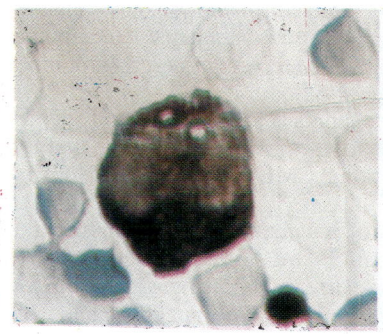

Fig. 29

MYELOPEROXIDASE[MP] is normally confined to primary granules of myeloid and monocytoid cells. However, primative blasts committed to myeloid path exhibit MP activity in the endoplasmic reticulum, paranuclear area and Golgi apparatus.

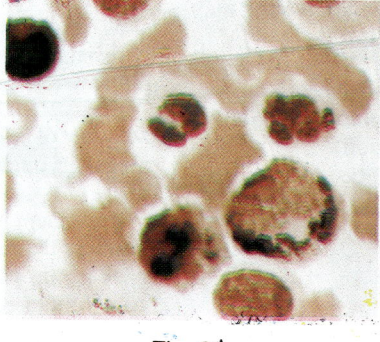

Fig. 30

SUDAN BLACK B [SB] reacts with lipid deposits in cells, paralleling the MP pattern of cellular distribution. The parallelism in not invariant since SB-positive blasts sometimes exceed those exhibiting MP. SB-positive and MP-negative blasts have been reported.

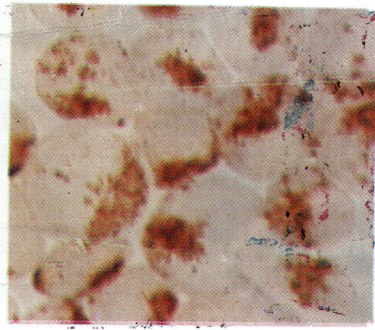

Fig. 31

ACID PHOSPHATASE[AP] is useful for differentiating sub-groups of acute lymphoblastic leukemia and delineating hairy cell leukemia from other chronic lymphoid neoplasias.

PERIODIC ACID-SCHIFF [PAS] stains glycogen and other 1, 2-glycol-containing carbohydrates. The earliest myeloid precursors are not PAS reactive, but staining increases with maturation along myeloid pathways. Normal erythroid precursors are negative while megakaryoblasts, megakaryocytes and platelets stain intensely. Diffuse or granular PAS patterns are exhibited by monocytes.

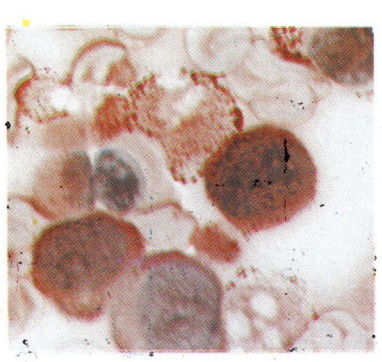

Fig. 32

I.1. Chronic Myeloid (Granulocytic) Leukaemia

Malignant clone derives from a committed stem cell and differentiates along myeloid lines. In 95% of cases the Philadelphia chromosome (Ph[1]), a number 22 chromosome missing part of its long arm which has become attached to chromosome 9 [t(22;9)], is present in the affected clone in bone marrow and blood. Myeloid. erythroid, megakaryocytic and some lymphoid cells carry the Ph[1] chromosome.

Clinical presentation

1. Typically middle age, but seen in all age groups.
2. Enlarged spleen and liver (splenomegaly may be massive and cause discomfort).
3. May present asymptomatically on routine blood count.
4. Symptoms of anaemia.
5. Abnormal bleeding.
6. Weight loss, anorexia, sweats, fever, 2° amenorrhoea.
7. Hyperviscosity syndrome from leucostasis.
8. Gout.
9. De novo 'blast transformation' clinically indistinguishable from acute leukaemia.

Severe infection is rare in untreated CGL (unlike all other types of leukaemia) as the relatively mature myeloid cells seen in the blood have some bacteriocidal capabilities.

Clinical signs

1. Splenomegaly; may vary from just palpable to massive and may have audible rub or bruit.
2. Hepatomegaly.
3. Pallor, emaciation (if advanced).
4. Bruising (seldom petechial, except in blast transformation)
5. Fever (low grade, even in absence of infection)
6. Fundal haemorrhages, tortuous veins, papilloedema (leucostasis).
7. Bone tenderness, especially sternum.
8. Lymphadenopathy (rare).
9. Skin infiltration (uncommon).

Investigations

Blood count
1. Leucocytosis may be very marked, often well over $100 \times 10^9/1$. Height of leucocytosis tends to correlate with size of spleen and degree of anaemia.
2. Differential leucocyte count: whole spectrum from neutrophils (around 50%) to blasts (usually > 5%). Myelocytes common. Eosinophils and basophils increased. Nucleated RBCs often seen.
3. Anaemia: normochromic, normocytic, may be mild or severe.
4. Thrombocytosis sometimes > $1000 \times 10^9/1$. Platelets occasionally low — may herald blast transformation.

The diagnosis is often obvious from the clinical signs and the blood count alone, in classical CGL.

Bone marrow

1. Grossly hypercellular.
2. May be difficult to aspirate.
3. Gross granulocytic hyperplasia with all degrees of differentiation seen, and increased megakaryocytes.
4. Send sample for examination for Ph[1] and other chromosome anomalies (liaise with laboratory about sample — marrow or blood anticoagulated with heparin is suitable).
5. Marrow trephine to assess fibrosis; may also show pockets of blasts not detected on aspirate, in early transformation.

Note: If Ph[1] chromosome detected in peripheral blood cells it may not always be necessary to perform a bone marrow.

Additional investigations (once diagnosis made or suspected)
1. Urate — often very high.
2. NAP score — neutrophil alkaline phosphatase zero or very low in untreated CML, in contrast to other causes of leucocytosis. Tends to rise after control of WBC, or before blast transformation.
3. Liver function — deranged enzymes and mildly raised bilirubin common.
4. Renal function — as baseline.
5. Serum vitamin B_{12} level and binding proteins if available. (Transcobalamin secreted by leucocytes is raised in CML and other myeloproliferative diseases, giving rise to high serum vitamin B_{12} level.)

Disease progression

At present time CML is incurable by conventional techniques. Median survival is approximately three years. After the initial chronic phase disease in which the patient is clinically well, one of two main terminal states develop:

1. *Blast transformation:* a more malignant clone appears which gives rise to progeny which are primitive blast cells. The result is a slow or abrupt transformation to an acute leukaemia of particularly resistant type, with appearance of increased number of blasts in marrow and peripheral blood.

Blasts often have additional chromosome anomalies as well as Ph[1] May be of any phenotype: i.e. AML, ALL. undifferentiated or megakaryoblastic. Some CML patients present for first time in this phase.

Treatment is that of acute leukaemia. Remission rates and duration less than straightforward AL, and patients who respond revert back to chronic phase disease. Grafting with autologous buffy coat cells (obtained at diagnosis by leucapheresis and cryopreserved), after intensive chemotherapy or radiotherapy, has been used, but long term results poor.

2. *Bone marrow failure*: Some patients do not enter a discernible blast crisis but develop insidious marrow failure with progressive anaemia, thrombocytopenia and splenomegaly. Marrow often very fibrotic. May be natural disease process or related to chemotherapy, particularly busulphan. Patients often emaciated and hypercatabolic. Treatment is supportive only.

Juvenile Chronic Myeloid Leukaemia

Adult-type CGL does occur occasionally in childhood, usually in older age group. Juvenile chronic myeloid leukaemia is a distinct rare disease.

Clinical features

1. Age < 2 years.
2. Mild splenomegaly.
3. Lymphadenopathy.
4. Facial rash.

Laboratory features

1. Thrombocytopenia.

2. Increased monocytes and blasts in blood and marrow.
3. Many nucleated RBC.
4. High Hb F level.
5. Absence of Ph[1] chromosome.

I.2. Chronic Myelomonocytic Leukaemia

May be classified either as a type of myelogenous leukaemia or as a myelodysplastic syndrome

Clinical and laboratory features

1. Elderly patient.
2. Chronic course often over several years.
3. Leucocytosis with absolute increase in monocytes and some abnormal forms in blood and bone marrow.
4. Splenomegaly.
5. Anaemia and thrombocytopenia.

Treatment

1. Treatment is generally supportive, and many patients do relatively well.
2. Gentle chemotherapy e.g. 6-mercaptopurine or hydroxyurea may be useful in controlling very high WBC count and splenomegaly, and may improve anaemia and thrombocytopenia.

I.3. Chronic Erythroleukaemia (syn. Di Guglielmo's syndrome, chronic erythraemic myelosis)

A chronic variation of which the acute counterpart is M6 AML.

Clinical features

Chronic form usually presents with anaemia and runs a course over months and years. Splenomegaly may be present.

Laboratory features

1. Anaemia.
2. Increased reticulocytes.
3. Numerous nucleated RBC in blood.
4. Gross erythroid hyperplasia in marrow.
5. PAS + ve erythroblasts in marrow.
6. Variable dysmyelopoiesis.
7. May terminate as AML.

II. Chronic Lymphoid Leukaemias

Can be classified:
1. Clinically.
2. Morphologically.
3. Immunologically.
Generally the malignant clone has a normal counterpart in lymphocyte development, but the cells have aberrant features and are functionally defective.

II.1. B-Cell Chronic Lymphocytic Leukaemia (B-CLL)

Commonest form of leukaemia in United Kingdom. Affects mainly elderly — very rare below thirty. Often detected on routine blood count as an absolute lymphocytosis. CLL is the most common cause of persistent lymphocytosis in a middle aged or elderly patient.

Clinical features

1. Often asymptomatic with no abnormal physical signs.

2. Lymphadenopathy — all areas, soft, may be very extensive.
3. Hepatosplenomegaly.
4. Weight loss, night sweats, fatigue, recurrent infections.

Laboratory features

1. Absolute lymphocytosis $> 15 \times 10^9/1$. WBC may be very high $500–600 \times 10^9/1$.
2. 'Smudge' cells or 'smear' cells (lymphocytes ruptured on spreading film) characteristic.
3. Anaemia, neutropenia and thrombocytopenia develop as the disease progresses.

Staging

Three main staging systems based on clinical and haematological parameters. All assume diagnosis based on minimum criteria of:
1. Peripheral blood lymphocytosis $> 15 \times 10^9/1$.
2. Bone marrow lymphocytosis $> 40\%$.
Simplest classification is as follows:
Stage A: Hb >10 g/dl. Platelets $> 100 \times 10^9/1$
       < 3 lymphoid areas involved.
Stage B: Hb >10g/dl. Platelets $>100 \times 10^9/1$
       3 or more lymphoid areas involved.
Stage C: Hb <10g per dl. or Platelets
       $<100 \times 10^9/1$. Regardless of lymphoid areas involved.
NB: 1. A lymphoid area includes liver, or spleen or a single group of nodes e.g. neck. axillae, groins.
    2. Level of lymphocyte count not considered prognostically important although counts tend to rise as disease progresses.
    3. Anaemia and thrombocytopenia excludes that caused by a definite auto-immune process.

Investigations

1. Full blood count and reticulocytes, film, direct antiglobulin test.
2. Peripheral blood for lymphocyte markers, "mouse rosettes" and 'slg' (surface immunoglobulin) if available.
3. Bone marrow aspirate and trephine. A 'nodular' pattern of lymphocyte infiltration on trephine may suggest better prognosis than diffuse infiltrate.
4. Renal and liver function.
5. Uric acid.
6. Protein electrophoresis and immunoglobulin levels.
7. Chest X-ray.

Prognosis

1. Related to stage of disease.
2. Overall median survival six years.
3. Death usually associated with bone marrow failure or infection.
4. Acute transformation analogous to CGL is very rare.

T-cell chronic lymphocytic leukaemia (T-CLL)

Much less common than B-CLL in United Kingdom. Generally greater splenomegaly for same stage of disease. May occur in younger age group.

II.2. Prolymphocytic Leukaemia

Less common than CLL.

May have B or T cell characteristics.

Diagnosis based on peripheral blood appearances and immunology.

Clinical and laboratory features

1. Splenomegaly prominent.
2. Lymphadenopathy slight or absent.
3. Elderly males predominate.
4. Often very high WBC.

Prognosis

Much worse than CLL.

II.3. Hairy Cell Leukaemia (leukaemic reticuloendotheliosis)

Typically 'hairy cells' are found in peripheral blood, but may not always be apparent on light microscopy.

Clinical features

1. Usually elderly — male > female.
2. Pancytopenia.
3. Splenomegaly prominent.
4. Recurrent infections common.

Laboratory features

1. 'Hairy cells' — lymphocytes with spiky projections from cytoplasm.
2. Pancytopenia and especially monocytopenia.
3. Bone marrow aspiration often difficult. Usually hypocellular with lymphoid cells showing staining with tartrate resistant acid phosphatase.
4. Trephine biopsy often needed for diagnosis and shows excess fibrosis.

ALEUKEMIC LEUKEMIA AND LEUKEMOID REACTIONS

Aleukemic Leukemia

Aleukemic leukemia is also referred to as aleukemic lymphadenosis and aleukemic myelosis.

Aleukemic leukemia means white blood without white blood. It is a phase of leukemia in which the white cell count is normal or below normal and the differential white cell count may show only a few immature white cells.

Aleukemic leukemia occurs in 10 to 20% of all cases of leukemia. Its significance lies in the fact that, during this phase, the disease may easily by confused with other diseases such as aplastic anaemia or agranulocytosis.

With the exception of the white cells, the laboratory findings and clinical picture are the same as those which have just been described for the various leukemias.

Because the white cell count is normal or below normal, the white cells in the differential white cell count are relatively few. These white cells may be concentrated, however, and the differential white cell count run on the concentrated specimen. The concentrated specimen of white cells is called buffy coat preparation.

As previously stated, in aleukemic leukemia, the differential white cell count may not show many immature white cells. A bone marrow examination then becomes the more significant laboratory examination. This examination usually reveals large numbers of immature white cells.

Leukemoid Reactions

Leukemoid reactions are reactions which resemble leukemia. Thus, the white cell count is high and the differential white cell count shows immature white cells. But the patient does not have leukemia.

The distinction between a leukemoid reaction and true leukemia is usually made by (1) careful clinical observations of the patient, (2) a continual check for changes in laboratory examinations, and (3) a bone marrow examination.

The more commonly encountered leukemoid reactions are neutrophilic leukemoid reactions and lymphocytic leukemoid reactions. These reactions are briefly discussed below:

Neutrophilic Leukemoid Reactions

A neutrophilic leukemoid reaction is accompanied by a white cell count of 20,000 to 100,000 per cubic millimeter and a differential white cell count showing immature neutrophils such as neutrophilic metamyelocytes and neutrophilic myelocytes.

Thus, from a laboratory viewpoint, a neutrophilic leukemoid reaction may resemble granulocytic leukemia.

A neutrophilic leukemoid reaction may be found in the following conditions: tuberculosis, meningitis, diphtheria, lobar pneumonia, malaria, syphilis, haemorrhage, haemolytic anaemia, severe burns, tumors, Hodgkin's disease, myeloid metaplasia, mercury poisoning, and eclampsia.

If it is difficult to distinguish between a neutrophilic leukemoid reaction and granulocytic leukemia, the alkaline phosphatase stain may be used.

The alkaline phosphatase stain reveals values above normal in a neutrophilic leukemoid reaction and values below normal in granulocytic leukemia.

Lymphocytic Leukemoid Reactions

A lymphocytic leukemoid reaction is accompanied by a white cell count of 20,000 to 150,000 per cubic millimeter and a differential white cell count showing 35 to 95% lymphocytes.

Thus, from a laboratory viewpoint, a lymphocytic leukemoid reaction may resemble lymphocytic leukemia.

A lymphocytic leukemoid reaction may be found in the following conditions: mumps, measles, chickenpox, whooping cough, infectious lymphocytosis, and infectious mononucleosis.

Of the above conditions, infectious mononucleosis probably gives the most trouble, for it is often difficult to differentiate between infectious mononucleosis and lymphocytic leukemia.

The distinction between infectious mononucleosis and lymphocytic leukemia can usually be made by the heterophil agglutination test.

The heterophil agglutination test is usually positive in infectious mononucleosis and negative in lymphocytic leukemia.

Myelodysplastic syndromes (MDS)

Precise diagnostic criteria for the MDS were recently proposed by the FAB group. All of them are characterized by hypercellular bone marrows. Five conditions are included under the broad term MDS.

1. Refractory anaemia (RA), with erythroid hyperplasia and/or dyserythropoiesis.

2. RA with ring sideroblasts, also designated as acquired idiopathic sideroblastic anaemia (AISA), the main feature being the presence of ring sideroblasts in at least 15% of erythroblasts.

3. RA with excess of blasts (RAEB) which shows dyspoiesis in the three bone-marrrow cell lineages, dysgranulopoiesis being always conspicuous. The percentage of bone-marrow blasts is between 5 and 20%; these cells may have a few or no azurophil granules.

4. Chronic myelomonocytic leukaemia (CMML), with many features of RAEB plus a significant peripheral blood moncytosis (usually over 1×10^9/l).

5. RAEB in transformation, a group close to AML, and defined by the presence of blasts in the peripheral blood (over 5%) and between 20 and 30% in the bone marrow.

In addition to staining for iron, the other cytochemi methods used in AML may be useful for the study of the MDS. They may help to define the monocytic component in CMML or the type of blasts in RAEB and they are particularly useful in demonstrating dysgranulopoiesis, e.g. by the presence of neutrophils negative for peroxidase and/or Sudan Black B reactions or giving extremely low NAP scores.

CHAPTER 7

DIAGNOSTIC SIGNIFICANCE OF PERIPHERAL BLOOD SMEARS

Apart from the search for blood parasites, examination of the stained smear is screening of formed elements of the blood. Valuable information can be collected in cases of anaemias and definite diagnosis can be established of the nature of some of them, like megaloblastic anaemia and sickle-cell anaemia. Infectious mononucleosis and frank leukaemias can also be easily spotted out. Lastly examination of the smear, used as a base-line study, can prompt one about further examinations to be undertaken for the diagnosis.

ABNORMALITIES OF ERYTHROCYTES

Size

With some experience it is possible to say if the red cells are of normal size (normocytosis), diminished in size (microcytosis) or increased in size (macrocytosis). One judges the size by the diameter (normal average: 7.2 microns). In severe anaemia there is variation in the size of cells; this is anisocytosis. Megalocytes are large oval cells found in megaloblastic anaemias.

Shape

Red cells with an irregular shape are called poikilocytes. The commonest irregularity is a pear-shaped cell. Poikilocytosis, like anisocytosis, is non-specific phenomenon found in all severe anaemias. In haemolytic anaemias the red cells are abnormally thick; they look like densely stained microcytes; the abnormality is known as microspherocytosis. Target cells are thin red cells with a relatively large diameter and resemble the concentric circles of a rifle target; they are seen in various anaemias, in obstructive jaundice and after splenectomy. Sickle-cells may be seen in stained smears; their presence, diagnostic of sickle-cell disease due to the abnormal haemoglobin S, is best demonstrated by a special in-vitro technique. Burr cells are red cells with a spiny periphery; they are seen in large numbers in uraemia. Schistocytes are red cell fragments found in many blood diseases with increased haemolysis.

Colour

The intensity of the red colour of the erythrocyte in a stained smear is a rough indication of corpuscular haemoglobin concentration. In a hypochromic red cell the normal central pallor is increased. Hypochromasia indicates iron-deficiency.

Immature red cells

Immature red cells in the peripheral blood can only come from the marrow. The correct significance of immature red cells in the peripheral blood can be best realised by studying their source —

erythropoiesis in the marrow by means of marrow biopsy. Normal erythropoiesis is described as "normoblastic". Abnormal erythropoiesis is called "megaloblastic" and is due to the deficiency of vitamin B_{12}, or folic acid, or both.

Abnormalities of Leucocytes

These mainly consist of the presence of immature leucocytes and of granulocytes with toxic granulations. Normally an occasional metamyelocyte or juvenile (about 1 per cent) are present. In pyogenic infections (with leucocytosis) their count goes up. A few myelocytes are common in the blood of infants and children. In adults a few myelocytes and an occasional myeloblast (without leucocytosis) may be found in severe anaemias and when the marrow is the seat of metastatic deposits of a carcinoma. However, in chronic myeloid leukaemia, the blood shows a large number of myelocytes (10 to 50 per cent) and fewer myeloblasts (2 to 5 per cent). In acute myeloid leukaemia the myeloblast is the predominant cell in the blood (upto 90 per cent). In chronic lymphatic leukaemia the predominant cell in the blood is the small lymphocyte, forming 85 to 99 per cent of leucoctyes; lymphoblasts are rare. In acute lymphatic leukaemia the lymphoblast is the predominant cell. In monocytic leukaemia 50 to 90 per cent of leucocytes are monocytes and their precursors (monoblasts); a few myelocytes and myeloblasts are also encountered. In infectious mononucleosis (glandular fever) 40 to 80 per cents of leucocytes are ordinary lymphocytes, ordinary "abnormal cells". The last are primitive monocytes. Morphologically infectious mononucleosis can be confused with monocytic leukaemia; in the former the patient's serum contains agglutinins for sheep's red cells (Paul-Bunnel's test).

In severe acute infections neutrophils may show vacuolation of the cytoplasm and their granules become coarse and blue-stained. These, "toxic granules" are indicative of severe toxaemia. Heavy granulation is also seen in aplastic anaemias.

ABNORMALITIES OF PLATELETS

A significant reduction of platelets (thromobocytopenia) can be judged in the smear. In essential thromocytopenia platelets may in addition show morphological abnormalities in the forms of small size, giant forms or non-granularity of their cytoplasm. Abnormal variation in the size of platelets is a feature of myelosclerosis.

PARASITES IN BLOOD

The malarial parasite and microfilariae are the commonest in our country. The former is seen in the red cell and takes various forms, depending upon the species and the stage of development. The latter is found free in the blood and a special technique has to be followed for its demonstration. The other blood parasites are the Leishman-Donovan bodies (in kala-azar), trypanosomes (in sleeping sickness of Africa) and spirochaetes (in relapsing fever). You will be learning about these parasites in detail in parasitology chapter.

Only common findings are referred to in what follows. Polychromasia (polychromatophilia) is diffuse bluish-grey staining of the red cell. Basophil stippling is the presence of multiple coarse granules in the red cell. Cells which show polychromatophilia and basophil stippling are reticulocytes and their presence is indicative of active erythropoiesis, as in haemolytic anaemias. Pappenheimer bodies are small scanty basophilic granules in the red cell; unlike the granules of basophilic stippling, these bodies give a positive prussian blue reaction; they are siderophilic granules. Pappenheimer bodies are characteristically present after splenectomy. Cells with Pappenheimer bodies or siderophil granules are known as siderocytes. Cabbot's rings are reddish purple rings or like the figure of eight. Howell-Jolly bodies are reddish blue nucleated fragments. Cabbot's rings and Howell-Jolly bodies are seen in severe anaemias and after splenectomy. They have no specific significance.

The nucleated red cell commonly encountered in the peripheral blood is the normoblast. An occasional normoblast is a normal finding in the newborn. A few normoblasts — 2 to 5 per 100 leucocytes — may be persent in any severe anaemia. If present in large numbers, a haemolytic anaemia with an actively regenerating marrow is suspected. The presence of a megaloblast in the peripheral blood means that erythropoiesis must be megaloblastic and that the patient must be suffering from a megaloblastic anaemia. The common red cell abnormalities are summarised in Table 17.

Table 17. *Red Blood Cell Abnormalities Seen on stained Smear*

Descriptive term	Observation	Importance
Macrocytosis	Cell diameter>8μm MCV>96fl.	Megaloblastic anaemias, severe liver disease. Hypothyroidism.
Microcytosis	Cell diameter<6μm MCV<76fl MCHC<27	Iron deficiency anaemia. Anaemia of chronic disease. Thalassemias.
Hypochromia	Increased zone of central pallor	Reduced Hb content.

Polychromatophilia	Presence of red cells not fully hemoglobinized	Reticulocytosis.
Poikilocytosis	Variability of cell shape	Sickle cell disease. Microangiopathic hemolysis. Leukemias. Extramedullary hematopoiesis. Marrow stress of any cause.
Anisocytosis	Variability in cell size	Reticulocytosis. Transfusing normal blood into microcytic or macrocytic cell population.
Leptocytosis	Hypochromic cells with small central zone of Hb (target cells)	Thalassemias. Iron deficiency anaemia. obstructive jaundice.
Spherocytosis	Cells without central pallor, loss of biconcave shape MCHC high	Loss of membrane relative to cell volume. Hereditary spherocytosis Accelerated RBCs destruction by reticuloendothelial system.
Schistocytosis	Presence of cell fragments in circulation	Increased intravascular mechanical trauma. Microangiopathic hemolysis.
Acanthocytosis	Irregularly spiculated surface	Irreversibly abnormal membrane lipid content. Liver disease. betaliporoteinemia.
Echinocytosis	Regularly spiculated cell surface	Reversible abnormalities of membrane lipid content. High plasma free fatty acids. Bile acid abnormalities. Effects of barbiturates, salicylates, etc.
Stomatocytosis	Elongated, slit-like zone of central pallor	Hereditary defect in membrane sodium metabolism. Severe liver disease.
Elliptocytosis	Oval cells	Hereditary anomally, usually harmless.

CHAPTER 8

HAEMORRHAGIC DISORDERS

Haemorrhagic disorders are characterised by bleeding into tissues, either spontaneous or after slight injury. They are due to failure of the normal haemostatic mechanism.

Haemostasis

Spontaneous arrest of bleeding is a complicated process. The first event after injury to a vessel is bleeding for some time. This is followed by prompt retraction and reflex vasoconstriction of damaged vessels lasting for a few minutes; simultaneously the normal tissue tone and the increased pressure on the vessel wall from without by the extravasated blood tend to halt the further escape of blood. The third event is the settling of platelets on damaged sites in the vessel wall and their agglutination. Agglutinated platelets release serotonin which causes a prolonged vasoconstriction of both damaged and surrounding vessels. Meanwhile a firm fibrin clot has formed in the wound and seals the vessel so that even with dilatation of the vessel, there is no further bleeding. Later the clot is dissolved through organisation and repair is complete.

Defective haemostasis may be due to : (1) defects in capillaries, (2) defects in platelets, (3) defects in plasma factors responsible for the clotting of blood and, (4) presence of circulating anticoagulants which may be normal protective factors in excess or abnormal factors. The first and the second mechanism may be combined, as also, the second and the third mechanism.

Defects in Capillaries

These are: (a) anatomical malformations, (b) defective contractility, (c) degenerative changes in the wall produced by old age and (d) damage to the wall caused by deficiency of vitamins C and P, bacterial toxins, chemicals, drugs and products generated during hyper-sensitivity reactions. The manifestations of capillary damage may be purpura (spontaneous pin-point haemorrhages in the skin and mucous membranes), ecchymosis (large purple areas of haemorrhage, which later become bluish, in the skin) and haemorrhages into tissues of internal organs. Hess' capillary resistance test (described below) is used to demonstrate capillary defects.

Defects in Platelets

Normally the platelet number is 250,000 to 500,000 per c.mm. The life-span of the platelet is 3 to 4 days. The spleen is their main graveyard but some destruction also occurs all over the reticuo-endothelial system. Possibly they have many functions, the chief one being haemostasis. They mechanically seal off defects in vascular endothelium. On coming into contact with a water-wettable surface larger than themselves, they adhere to it and disintegrate (only in the presence of Ca ions) liberating thrombo-plastin (ethanolamine-phosphatid) which converts prothrombin into thrombin. A small number of platelets suffices for this reaction. However, plentiful platelets must be present to cause retrac-

tion of the fibrin clot. Platelets also contain serotonin (5 hydroxy-tryptamine) and epinephrine and norepinephrine which can cause vasoconstriction of small vessels. A heparin-neutralising factor has also been demonstrated in them.

Defects in platelets may be quantitative or qualitative. Reduction in platelets (thrombocytopenia) below 40,000 is usually associated with purpura; there is also an increase in the bleeding time and the capillary resistance test is positive, but the coagulation time is not altered unless the reduction is extreme. The clot, however, will not retract well. The decrease in the number may be due to insufficient production in the marrow (hypoplasia or aplasia of the marrow) or due to splenic action (hypersplenism) restricting their release into circulation, or due to consumption of a large number in closing gaps in bleeding blood vessels, or due to an antiplatelet antibody (produced as an immunologic response) destroying platelets rapidly. The qualitative defect consists of an undue stability (thrombasthenia) which will lengthen the coagulation time, or of reduction in their adhesive property (possibly due to the splenic influence).

Defects in Plasma Factors Responsible for Clotting of Blood

Coagulation of blood is a chain reaction in which many different factors are involved. The nomenclature of these factors is confusing. The following table from Dacie gives the recommendations of the International Nomenclature Committee.

Nomenclature for Blood Coagulation Factors

Factor	Synonym
I	Fibrinogen
II	Prothrombin
III	Thromboplastin (Tissue)
IV	Calcium
V	Proaccelerin, labile factor
VI	(Entity not defined)
VII	Proconvertin
VIII	Antihaemophilic factor (AHF)
IX	Christmas factor, plasma thromboplastic component (PTC)
X	Stuart-Power factor
XI	Plasma thromboplastin antecedent (PTA)
XII	Hageman factor
XIII	Fibrin stabilising factor, Laki-Lorand factor

Theories of coagulation of blood will have to be read from text books of physiology or haematology; the following is a general outline of various factors concerned, as given by Leavell and Thorup.

I. The development of thromboplastic activity:

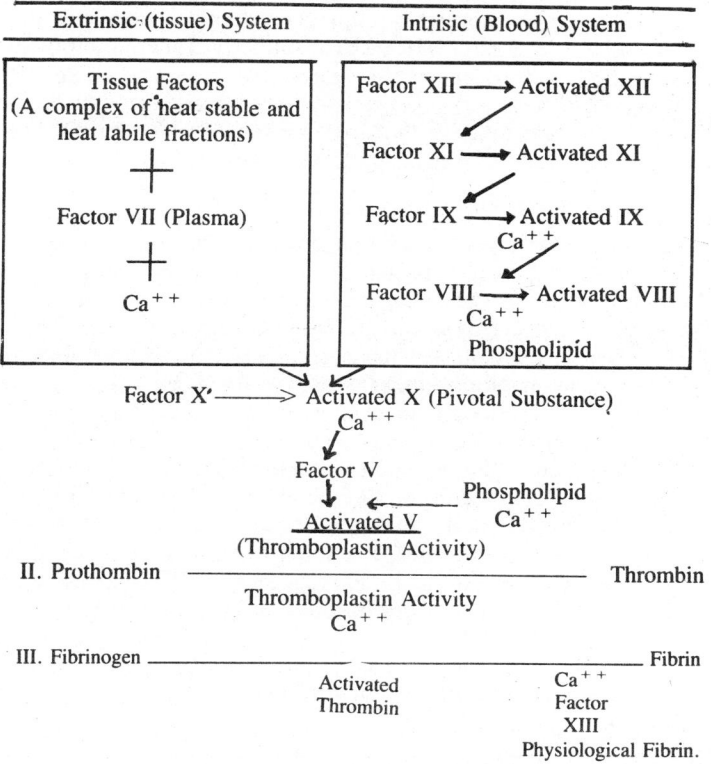

Extrinsic (tissue) System	Intrisic (Blood) System

Tissue Factors
(A complex of heat stable and
heat labile fractions)

$+$

Factor VII (Plasma)

$+$

Ca^{++}

Factor XII $\longrightarrow$ Activated XII

Factor XI $\longrightarrow$ Activated XI

Factor IX $\longrightarrow$ Activated IX
Ca^{++}

Factor VIII $\longrightarrow$ Activated VIII
Ca^{++}
Phospholipid

Factor X' $\longrightarrow$ Activated X (Pivotal Substance)
Ca^{++}

Factor V
$\downarrow$ $\longleftarrow$ Phospholipid
Activated V Ca^{++}
(Thromboplastin Activity)

II. Prothombin $\underline{}$ Thrombin
Thromboplastin Activity
Ca^{++}

III. Fibrinogen $\underline{}$ Fibrin
Activated Ca^{++}
Thrombin   Factor
XIII
Physiological Fibrin.

IV. Accelerating and inhibiting mechanisms: Blood must be kept fluid in the vascular system yet clot quickly whenever necessary. Further, there must be a mechanism to dispose off a clot once the damaged vessel has been repaired. Thrombin is supposed to accelerate coagulation when it is in a nascent state through an autocatalytic or chain reaction, possibly by causing lysis of platelets. The inhibitors of coagulation in the plasma are: anti-cephalin (neutralises thromboplastin), anti-thrombin and heparin which interferes with the development of thromboplastin activity, possibly by acting in co-operation with a heparin-co-factor. The removal of the clot, once it has served its purpose, is done by the proteolytic enzyme fibrinolysin or plasmin. Plasmin exists in plasma in an inactive state (plasminogen).

Investigations In Cases Of Haemorrhagic Disorders

The underlying basis for the patient's symptoms and complaints is abnormal bleeding. The objectives behind the investigations are: (1) to establish the presence of an abnormality and (2) to determine the specific defect and its cause. Screening tests are enough for the first objective; the second objective can only be realised by employing elaborate specific tests.

History: This is an important preliminary. Is there history of bleeding from different sites or does the bleeding occur from the same site but without an organic cause? In the past history the following points are important. Is there history of bleeding from the umbilical cord, after loss of a tooth or after an operation? In the adult life and in a female patient, is there history of excessive menstruation or abnormal bleeding during pregnancy and delivery? At all period of life a history of bleeding profusely after a minor trauma is most suggestive of an disorder of coagulation. The family history — enquiry for the existence of bleeders in the family

— should extend upto the patient's grandfather. It is necessary to note whether the bleeders in the family are all males or whether they belong to either sex.

The physical examination: Petechiae and ecchymyosis in the skin over pressure points indicate vascular defect. The location of bleeding spots has a characteristic distribution in different purpuras. On the other hand, haemorrhage in joints, large haematomas or post-traumatic haemorrhages suggest a disorder of coagulation.

Laboratory Investigations

To detect the specific defect a number of investigations may have to be carried out; some are simple and within the reach of every laboratory, others so complex that only specialised laboratories can undertake them.

Base-line Studies

Haemoglobin estimation and examination of the stained smear.

Simple and Basic Laboratory Investigations

(a) Hess' capillary resistance test (tourniquet test): A circle of 6 cm diameter is marked out in the antecubital fossa and the skin in that area is examined for petechiae; these are marked out. Apply the sphygmomanometer cuff at least 1 inch above the circle and keep the pressure at 50 mm. for 15 minutes or at 80 mm for 5 minutes. Now count the number of petechiae in the circle in light (300 wattlamp kept 2 feet from the arm). More than 8 petechiae are considered abnormal and the test is declared positive.

(b) Bleeding time (Duke method): Make a skin puncture, preferably in the lobe of the ear with a straight needle and note the time. Every half a minute blot the drop of blood with filter paper without touching the skin till the bleeding stops, and note the time. The interval between the time of the puncture and the time of stoppage of bleeding, or the number of drops on the paper divided by 2 gives the bleeding time in minutes. the normal range is 1 to 5 minutes.

(c) Coagulation time (Lee and White method): Collect with a dry (preferably siliconised) syringe 5 ml of blood from a vein; the venepuncture should be quick and neat, otherwise much tissue juice will get mixed with the blood. Start a stop watch the moment the blood enters the syringe. Detach the needle and gently deliver 1 ml of the blood in each of four clean and dry tubes (75×8 mm). The tubes are previously warmed at 37°C and kept in a water-bath at that temperature. At every half a minute tilt the tubes in turn untill each can be tilted through an angle greater than 90 without spilling the contents. Note the time. The clotting time of each tube is measured separately. Take the average of the four readings. The normal clotting time is 4 to 10 minutes.

(d) Clot retraction time: The clot in one of the tubes for the coagulation time is separated from the wall of the tube by gently rimming the top of the clot with glass applicator. The tube is stoppered and kept in a water-bath at 37°C. Inspect at ½, 1, 2, 4, and 24 hours for signs of retraction (separation of clot with expression of serum). Normally retraction of the clot from the walls of the tube starts in 30 minutes, is appreciable in 1 hour and is complete in 24 hours. In abnormal conditions there is no retraction even after 24 hours. Clot retraction is delayed in cases of thrombocytopenia (below 100,000 per c.mm), in fibrinogenopenia and in some cases of hypoprothrombinaemia.

(e) Platelet Count Direct method: As described earlier.

(f) Prothrombin Time (one stage)

1. Collect the blood from a vein taking care to avoid tissue injury. The blood is collected in citrate solution in the proportion of 9 parts of the blood to 1 part of 3.8 per cent citrate solution.

2. Centrifuge the mixture and separate out the plasma immediately. This may be stored in a refrigerator for not more than 4 hours. Haemolysed specimens should be discarded.

3. Normal plasma, collected in a similar manner, must also be available (control). Both this and the patient's plasma are treated in the same manner.

4. In a tube (75 × 8 mm) pipette 0.1 ml of the plasma and 0.1 ml of thromboplastin solution (Thromboplastin is prepared from human brain).

5. Place the tube in water-bath at 37°C for 2 minutes.

6. Add 0.1 ml. of warmed M/40 calcium chloride solution. Mix the contents gently. Start a stopwatch. Shake the tube gently in the bath for 3–4 minutes. Now take it out and tilt almost horizontally to allow the contents to run back and forth. Note the appearance of fibrin clot; this is the end point. Note the time.

The normal prothrombin time is about 12 to 14 seconds. The principle of this method is that all substances required for clotting — thromboplastin, calcium and fibrinogen — with the exceptin of prothrombin are supplied in optimum quanties and the clotting time becomes a measure of the prothrombin content of the plasma tested. However, it is not realised that the prothrombin is affected by firinogen, prothrombin, Factor V, Factor VII and Factor X.

(g) Prothrombin Consumption Test: In normal coagulation thrombin production and prothrombin utilization go on even after the blood or the plasma has clotted. The prothrombin consumption test finds out the prothrombin time of serum one hour after coagulation has occurred to measure the amount of prothrombin consumed in reacting with the plasma thromboplastin. Deficiency of coagulation factors leads to incomplete consumption of prothrombin. It is more sensitive test in detecting of AHF and platelets, than the whole blood clotting time.

Special Tests

These can only be undertaken by laboratories specialised in work on coagulation disorders. Therefore only the principles of the tests and their significance will be mentioned below:

(a) Thromboplastin Generation Test: The reagents used are: (1) Absorbed plasma (adsorbed by aluminium hydroxide gel)· which contains Factors V, VII, XI, and XII; (2) Serum which contains Factors IX, X, XI and XII; (3) Platelets or cephalin substitute; and (4) Ca. If a mixture of these four reagents is incubated and if at one minute intervals a portion of the incubation mixture is added to normal platelet-free citrated plasma, the coagulation time of the latter becomes a measure of the intrinsic thromboplastin generated in the incubation mixture. If the test gives abnormal results, it is repeated by serially substituting the patient's plasma, serum and platelts by the normal counterpart. The defect can thus be localised; if the defect is in the patients' adsorbed plasma, the deficiency involves Factors V and VIII; if in the patient's serum, it involves Factors IX and X; and if in both the plasma and the serum, circulating anticoagulants are suspected. If one stage prothrombin time is combined with thromboplastin genera-

tion test, it becomes possible to track down the defect still further: In the face of a normal prothrombin time a plasma defect in the thromboplastin generation test indicates deficiency of Factor VIII (AHF); similarly if the prothrombin time is normal, the serum defect is deficiency of Factor IX (PTC).

(b) Circulating anticoagulants: The clotting time of normal blood is lengthened by the patient's platelet-free plasma. To determine the nature of the anticoagulant further tests are necessary. Heparin is neutralised by protamine sulphate or toludine blue; if the anticoagulant is an inhibitor of thromboplastin, or of AHF, further tests with mixtures of patient's plasma and normal plasma are recurred. Circulating anticoagulants may be spontaneously occurring (as in haemophilia, Christmas, disease, disseminated lupus erythematosus and pregnancy) or of the nature of drugs.

(c) Tests for Fibrinogen concentration: These are meant to detect hereditary hypofibrinogenaemia and acquired hypofibronogenaemia (defibrination syndrome of late pregnancy). The clotting time and the prothrombin time are raised: the thrombin generation test gives normal results. The thrombin time— the ability of a standard solution of thrombnin to clot the citrated plasma of the patient — can be used as a measure of the concentration of fibrinogen. Fibrinogen can also be estimated chemically.

The following table summarises the significance of the various laboratory tests in haemorrhagic disorders:

Table 18

Laboratory test	Conditions in which it is abnormal
1. Clotting time (prolonged)	Haemophilia (AHF, VIII deficiency), PTC deficiency (IX, Christmas disease) PTA, (XI) deficiency, circulatory anticoagulants, hypofibrinogenaemia, sometimes in vitamin K deficiency (hypoprothrombinaemia).
2. Bleeding time (prolonged)	Thrombocytopenia, thrombasthenia, vascular purpura and conditions listed under 1, if severe.
3. Platelet count (reduced)	Abnormality affecting haemopoiesis or haemopoietic tissues.
4. Clot retraction (poor)	Thrombocytopenia (primary or secondary), thrombasthenia, fibrinogen deficiency and prothrombin deficiency.
5. Prothrombin time (one stage) (prolonged)	Deficiency of prothrombin, deficiency of fibrinogen, deficiency of Factors V, VII and X decumarol or tromexan therapy, vitamin K' deficiency, liver disease (impaired formation of prothrombin and Factors V and VII) hyperheparinaemia.
6. Prothrombin consumption (reduced)	Deficiencies of AHF, PTC and PTA, thrombocytopenia, thrombasthenia., circulating antithromboplastin.
7. Tourniquet test (positive)	Thrombocytopenic purpuras, non-thrombocytopenic purpura (vascular purpura scurvy, thrombasthenia).
8. Thromboplastin generation test: Al(OH)₃ plasma deficiency Serum deticiency'	AHF (VIII) deficiency, Factor V deficiency, anti-thromboplastin. PTC (IX) deficiency, Factor X deficiency.
Deficiency of both adsorbed plasma and serum	Deficiency of Factors XI and XII.
Platelet deficiency	Thrombasthenia.

40

CHAPTER 9

SPECIAL NOTE ON L.E. CELL PHENOMENON

Systemic lupus erythematosus affects women most commonly and is characterized by a skin rash, arthralgia, fever, renal, cardiac, and vascular lesions, anaemia, leukopenia, and often thrombocytopenia. There is a factor in the serum that has the ability to cause depolymerization of the nuclear chromatin of polymorphonuclear leucocytes and this depolymerized material is subsequently phagocytosed by an intact polymorph, giving rise to the "LE Cell". This antinuclear material may be found in other collagen disorders, in some cases of rheumatoid arthritis, and in some cases of chronic discoid lupus erythematosus, which is a relatively benign form of the disease limited to the skin. The serum factor is an immunoglobulin and may be of the IgG, IgM, or IgA class, or combinations of them. IgG is most commonly present. There does not appear to be any relationship between the immunoglobulin class and the clinical status.

Demonstration of LE Cells

A variety of methods exist, all of which can be used. The rotary technique is considered the most sensitive cellular technique. In practice, most laboratories perform a latex test and anti DNA antibody test. If these are both negative, the LE cell preparation is not performed (vide infra).

Clotted Blood

This is the simplest method and gives good results. 10 ml of clotted blood is placed in the water bath at 37°C for 1 to 2 hrs. After incubation the supernatant and loose cells are withdrawn (the clot may first have to be "ringed" or separated) and buffy coat smears made.

Alternatively, the whole clotted specimen after incubation may be mashed through a fine wire sieve and buffy coat smears made from the resultant cell suspension.

Defibrinated Blood

Defibrinated blood gives good preparations. The blood is defibrinated immediately after withdrawal and the blood incubated for 2 hours at 37°C. Smears are made as with clotted blood.

Citrated or Heparinized Blood

Citrated or hepainized blood may be used and incubated, as for clotted and defibrinated blood. The preparations obtained in this manner are satisfactory, but inferior to those from clotted or defibrinated blood. Also, heparin tends to produce bluish staining.

Incubated Serum

The patient's serum may be incubated with washed normal leucocytes, even after storage of the serum at 20°C for months.

Rotary Method

Five glass beads 3 mm in diameter are added to a heparinized sample of blood. The tube is then rotated at 50 rpm for 30 minutes at 37°C. Buffy coat smears are subsequently prepared.

The LE Cell

This is usually a neutrophil polymorph (Occasionally a monocyte or eosinophil) that has ingested the altered nucleus of another polymorph. The bulk of the cell is occupied by a spherical, homogeneous mass that stains purplish-brown. The lobes of the polymorph are usually seen at the periphery of the mass. The smears, (LE cell are most numerous at the edges and end of the smear), are searched and a minimum of 500 polymorphs are counted before a negative result is given. Frequently, dead nuclei will be seen lying free; if numerous, these may heighten suspicion, but they are never diagnostic. Occasionally a group of polymorphs will collect around altered nuclear material and will form a "Rosette" (Fig. 33).

With the rotary technique, free extracellular altered nucleoprotein may be seen and this again will increase the suspicion of LE cells being present. LE cells must be differentiated from "Tart" cells which are usually monocytes that have phagocytosed another whole cell or nucleus (often a lymphocyte). The ingested nuclear material is well preserved in contrast to the LE cell inclusion body, and may be found in normal people. Its significance, if any, is unknown.

Sensitivity and Specificity of LE Tests

The simplest test to perform is the latex nucleo protein test. This test is specific when positive, but will detect only 45 to 50% of possible positives. The LE cell test is moderately sensitive and specific but both false positive and false negative results can occur. Attention to technique is important and serial examinations should be performed before a patient can be considered as negative for LE. The fluorescent technique for antinuclear antibody (ANA) is a highly suitable screening procedure because of its sensitivity. It does, however, lack specificity and positive results can be obtained in other autoimmune and collagen diseases. A negative ANA virtually eliminates a diagnosis of LE.

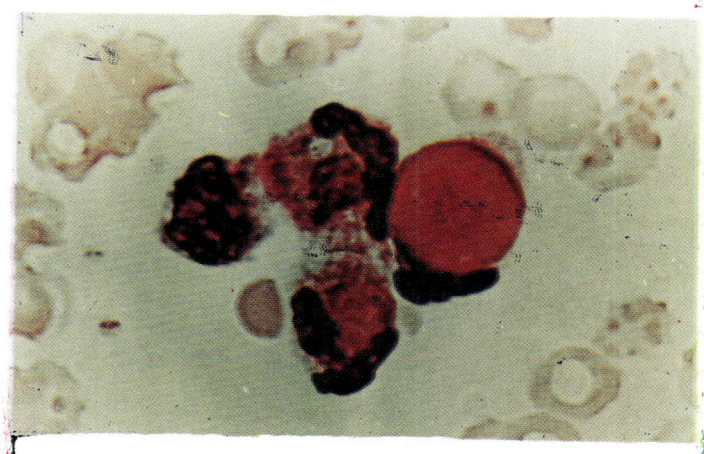

Fig. 33 Showing L.E. cells

SECTION II

URINE ANALYSIS; CEREBROSPINAL FLUID; OTHER BODY FLUIDS AND STOOL EXAMINATION

CHAPTER 10

URINE ANALYSIS

INDICATION FOR EXAMINATION OF URINE

Examination of the urine is an invaluable procedure in the detection of anatomical and functional abnormalities of the kidney and the 'urinary tract'. It is one of the most important screening procedure in clinical medicine because it can give diagnostically important information about the presence of diseased states even outside the urinary tract. For example, the presence of diabetes mellitus, acidosis or jaundice can be so easily detected. Urinalysis becomes a basic investigation in conditions characterised by derangements of metabolism. Cultural examination of the urine is done for the diagnosis of enteric fevers, as also, for the detection of urinary carriers of these infections. So widespread is the utility that basic examination of the urine may be considered as part of the physical examination of a patient.

COMPOSITION OF URINE

Although about 98 to 99 per cent of the water in the glomerular filtrate is reabsorbed in the tubules, it still constitutes about 95 per cent of the urine. The other 5 per cent (Table 19) is 2 per cent urea, and the remaining 3 per cent is divided into small amounts between a number of inorganic and organic substances — principally sodium chloride, potassium, calcium, magnesium, ammonia, uric acid, phosphates, sulfates and creatinine. Variations in diet, work and exercise influence the relative amounts of these various constituents to a considerable degree. The blood serum level of many of these materials is preferred clinically. Therefore, the chemical determination of only those materials that are clinically significant will be considered in the examination of urine. Also, as previously indicated, the chemical composition of an individual's urine varies during different parts of the day, in relation to meals, work and sleep. Normally the total solids excreted in the urine vary from 60 to 75 gm with no sugar and no protein.

A rough but valuable estimation of the total solids can be made by the following technique:
1. The last two figures of the 24-hours specimen specific gravity × 2.33.
2. This figure × the number of ml in the 24-hour specimen.
3. This figure divided by 1000 = total solids in gm.

Collection of Urine

The sample should be fresh and should be examined immediately. This is because, on keeping at room temperature, the reaction might change (from acidic to alkaline), casts might disintegrate, crystalline precipitate — not originally present — may appear and bacterial growth may make the specimen turbid. General preserva-

Table 19 *Average Normal Composition of Urine*

Constituents	Grams/Liter
Inorganic	
Chloride (as NaCl)	9.0
Phosphorus (as P_2O_5)	2.0
Total sulfur (as SO_3)	1.5
Sodium (as Na_2O)	4.0
Potassium (as K_2O)	2.0
Calcium (as CaO)	0.2
Magnesium (as MgO)	0.2
Iron	0.003
Organic	
Urea	25.0
Uric acid	0.6
Creatinine	1.5
Ammonia	0.6
Undetermined N	0.6
Sugar (insufficient for positive Benedict's test)	Trace
Ketone bodies	Trace
Carbonates, bicarbonates, and free carbonic acid	Trace
Pigments	
Mucin and mucin-like substances	
Diastase	

tion of the specimen, is done by addition of chemicals (Boric acid 0.5 g per 60 ml; formaldehyde, 2 to 4 drops per 30 ml; thymol, 0.1 g per 100 ml; and toluol, enough to cover the surface on which it floats) or by keeping the specimen in a refrigerator. Special preservatives are to be used for special tests; for example, concentrated hydrochloric acid in estimations of calcium and nitrogen. Obviously, no preservatives can be added if a bacteriological (culture or animal inoculation) examination is to be done. Specimen meant for examinations, other than bacteriological, can be collected in a bottle of suitable size, cleaned with soap & water. The specimen must be properly labelled.

(1) For routine examination the usual practice is to collect the early morning sample, the quantity required being about 100 ml. This sample, being the night's collection, is the most concentrated and will show casts best. On the other hand, if the objective is to determine the presence of albumin or sugar, a specimen collected 2–3 hours after a meal is preferable.

(2) For any quantitative test a specimen obtained from a mixed 24 hours collection is absolutely necessary; a quantitative estimation on a random sample has no meaning.

The patient empties the bladder (say at 8 a.m.) and this sample is discarded. Thereafter he preserves all the urine he voids till 8 a.m.

the next day; he must empty the bladder at this time (8 a.m.) and this sample must be added to the total collection. The collection is done in a large bottle of suitable size; a preservative may be added. The whole quantity is thoroughly mixed, its volume measured and about 150 to 200 ml submitted for examinaiton.

Preservation of specimen

Urinary decomposition occurs quickly in warm temperatures. Hence fresh specimens should be examined, if not, then it should be refrigerated. As far as possible the need for preservation should not arise. However the following presevatives can be used:

1. *Toluol*— best for preservation of chemical constituents. Add 2 ml toluol/100 ml urine.
2. *Thymol*— a small floating lump of thymol can preserve the urine for several days in a bottle. Thymol may, however, cause a false positive reaction for protein.
3. *Formalin*— 1 drop/30 ml urine is good for preserving formed elements. It can precipitate proteins and can reduce Benedict's solution.
4. *Boric acid*— 0.3 gm/120 ml of urine. However, yeasts can still grow and urine acid crystals get precipitated.

Routine Examination of Urine

Physical Examination

1. *Total volume*: The quantity of the urine passed in 24 hours varies inversely with the amount of fluid eliminated by the lungs, the skin and the bowels, and is influenced by physiological factors like fluid intake; diet (a high protein diet having a diuretic effect), exercise, environmental temperature and humidity, body-weight and age. Infants and children excrete for their weight, 3–4 times more urine than adults.

Polyuria is increase in the output of urine and is seen in diabetes mellitus, diabetes insipidus, early stage of chronic nephritis and during recovery from oedema. In renal insufficiency the night urine may exceed the day urine (nocturia). *Oliguria* is diminution in the urinary output; this is seen in acute and chronic glomerulonephiritis, congestive cardiac failure, shock fevers and dehydration from any cause. *Anuria* is supression of urine formation, the output fa lling to less than 100 ml. It is seen commonly in acute glomerulonephiritis, in chronic renal disease (terminally), crushed injury and after a mismatched blood transfusion.

Serial measurement of the total urinary excretion is an important procedure in gauging the efficacy of the treatment of oedema.

2. *Specific Gravity*: A twenty-four hours sample is to be preferred. The urine should be taken in a cylindrical or conical urine-glass and the urinometer floated in it freely. Urinometers are usually calibrated for 20°C. So the observed figure has to be corrected for the difference between this temperature and the room temperature in the proportion of 0.001 to every 3°C.

In health the specific gravity of urine is directly proportional to the concentration of dissolved solids and inversely to the volume. This relationship between the volume and the specific gravity is lost in disease; in diabtes mellitus the volume is increased as also the specific gravity over (1040) due to presence of sugar), while in the late stage of chronic glomernephritis the urine passed is of low specific gravity (below 1010) despite the low total volume. Proteinuria (albuminuria) raises the specific gravity (as in the nephrotic syndrome). The fixity of the specific gravity round about 1010

— inability of the kidney to lower the specific gravity (or raise the volume) on a high fluid intake, or raise the specific gravity (or lower the volume) on a restricted fluid intake — is an indication of renal insufficiency or defective resorptive power of the renal tubule. The dilution and concentraton tests for renal efficiency are based on this principle.

3. *Color*: Under normal conditions the color of the urine varies directly with the concentration because *urochrome*, the chief normal pigment, is a product of endogenous metabolism and excreted in constant quantities independent of the diet. Another yellow pigment normally present in the urine, *urobilin*, is derived from the urobilinogen formed in the intestinal tract and absorbed into the blood stream. With increased blood destruction, as in pernicious anaemia or hemolytic icterus, increased quantities of urobilin are formed, resorbed, escape from the liver into the general circulation and are excreted in the urine. In liver damage increased amounts of urobilin likewise may appear in the urine. A positive test for urobilin, therefore, indicates increased blood destruction or pathologic changes in the liver.

Other pigments (Table 20) that may color the urine include *bilirubin* or its oxidation product *biliverdin*. Bile pigments are present in the urine only when some obstruction within the duct system or hepatocellular damage prevents their normal excretion by the liver.

4. *Turbidity*: Freshly voided acid urine is clear. However, when alkaline it may be cloudy due to the presence of phosphates. Pus

Table 20 *Abnormal Color of Urine*

Substance	Color	Pathological States Occuring in
Bilirubin	Yellowish foam	Obstructive lesion of bile duct system or severe hepatocellular damage
Biliverdin	Greenish foam	Oxidation product from bilirubin
Increased urobilin	Yellow to amber	Increased blood destruction or pathological changes in liver
Porphyrins	Reddish	Congenital porphyria, lead and barbital poisoning, pernicious anaemia, and hemolytic jaundice
Hemoglobin	Clear red to reddish brown	Paroxysmal hemoglobinuria, malaria, transfusion reaction, arsenic poisoning
Blood	Smoky red to brown	Acute nephritis, intarenicts in kidneys, bleeding lesions in urogenital tract
Melanin	Brown to black	Malignant melanoma, leukemia, ochronosis, and carcinoma of liver
Homogentisic acid	Black	A congenital anomaly, alkaptonuria
Methylene blue	Blue	Administered for renal function test
Pyridium	Orange to red	Administreed as urinary analgesic
Acriflavine	Greenish fluorescence	Administered as urinary antiseptic
Phenol	Dark, smoky	Poisoning
Phenol-sulfonphthalein	Red in alkaline urine	Adminsitration as laxative or for renal function test
Bromsulfalein	Red in alkaline urine	Adminstration as liver function test

and blood also may cause turbidity, the former being white whereas the latter produces a red smoky appearance. Upon standing urine may show clouding to the point of sediment formation from bacterial decomposition or precipitation of alkaline salts, mostly amorphous phosphates, or a white to pinkish sediment of amorphous urates in acid urine. A faint cloud of mucus, leukocytes and epithelial cells may become visible. All these must be differentiated by microscopic examination.

5. *Odour*: The normal odour is due to volatile aromatic acids and urinoid. An ammoniacal odour, in a freshly passed sample, is due to decomposition from stasis in the bladder, and is present in cystitis. Fruity odour is present when the urine contains acetone bodies.

Chemical Examination

Reaction: This is tested by means of red and blue litmus papers. It is recorded as acidic, alkaline or amphoteric. The reaction has diagnostic significance. The *pH* of the urine in health varies between 5 and 7.5. This can also be tested by *pH*-Papers.

Qualitative Tests For Proteins In Urine

Heat and Acetic Acid Test

Procedure: In a 6 × 5/8 inch test tube place about 10 ml of urine; make acidic with a few drops of 30% v/v acetic acid. Heat the top inch of the urine in a small Bunsen flame. If a cloudy precipitate appears in the heated portion of the urine, add a few more drops of 30% v/v acetic acid and reheat. If the precipitate persists, proteins are present.

Methods for Recording Reactions: A wide diversity of methods for reporting qualitative tests is in use which accounts, in large part, for discrepancies in reports from different laboratories. A uniform method and terminology are urgently needed. The following are recommended:

    − = *negative*

    ± = *very slight trace*. Cloudiness or ring can just be seen against a black background (0.01 per cent or less).

  + (1) = *slight trace*. Cloud is distinct but not granular; no definite flocculation. or the ring is sufficiently definite to be seen without a black background (0.01 to 0.05 per cent).

  + + (2) = *moderate trace*. Cloud is distinct and granular without definite flocculation. or the ring is dense but not wholly opaque when viewed from above (0.05 to 0.2 per cent).

 + + + (3) = *heavy cloud*. Cloud is dense with marked flocculation or the ring is heavy, wholly opaque and sometimes curdy (0.2 to 0.5 per cent).

+ + + + (4) = *very heavy cloud*. Heavy precipitate to boiling solid; or very dense ring. Represents 0.5 or higher per cent of albumin; 3 per cent albumin boils solid.

Sulfosalicylic Acid Test

Procedure: Layer onto about 3 ml of urine in a test tube an equal quantity of 10% w/v sulfosalicylic acid in 50% methanol. If proteins are present, a cloudy precipitate will appear at the junction of the two fluids.

Heller's Ring Test

Reagent: Nitric acid, concentrated, or 1 part of concentrated nitric acid + 5 parts of a saturated aqueous solution of magnesium sulfate (Robert's Reagent).

Take 2 to 3 ml of the reagent in a test tube, and allow filtered urine to run slowly down the inside of the tube from a pipette so as to form a layer on top of the acid. Note whether a ring appears or not.

When the test is positive, a sharply defined white ring of varying density appears where the two fluids come into contact. If only trace of albumin is present, the ring appears after a few minutes.

Uric acid, urea, thymol, and resinous drugs, when present in urine in high concentrations, may give a white crystalline precipitate which however disappears on dilution, and when due to resinous drugs, dissolves in alcohol.

Robert's Test

Reagent: To 5 parts of a saturated solution of magnesium sulphate add one part of pure nitric acid.

Place few ml of the reagent in a test tube and gently layer the urine on the reagent. Albumin gives a white ring which varies in density with the amount of albumin present. When only traces of albumin are present, the white ring may not appear 2 to 3 minutes.

Quantitative Tests for Albumin

Esbach's Test

Prepare the reagent by dissolving 5 g of picric acid and 10 g of citric acid in 500 ml of water. Or, the reagent may be prepared by diluting 100 ml of trichloracetic acid with 900 ml of water.

Fill an Esbach's albuminometer with urine to the mark "U". Add reagent to the mark "R". Close with a rubber stopper, invert several times and set aside in a cool place for 18 to 24 hours. Read off the results according to the markings on the tube which show albumin in grams per litre; to express the per cent, divide by 10.

Bence-Jones Protein Test

(1) Bence-Jones protein is particularly pathognomic of multiple myeloma. Proteins with somewhat similar characteristics have been observed in leukaemia, osteomalacia and in young persons with high blood pressure. The protein is characterized by the formation of a precipitate when urine is heated at 50° to 60°C. It disappears wholly or partially as the temperature approaches the boiling point and reappears upon cooling. It is markedly influenced by the acidity and salt-concentration.

Technique: It is advisable to put up three tubes of different acidity. Filter the urine if it is not clear, and adjust to a *pH* just faintly acid to litmus. Put a few ml. of this urine into each of three tubes. To the second and third add respectively 1 and 2 drops of 33% acetic acid. Place the tubes in a waterbath with a thermometer and heat very slowly and gently. Turbidity will begin to appear at about 40°C and precipitates will be visible at 60°C. Now raise the temperature to 100°C. The precipitate now partly or totally disappears. Allow to cool, and the precipitate will reappear.

Urine containing albumin should be filtered at or near the boiling point, and the filtrate is tested for Bence-Jones protein.

When only small amount of Bence-Jones protein is present *electrophoresis* is particularly useful.

(2) *Toluenesulfonic acid test*: Add 1 ml of TSA reagent to 2 ml of urine, let the reagent flow slowly by the side of the test tube. Mix. A precipitate appearing within 5 mts, indicates presence of Bence Jones Protein. A negative test excludes.

Bence-Jones proteins are microglobulins and like haemoglobin are synthesised by plasma cells, both normal and neoplastic (myeloma cells). Bence-Jones proteinuria is seen most commonly in multiple myelomatosis (in 50 per cent of cases); uncommonly it is also seen in leukaemias and other malignant lymphomas, metastatic carcinoma of bone, senile osteomalacia and primary amyloidosis. In multiple myelomatosis combined serum and urine electrophoresis for Bence-Jones protein is the procedure of choice.

Test For Mucin

Principle: The exact chemical nature of mucin has not been determined but it appears to be a glycoprotein. Traces may be present in normal urine. It is frequently increased in irritations and inflammations of the mucous membrane of the urinary tract or vagina. Upon boiling with an acid or alkali, as in Fehling test, it may yield a carbohydrate which reduces copper. Mucin must be differentiated from the Bence-Jones protein.

Procedure: 1. Dilute the urine with about 3 volumes of water and make strongly acid with glacial acetic acid. Do not heat.

2. The presence of turbidity indicates a positive reaction. Albumin is not precipitated by this concentration of acetic acid.

Reducing Substances In Urine

Normally, detectable amounts of reducing substances are not found in urine, except in renal glycosuria. The reducing substance most commonly found in urine is glucose, and its presence there indicates either renal glycosuria, diabetes mellitus, miscellaneous endocrine disorders, intravenous infusion of glucose, or increased intracranial pressure. Other sugars sometimes appears in the urine. e.g., lactose, fructose, pentose, and galactose.

In pregnancy lactosuria occurs at some time in about one-half, glycosuria in about one-fifth, and both sugars together in about one-sixth of the patients, on the average.

Other Reducing Substances

A number of reducing substances other than sugars may be present in urine. Dextrins from ingested pastry, homogentisic acid, and glucuronates reduce Benedict's reagent, although the reduction by homogentisic acid is atypical, ultimately forming a black color. Preservatives, such as chloroform and formaldehyde, indican, santonin, rhubarb, ascorbic acid, creatinine, and protein may react with Benedict's reagent producing a false positive reaction.

Tests for Reducing Substances in Urine

Benedict's Qualitative Test

This test is not specific for sugars and is affected by most reducing substances if they occur in large quantities.

Procedure: In a Pyrex test tube place 0.5 ml (10 drops) of urine and 5.0 ml of Benedict's qualitative reagent. Mix and place in a boiling water bath for five minutes. Allow to cool to room temperature and read as follows:

Color		Result
Blue	—	Negative
Greenish blue	Tr.	Trace
Green	+	Approximately 0.5% reducing substance
Greenish brown	+ +	Approximately 1.0% reducing substance
Yellow	+ + +	Approximately 1.5% reducing substance
Brick red	+ + + +	Approximately 2.0% reducing substance

Benedict's Quantitative Method

Reagents:

Copper sulphate (pure crystallized)	.... 18 g.
Sodium carbonate (crystallized)	.... 200 g.
Sodium or potassium citrate	... 200 g.
Potassium ferrocyanide solution (5 per cent)	.... 5 ml.
Potassium sulfocyanate	.... 125 g.
Distilled water, to make	.... 1000 ml.

With the aid of heat dissolve the carbonate, citrate, and sulphocyanate in about 700 ml. of water and filter. Dissolve the copper sulphate in 100 ml. of water stirring constantly. Add the ferrocyanide solution, cool and dilute to 1 litre. The solution now is of such strength that the copper sulphate in 25 ml is reduced by 0.05 g of dextrose.

Technique: Take 25 ml of the reagent in a small flask, add 10 to 20 g of sodium carbonate crystals, and a small quantity of powdered pumice stone. Boil and add the urine a little at a time, but rapidly, from a burette until a chalk-white precipitate forms and the blue colour of the reagent begins to fade. At this point, add urine in drops, until the last trace of blue just disappears. During the period of titration, the mixture must be kept boiling vigorously. Loss of evaporation must be made good by adding sufficient water. Note the quantity of urine required to discharge the blue colour; this amount of urine contains exactly 0.05 g. of dextrose.

Thus if 'x' ml of urine is required to reduce 25 ml of Benedict's solution, 0.05 g. of dextrose is then present in 'x' ml. of urine. Or, 100 ml of urine contains $(0.05/x) \times 100$g. of dextrose, i.e., $(5/x)$ g.

If the sugar is shown to be mainly lactose, the following figure may be used in the calculations:

25 ml of reagent = 67 mg of lactose.

Acetone Bodies (Ketone bodies)

The acetone bodies are acetoacetic acid (diacetic acid), acetone, and β-hydroxybutyric acid. A state in which these substances are present in increased amounts in the blood and urine is called *ketosis* and is one type of acidosis. Ketonuria indicates abnormal fat metabolism. Acetoacetic acid and β-hydroxybutyric acid, from which acetone is derived, are normal intermediate products of fat metabolism. When greater amounts of fatty acids are utilized with the production of more acetoacetic acid and β-hydroxybutyric acid than can be oxidized by the tissues, these materials accumulate in the blood and are excreted in the urine. Thus ketosis develops in any of the clinical states of deficient carbohydrate metabolism. The most important of these is diabetes mellitus. A ketosis develops with starvation as the carbohydrate stores are depleted and metabolism of fat predominates. A special type of starvation ketosis develops with prolonged vomiting or diarrhea. An interesting but rare condition described by Van Crevald associated with a ketosis is Von Gierke's diseases, in which carbohydrate is stored to an excessive degree in the liver and other organs, but the mobilization is poor. The level of blood sugar is subnormal.

Tests for Acetone Bodies in Urine

Rothera's Test for Acetone and Acetoacetic (Diacetic) Acid

Principle: Both acetone and diacetic acid give a purple color with alkaline sodium nitroprusside. The test will detect acetone in a dilution of 1 in 10,000 and diacetic acid in a dilution of 1 in 125,000.

Procedure: In a test tube place a small crystal of sodium nitroprusside; add about 2 g of ammonium sulfate and about 10 ml of the urine under examination. After shaking well, add about 2 ml of concentrated ammonium hydroxide solution (sp gr 0.88). A deep purple color indicates the presence of excessive amounts of acetone or diacetic acid or both. A pale purple color or no color at all is a negative reaction.

Gerhard's Test for Acetoacetic (Diacetic) Acid

Principle: Diacetic acid gives a Bordeaux red color with ferric chloride solution. Many other substances give colored products with this reagent. and it is important to determine whether the color obtained with a particular urine is the result of the presence of diacetic acid or of some other substance. The excreted derivatives of aspirin are the most common substances that interfere with this test.

Procedure: Place about 5 ml of urine in a test tube and to it add drop by drop, 10% w/v ferric chloride solution until no more precipitate forms; then add two more drops. In the presence of excessive quantities of diacetic acid a Bordeaux red color will develop. Aspirin gives a purple color with this reagent, but it may be confused with the diacetic acid reaction. Therefore, the presence of diacetic acid must be confirmed as follows: Place about 5 ml of urine in a Pyrex test tube and boil it over a Bunsen flame for 3 minutes, or place it in a boiling water bath for 15 minutes. This will convert all the diacetic acid to acetone which will then be volatilized. After it cools, the urine is treated as before with ferric chloride solution. If diacetic acid was present, the test will now be negative. If aspirin or other similar drugs are present, the test will still be positive.

Causes of Ketonuria

1. *Diabetic*: Ketonuria indicates ketoacidosis and if unchecked may go on to coma. Juvenile diabetics are more susceptible to develop this. Whenever glycosuria is more then 2 +, always test for ketone bodies also.
2. *Non diabetic*: In infants and children in.
— Acute febrile states.
— Toxic states with vomiting, diarrhoea etc.
— Hyperemesis gravidarum.
— Cachexia with vomiting.
— Post-anaesthesia vomiting.
— Conditions where there is limited availability of glucose e.g., glycogen storage disease.
— Sometimes following exposure to cold or severe exercise.

Urobilin and Urobilinogen

Urobilinogen, urobilin, stercobilinogen, and stercobilin are decomposition products of bilirubin, normally present in the faeces. In conditions in which there is increased excretion of bile by the liver, e.g., hemolytic jaundice, increased amounts of these substances are absorbed from the intestine and are excreted in the urine. Although it is customary to refer to the substances in the urine as urobilinogen and urobilin, stercobilinogen and stercobilin are usually present in higher concentrations than the former.

Schlesinger's Test for Total Urobilinogen and Urobilin

Principle: Urobilinogen is oxidized with iodine to urobilin. The urobilin is then reacted with an alcoholic solution of zinc acetate and a green fluorescent complex is formed.

Procedure: If bilirubin is present, it is removed by adding a few ml of 10% w/v barium chloride solution to about 20 ml of urine and filtering. Place about 10 ml of urine or bilirubin-free filtrate of urine in a test tube and add two or three drops of Lugol's iodine solution. In another test tube place about 1 g of solid zinc acetate and add about 10 ml of ethyl alcohol; mix by shaking. Pour the urine into the zinc acetate solution and shake thoroughly. Filter through a Whatman No. 1 filter paper into a clean dry test tube. Examine the filtrate for green fluorescence, using either daylight or an ultraviolet lamp. Normal urine shows a faint green fluorescence. A definite green fluorescence indicates an increased output of urobilin(ogen).

Ehrlich's test: Nitrites and bilirubin interfere with this test. Sulfonamide and procaine cause yellowish colour reactions. Pyridium, indole, porphobilinogen and PAS yield pink-red colour not different from that produced by urobilinogen.

To 10 ml of fresh sample at room temperature add 1 ml of Ehrlich's reagent, invert several times and let stand for 5 minutes. A pink colour is normal; cherry or darker red colour indicate abnormal amount of urobilinogen. Dilutions may be used. Colour reactions are normal in dilutions upto 1:20.

(Sensitivity ≥ 1.3 mgm%).

Bile

The constituents or derivatives of bile that may appear in the urine are the bile pigments bilirubin and biliverdin; bile acids, chiefly glycocholic acid; urobilin and urobilinogen. The presence of bile pigments and acids together is associated with obstruction to the outflow of bile from the liver. This may be either intra or extra hepatic. Urinary excretion of bilirubin alone is seen in conditions of excessive hemolysis. Increased amounts of urobilin point to functional incapacity of the liver. Urobilinogen normally is present in the urine in amounts sufficient to give a positive test in dilutions of 1:10 to 1:20. Its absence indicates complete biliary obstruction while increased amounts are associated with excessive blood destruction.

Detection of bile pigment (bilrubin and biliverdin)

Foam test: A yellow or brownish color of the foam produced by vigorous shaking of a sample of urine is suggestive evidence of the presence of bilirubin and usually bile acids in the urine.

Gmelin's test: To a few ml of urine in a test tube add a small amount of concentrated nitric acid in such a manner that two layers are formed. The formation of a rainbow band of colors at the junction of the layers shows the presence of bilirubin. The colors result from the oxidation of bilirubin.

Iodine ring test: A sensitive cum reliable test. Layer a solution 10%, alcoholic iodine on urine in a test tube. A green ring indicates presence of bile.

Fouchet's Test

Principle: Barium chloride solution is added to the urine. A precipitate of barium sulfate is produced onto which the bilirubin is adsorbed. The barium sulfate adsorbed bilirubin is filtered off and a drop of Fouchet's ferric chloride solution added to the precipitate. The ferric chloride oxidizes the bilirubin to biliverdin, producing a greenish blue spot.

Procedure

Take 10 ml of the urine in a test tube and add 5 ml of barium chloride solution (10% aqueous) to precipitate bilirubin. Mix and filter through Whatman No. 2 filter paper, unfold the paper and invert it on another paper to gently transfer the precipitate. To the second paper now add 1–2 drops of Fouchet's reagent (25 g of trichloracetic acid, 100 ml of water and 10 ml of 10% feric chloride solution). Fouchet's reagent oxidises bilirubin to produce a green or blue colour.

Test for Bile Salts (Hay's Sulpher Test)

Take 5 ml of the urine in a test tube and sprinkle on the surface flowers of sulpher. If bile salts are present, sulphur particles sink to the bottom of the tube because bile salts have lowered the surface tension. The urine sample must be fresh & a control with the normal urine should also be done.

In hepatocellular jaundice (infectious hepatitis) there are bile pigments in urine even before jaundice becomes clinically detectable choluria is also present in obstructive jaundice. In haemolytic jaundice there is acholuria, though the urinary urobilinogen is raised.

Blood

Blood present in the urine may be in the form of either intact cells, *haematuria*, or hemoglobin, *hemoglobinuria*. Haematuria may be detected by microscopic examination and hemoglobinuria by chemical test.

Hemoglobin, unaccompanied by red cells, appears in the urine with excessive hemolysis in a number of toxic states; notably, in mushroom poisoning, in poisoning by beans of the species *Vicia fava* (favism), following severe burns, in the black-water fever of falciparum malaria, and following reaction from mismatched transfusion. Poisoning by certain chemicals, notably arsine potassium chlorate and pyrogallic acid produce hemolysis with presence of hemoglobin in the urine. *Paroxysmal* hemoglobinuria may occur with exposure to cold and is associated usually with syphilis and the development of specific hemolysins as shown by the Donath-Landsteiner test. In a second type (nocturnal paroxysmal hemoglobinuria) the attacks are not associated with chilling and usually come on at night. In the march variety, hemoglobinuria appears with severe muscular exertion.

Detection of blood

Benzidine test: Dissolve a small amount (knife-point full) of benzidine base in 2 ml of glacial acetic acid and add an equal volume of 3 per cent hydrogen peroxide. Add 2 ml of urine and mix. The appearance of blue color indicates the presence of hemoglobin. Inferior grades of benzidine may require the addition of larger amounts to obtain a positive reaction.

Guaiac test: Acidify a portion of urine with glacial acetic acid. Add a fresh alcoholic solution of gum guaiac, drop by drop, until there is a slight turbidity. Add a few ml of 3 per cent hydrogen peroxide solution. Development of a blue color indicates the presence of hemoglobin.

Pus will produce the blue color but not if the urine is previously boiled.

A thin film of copper left in the tube after testing for sugar will give a positive reaction as will bromides and iodides.

If minute amounts of blood cells are present, the tests are best performed on the sediment from a centrifuged specimen.

Test for Homogentisic acid

Alcaptonuria is an inborn error of metabolism characterised by a failure to oxidise completely tyrosine and phenylalanine and the resulting excretion in the urine of homogentisic acid.

Technique: 1. Alkali test: Addition of 10 per cent. NaOH solution to alcaptonuric urine produces a brown color in 1 to 2 minutes.
2. Ferric chloride test: Upon the addition of dilute ferric chloride solution to the sample of urine, a deep blue colour appears for a moment until oxidation is complete.

Phenylketonuria

Phenylketonuria is a hereditary metabolic defect due to the lack of the enzyme phenylalanine hydroxylase. This results in blocking the conversion of phenylalanine, an essential amino acid, into tyrosine. The accumulation of phenylalanine and/or some of its abnormal metabolites early, perhaps by age 4 to 6 months, results in brain damage and mental retardation. The disease phenylpyruvic oliophrenia develops characterized by severe mental deficiency with elevated serum phenylalanine and large amounts of phenylpyruvic being excreted in the urine. Early detection and proper dietary regime can prevent the development of this disease.

Detection of phenylpyruvic acid

Ferric chloride diaper test: A drop of 5 or 10 per cent ferric chloride is placed on the diaper which is wet with urine. A gray-green or blue-green spot indicates phenylketonuria.
Ferric chloride tube test: Five drops of 5 per cent ferric chloride are added to acid urine or to urine which has been acidified with dilute sulfuric acid. A dark green color indicates phenylpyruvic acid.

Test for 5-Hydroxyindoloacetic acid (HIAA)

In the malignant carcinoid syndrome excessive amounts of 5-HIAA are excreted in the urine. This can be detected as follows:
Technique: 0.2 ml of urine, 0.8 ml of distilled water, and 0.5 ml of 1-nitroso-2-naphthol solution are mixed in a test tube. Add 0.5 ml. of freshly prepared nitrous acid solution and let stand for 10 minutes. Add 5 ml. of ethylene dichloride and shake.
Reagents: 1.1g of 1-nitroso-2-naphthol in 100 ml of 95 per cent ethyl alcohol.
2. Nitrous acid (0.2 ml of 2.5 per cent sodium nitrite added to 5.0 ml of 2 N H_2SO_4).

A normal urine should be tested as a control. A purple colour of the top layer indicates increased 5-HIAA excretion.

Calcium

Before the estimation of urinary calcium the patient should be on a low calcium diet for 3 days. An aliquot of a 24-hour urine collection is utilized.

Sulkowitch test

Reagent

Oxalic acid..2.5 gm
Ammonium oxalate...2.5 gm

Glacial acetic acid .... 5.0 ml
Distilled water q.s .... 150 ml

Procedure: To 3 ml of cleared urine are added 3 ml of Sulkowitch reagent and they are mixed. After 2 minutes the degree of turbidity is estimated by a scale of 0 (no precipitate) to 4 + (a flocculent precipitate).

Interpretation: A zero test indicates hypocalcemia with a serum level below 7.5 mg. per 100 ml, the renal threshold. With a normal serum calcium of 9.5 to 11.5 mg per 100 ml there is a moderate amount of turbidity. A 3 or 4 + test indicates hypercalcuria and suggests hypercalcemia, such as in hyperparathyroidism.

Cystine

To 5 ml of urine add 2 ml of 5% sodium cyanide solution and let them react for 10 minutes. Add 5 drops of 5% sodium nitroprusside solution and mix thoroughly. Cystine produces a magenta colour. If no cystine is present a pale brown or pale pink color results. All solutions should be freshly prepared. Also examine the urinary sediment for cystine crystals. Urinary cystine is raised in cystinurias.

Fat in urine

Take equal parts of urine and ether; coludiness due to fat disappears, decant ether onto a watch glass, evaporate; fat leaves a greasy deposit. Fat may be seen microscopically.

Porphyrins

The porphyrin nucleus is a structural component of hemoglobin, myoglobin, cytochromes, catalases, oxidases and peroxidases. Characteristic magenta fluorescence is seen when acidic solutions of porphyrins are irradiated with ultraviolet light.

In *porphyria* increased amounts of uroporphyrin or protoporphyrin are present in urine. Coproporphyrins also may be present. All are derived from prophobilinogen. The porphyrias are of two types, *porphyria erythropoietica* and *porphyria hepatica* depending upon the pathway of synthesis. Porphyria erythropoietica has its onset in infancy or childhood. Bullous skin lesions appear on exposure to light. The urine is a burgundy-red color which darkens with standing. Laboratory identification of uroporphyrins but no porphobilinogen confirms the diagnosis. Porphyria hepatica may be of the intermittent acute type, a chronic disease of adults in which gastrointestinal and neurological symptoms predominate; the cutanea tarda type, in which photosensitivity becomes manifest in adult life, and the mixed type in which symptoms of both are combined. Porphobilinogen is characteristic of the disease but its identification in the urine is difficult. Porphobilinogen in urine exposed to air will be converted into the dark red colored porphobilin.

In *porphyrinuria* coproporphyrins predominate in the urine. Coproporphyrinuria III may occur after exposure to metals (lead poisoning is a prominent example), sedatives, sulfonamides, alcohol and various organic substances; in hypermetabolic states; with hepatic disease; in various hematological conditions; and in pellagra and riboflavin deficiency. In lead poisoning the amount of coproporphyrin III excreted in the urine is markedly increased. Small or moderate increases are to be interpreted with caution.

Methods for identification and quantitative estimation of porphyrins are based upon solubility differences in organic solvents and chromatographic or spectrophotometric analysis. Qualitative testing of urine for porphobilinogen is simple procedure.

Watson-Schwartz porphobilinogen test

Ehrlich's reagent

Paradimethylamidobenzaldehyde .... 0.7 gm
Concentrated hydrochloric acid .... 150 ml
Distilled water .... 100 ml

Procedure: Add 3 ml of Ehrlich's reagent to 3 ml of urine and mix. Add 6 ml of saturated solution of sodium acetate. If a reddish color develops, add 3 ml. of chloroform. Shake for 2 minutes then let stand. Persistence of the reddish color in the aqueous supernatant indicates porphobilinogen. However, many substances can cause a false positive reaction. Notable are the anticonvulsant drugs, pyridium, urorosein or indoxyl.

Tests For Porphyrins

Principle: Porphyrins are substituted tetrapyrril methenes. Small amounts may be found in normal urine. Urine containing large amounts (*porphyrinuria*) may be dark red or a "port wine" color. Darkening of a light colored urine upon standing hours or longer is suggestive of porphyrinuria.

Procedure: 1. To 25 ml of urine in a separatory funnel add 10 ml of glacial acetic acid. Extract this mixture twice with 50 ml portions of ether and combine the extracts. Wash the combined extracts with 10 ml of 5 per cent hydrochloric acid.

2. Examine the washings under ultraviolet light. If there is a strong red fluorescence, a large amount of coproporphyrin is present, suggestive of porphyria. Examine the urine residue after ether extraction under ultraviolet light. A discernible red fluorescence is indicative of the presence of uroporphyrin. These tests should be confirmed spectroscopically as follows:

3. To 100 ml of urine add 20 ml of a 10 per cent solution of sodium hydroxide.

4. Filter or centrifugalize off the precipitate.

5. Wash the precipitate with water and with alcohol.

6. Add 5 ml of alcohol and 5 to 10 drops of concentrated hydrochloric acid.

7. Dissolve, filter until absolutely clear, and examine spectroscopically for the adsorption bands of acid haematoporphyrin (Chart 2).

An acetic acid test, which is much less reliable, consists in adding 5 ml of glacial acetic acid to 100 ml of urine and allowing the mixture to stand 48 hours. The pigment exists in the form of a precipitate.

Ferric Chloride Testing

Many amino acids react with ferric chloride to give distinctive colors. Ferric chloride testing is a screening test not only for aminoacidurias but also for many abnormal metabolites and drug excretion products. Definitive diagnosis requires specific identification and measurement of the relevant materials in blood or urine

Substance	Colour alteration
Amino acids	
α-Ketobutyric acid	Purple, fading to red brown
Homogentisic acid (alkaptonuria)	Rapidly fading blue or green
p-Hydroxyphenylpyruvic acid (tyrosinosis)	Rapidly fading green
Valine, leucine, and	Blue

isoleucine (maple syrup disease)

Phenyl pyruvic acid (phenylketonuria)	Stable green or blue green
Other metabolites	
Acetoacetic acid	Red or red-brown
Melanin	Gray, changing to black
Indican (Hartnup disease, intestinal stasis, malabsorption)	Violet or blue
Drugs	
Aspirin, salicylates	Stable red-wine colour
Phenothiazine derivatives	Immediate purple-pink
p-Aminosalicylic acid (PAS)	Red-brown
Phenol derivatives	Violet

Strip Technology

Now-a-days strips are available commercially which can be used for following tests — specific gravity, *p*H, Protein, Glucose, Ketone (Aceto-acetic acid), Bilirubin, Blood and Urobilnogen in urine. The strips are firm plastic strips to which are affixed various seperate reagent areas.

Principles of Procedures and their Limitations

1. **Specific Gravity:** This test is based on the pKa change of certain pretreated polyelectrolytes in relation to ionic concentration. In the

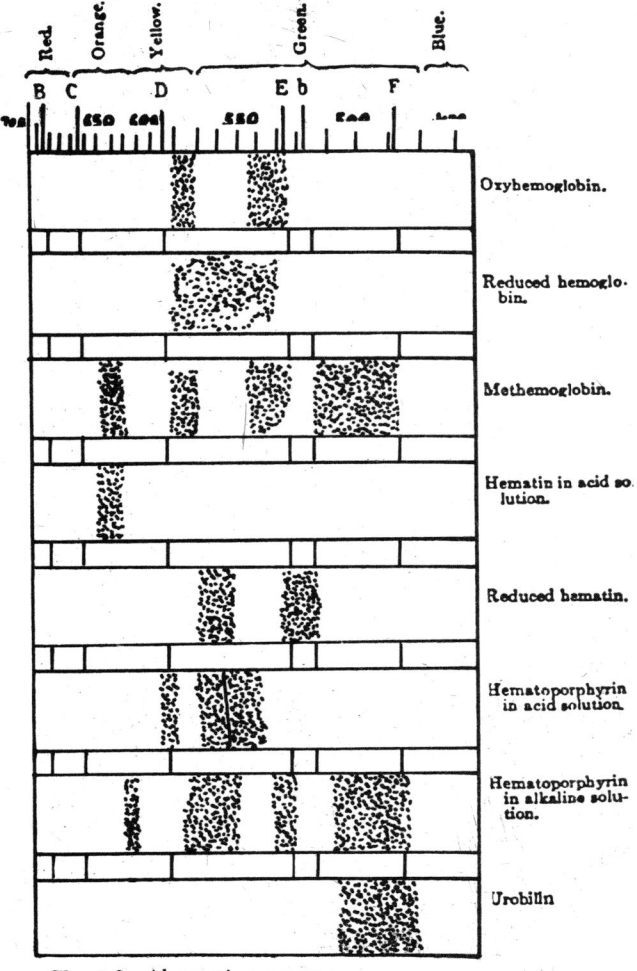

Chart 2. *Absorption spectra.*

presence of an indicator, colors, range from deep blue-green in urine of low ionic concentration through green & yellow-green in urines of increasing ionic concentration.

Limitations: Urine containing glucose or urea at concentratiopn greater than 1% may cause a low specific gravity reading relative to other methods. Highly buffered alkaline urines may also cause low readings. Elevated specific gravity reading may be obtained in the presence of moderate (100–750 mgm/dl) quantities of protein.

2. *p*H: This is based on double indicator principle which gives a broad range of colors covering the entire urinary *p*H range. Colors range from orange through yellow and green to blue.

3. **Protein:** At a constant buffered *p*H, the development of any green color is due to the presence of protein. Colours range from yellow for negative through yellow-green and green to green-blue for positive reactions.

Limitations: False positive results may be obtained with highly buffered, alkaline urine. Contaminating ammonium compounds may also cause false positive results.

4. **Glucose:** Glucose oxidase enzyme catalyzes the formation of gluconic acid and hydrogen peroxide from oxidation of glucose. Second enzyme peroxidase, catalyzes the reaction of hydrogen peroxide, with a potassium iodide chromogen to oxidize the chromogen to colors ranging from green to brown.

Limitations: Ascorbic acid concentration of 75 mgm/dl or greater may cause false negative results for specimen containing small amounts of glucose (100 mgm/dl)

5. **Ketone:** It is based on the development of colors ranging from buff-pink, for a negative reaching, to maroon when acetoacetic acid reacts with nitroprusside.

Limitations: False positive result may occur with highly pigmented urine.

6. **Bilirubin:** This is based on the coupling of bilirubin with diazotized dichloroaniline in a strongly acidic medium. The color ranges through various shades of tan.

Limitations: Metabolites of drugs which give a color at low *p*H may cause false positive results. Ascorbic acid may cause false negative results.

7. **Blood:** This is based on the peroxidase like activity of haemoglobin.

Limitations: Elevated specific gravity or proteins may reduce the activity of the test.

8. **Urobilinogen:** This is based on Ehrlich reaction in which paradimethylaminobenzaldehyde reacts with Urobilinogen in a strongly acidic medium to produce a brown orange color.

Procedure: 1. Collect fresh urine in a clean, dry container. 2. Remove strip from bottle and replace cap. Completely immerse reagent areas of the strip in fresh urine and remove immediately. 3. Remove excess of urine & hold the strip in horizontal position. 4. Compare test areas to corresponding color charts on the bottle label at the specified time, match carefully.

Microscopic Examination Of Urine

If possible, urine deposits should be examined within 8 hours of collection, preferably within 1 to 2 hours.

Procedure

1. Mix the urine thoroughly and place about 12 ml in a conical centrifuge tube. Centrifuge for 5 minutes at 1500 to 2500 rpm; pour off the supernatant fluid; resuspend the deposit in the few drops of urine that remain by flicking the end of the tube with the

52

finger; then place a drop on a microscope slide; cover with a cover glass.

2. Examine with the low power objective to obtain an over-all picture of the deposit. Use the higher power objectives to examine objects more closely. In order not to miss casts cut the light to a minimum by means of the rheostat, or by lowering the condenser, or by closing the iris diaphragm.

Substances appearing in the urine deposits are of three main types: cells, casts and crystals (including amorphous chemical deposits)

Cells

Epithelial Cells

Squamous Epithelial Cells: These large cells with small round or oval nuclei are derived from the ureters, bladder and urethra. In urine from female patients not obtained by catheterization, vagina epithelial cells may also be present. This is normal and of no significance.

Polyhedral Epithelial Cells: Small round cells slightly larger than leukocytes, and caudate epithelial cells, which are smaller than the squamous cells and have a tail-like process, may also be present. These are derived mainly from the upper tract.

Red Cells: In hypertonic urine the red cells may be crenated and smaller than normal. In hypotonic urine they are swollen and larer than usual, losing their typical "double ring" appearance. The presence of red cells in the urine indicates bleeding in some part of the urinary tract. It is important that contamination from menstrual flow be avoided when urine from females is to be examined.

Leukocytes: The normal excretion rate for leukocytes in the urine is up to 3 per μl i.e., 3000 per ml or up to about 200,000 per hour.

Microscopy of uncentrifuged urine is better, but the only accurate method is to make quantitative WBC counts on a timed (2–4 hour) specimen of urine, using a Fuchs-Rosenthal or equivalent, hemocytometer, and taking the average of four to six counts on the mixed, fresh specimen.

Spermatozoa: Spermatozoa may be present in the urine of a male after ejaculation or in female urine as a vaginal contaminant after coitus. They are easily recognized.

Bacteria: Bacteria are not normally present in urine. Contamination can easily occur if the urine is not collected by catheterization, however, and if the urine is allowed to stand at room temperature for any length of time, it may be swarming with bacteria. They are of no significance unless the urine has been collected by an aseptic technique and placed in a sterile container.

Casts

Casts are of many types; they are formed by the solidification of protein in the nephron tubule, often with trapped cells, granular debris, and so forth.

Hyaline Casts: Hyaline casts are cylindrical, transparent bodies that are difficult to see unless the illumination is cut a minimum.

Finely Granular Casts: These casts are similar to hyaline casts but contain fine granules.

Coarsely Granular Casts: These have larger granules than the finely granular casts but are similar in appearance.

Leukocyte Casts: Leukocyte casts are composed mainly of leukocytes.

Blood Casts: These are easily recognized because they are almost entirely composed of red cells and often have a bright orange color.

Fatty Casts: These casts are any casts that contain fat droplets. Examination by polarized light may show anisotropic lipids, especially in lipid nephrosis.

Waxy Casts: Waxy casts are similar to hyaline casts but are more opaque and often have a curled end or "tail"

Renal Failure Casts: In the late stages of many renal diseases residual nephrons often become dilated. Casts developing in these nephrons tend to have large diameters. If they are numerous they indicate a grave outlook or "end-state" kidney.

Cylindroids: Cylindroids are long ribbon-like formations that resemble hyaline casts but are much longer and are often tapered.

Mucus Threads: Mucus threads may be mistaken for hyaline casts, but they are usually much longer, less regular, and wavy, and they have tapered ends. Amorphous urates or phosphates may form aggregates on mucus threads which resemble casts but they seldom have the parallel sides and smooth ends of true casts.

The presence of casts in urine, especially if albumin is also present, usually indicates kidney disease.

Staining of Urine Sediment

This facilitates recognition of cells, especially for the inexperienced technologist. Wet preparations may be stained in several ways:

1. A drop of resuspended sediment on a slide is mixed with a small drop of a 1:2 to 1:4 dilution of Löffler's methylene blue.

2. Sternheimer-Malbin Stain

Solution A:

Crystal violet	3.0 g
95% alcohol	20 ml
Ammonium oxalate	0.8 g
Distilled water	80 ml

Solution B:

Safranin O	0.25 g
95% alcohol	10 ml
Distilled water	100 ml

Working Stain: Mix 3 volume of solution A with 97 volume of solution B and filter. This will last up to three months.

Procedure: To the resuspended sediment in a centrifuge tube add 1 drop of the working stain and let stand 3 minutes after mixing. Then place a drop on a microscope slide, cover and examine.

Results: Normal polymorphonuclear nuclei take up both dyes and stain orange-purple. Glitter cells tend to take only the crystal violet and appear pale blue or colorless. Hyaline casts are stained pink to purple; RBCs, lavender; cellular casts, dark purple; and *Trichomonas* and nuclei of bladder and vaginal epithelia, light blue, blue and purple, in that order.

3. Oil Red O. If a drop of sediment is mixed with a drop of saturated solution of oil red O in isopropanol, fatty casts and fat droplets will be stained, but most of the latter, if present, will be found floating on the surface of the urine.

Ova and Parasites in Urine

Trichomonas is occasionally seen, especially in fresh specimens. Ova in urine are usually derived from fecal contamination, except in cases of *Schistosoma haematobium* intestation.

Crystals

Crystals are not normally present in freshly passed urine and are precipitated from solution as the urine cools. Generally speaking, crystals in the urine are of no significance, except crystals of sulfonamides, cystine, oxalate in persons with a history of ureteral colic or stone formation, and, possibly, urates in those with gout.

Crystals Appearing in Acid Urine (Refer Table 21)

Calcium Oxalate: These are colorless, octahedral crystals and appear as small squares crossed by two diagonal lines. In another form calcium oxalate crystals are dumbbell-shaped. They vary greatly in size.

Uric Acid: Uric acid crystallizes in many forms (e.g., plates, prisms, sheaves, and hexagons). The crystals are usually colored and are easily dissolved by heating. They are soluble in sodium hydroxide but insoluble in hydrochloric acid.

Urates: Urates often appear as an amorphous sediment which dissolves when heated. Sodium urate crystals are often in the form of thorn apples.

Cystine: These crystals are highly refractile hexagonal plates, similar to the plate form of uric acid crystals; however, they may be differentiated from uric acid crystals by their solubility in hydrochloric acid. They are rarely found, but when present are diagnostic of a rare inborn error of metabolism termed cystinuria, in which the patient excretes excessive amounts of the amino acid in the urine. Cystine crystals are soluble in alkali and are not found in alkaline urine.

Tyrosine: Tyrosine is usually in the shape of fine needles or sheaves. The are seldom found except in acute liver failure.

Leucine: The occurrence of leucine crystals in urine is open to question.

Crystals Appearing in Alkaline Urine (Refer Table 21)

Phosphates: Phosphates often appear as an amorphous sediment which is soluble in acetic acid.

Triple Phosphates: The usual forms of these crystals are "prisms" and "coffin lids." They are soluble in acetic acid.

Calcium Carbonate: These crystals can appear as dumbbells, spheres, or amorphous granules. They are soluble in acetic acid.

Ammonium Urate: These crystals can appear in round, oval or thorn-apple form. They are soluble in acids.

Other Crystals

Sulfonamide: Crystals of the sulfonamides often appear in the urine after administration of these drugs. They are of many forms and may be confused with some of the naturally occurring crystals. If there is any doubt as to the identity of crystals, and if the patient is being treated with sulfonamides, the following test may be applied:

Test for Sulfonamides: Deposit the crystals by centrifuging the urine in a Pyrex centrifuge tube. Decant the supernatant urine and add to the deposit 0.5 ml of 50% v/v hydrochloric acid. Mix and place the tube in a boiling water bath for about 30 minutes. Cool the solution and then dilute to 10 ml with distilled water.

The presence in the urine of excreted radiographic contrast media, e.g., iodopyracet (Diodrast), occasionally will produce masses of neddle-like crystals accompanied by a very high specific gravity.

Table 21 *Chemical sediments in urine*

Reaction of urine	Character of sediment	Chemical composition of sediment
Acid	(i) Yellow or reddish-brown crystals, variable size & shape; most characteristic forms are rosette-like clusters of 'whetstones' or prisms; often rhombic(paler colour).	Uric acid; soluble in sodium hydroxide solution
	(ii) Colourless, glistening, octahedral crystals, so-called envelope crystals. Variable size. Unusual forms are: colorless dumb-bells, spheres. (May be encountered in alkaline urine).	Calcium oxalate; soluble in hydrochloric acid.
	(iii) Fine, yellowish granules, sometime colorless; rarely, slender prisms arranged in fanlike or sheaflike structure.	Sodium and potassium urates; heat-soluble.
Alkaline	(i) Colourless crystals, "coffin-lid" like; sometimes feathery, star-like or leaf-like.	Ammonio-magnesium phosphate; soluble in acetic acid.
	(ii) Colourless prisms, arranged in stars or rosettes (stellar phosphate).	Dicalcium phosphate; soluble in acetic acid.
	(iii) Colourless granules.	Amorphous phosphates; soluble in acetic acid.
	(iv) Colourless granules; rarely, spheres or dumb-bells.	Calcium carbonate; soluble in acetic acid with liberation of gas.
	(v) Opaque yellow crystals, usually spheres with fine or coarse spicules.	Ammonium biurate: soluble in acetic acid; (rhombic plates of uric acid appear on acidification).

For urinary sediments refer Fig. 34–42.

EVALUATION OF RENAL FUNCTION TESTS

General Considerations

A clear understanding of the mechanism of kidney function is essential for a complete appreciation of the significance of urinary findings and the renal function tests.

The kidneys, fortunately, have, like the liver, a tremendous reserve functional capacity. Normal life activities easily can be sustained by only one kidney and while many lesions, infections, tumors, or traumatic injuries may be unilateral, kidney disease, such as glomerulonephritis or nephrosclerosis, is bilateral. The functions of the kidneys are: (1) to rid the body of waste products of metabolism, (2) to rid the body of foreign and nonendogenous substances, (3) to maintain salt and water balance, and (4) to maintain the acid-base equilibrium of the body.

The formation of urine involves three separate activities of the nephron: (1) an adequate flow of blood to the nephron; (2) filtration of the plasma of this blood by the glomerulus; and (3) reabsorption and secretion of substances by the renal tubules.

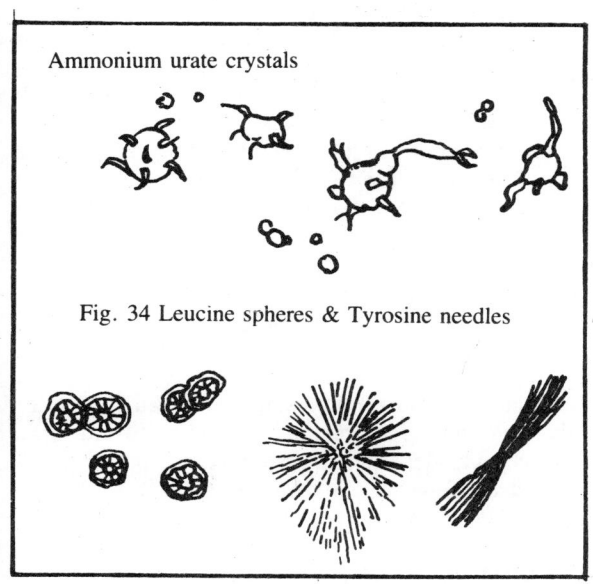

Ammonium urate crystals

Fig. 34 Leucine spheres & Tyrosine needles

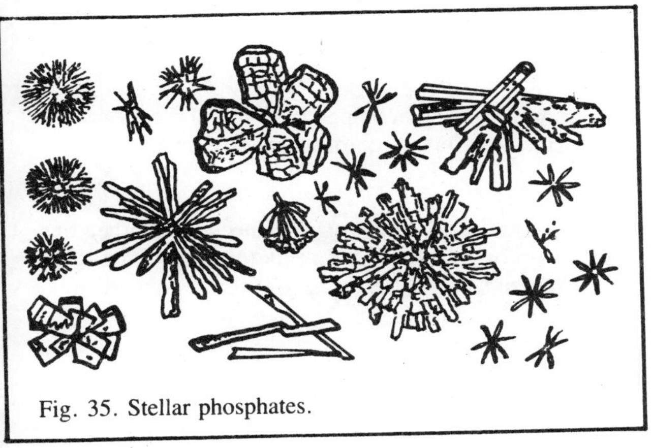

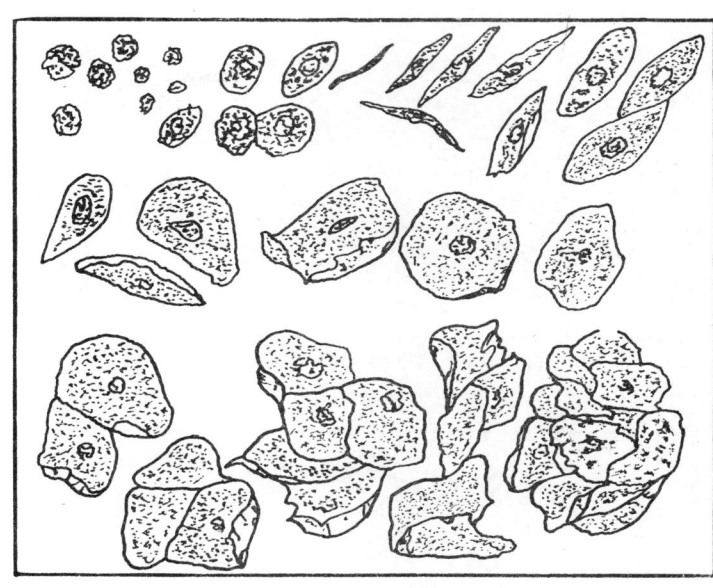

Fig. 37. Types of epithelial cells

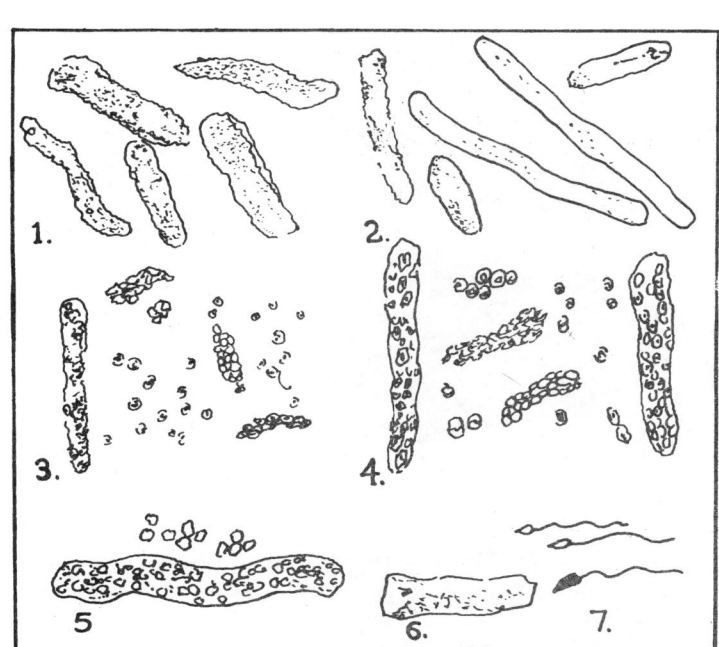

Fig. 35. Stellar phosphates.

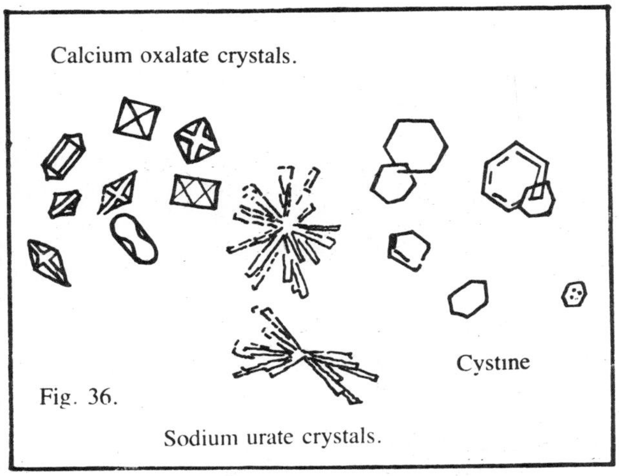

Calcium oxalate crystals.

Cystine

Fig. 36.

Sodium urate crystals.

Fig. 38 1. Fine and Coarse granular casts.
2. Hyaline casts.
3. Leucocyte casts.
4. Epithelial casts.

5. Blood casts.
6. Waxy casts.
7. Spermatozoa.

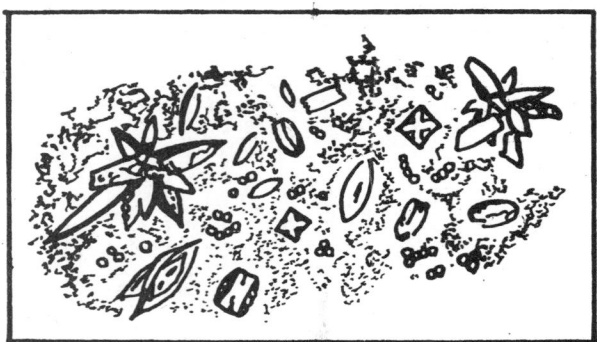

Fig. 39 Deposit in acid urine

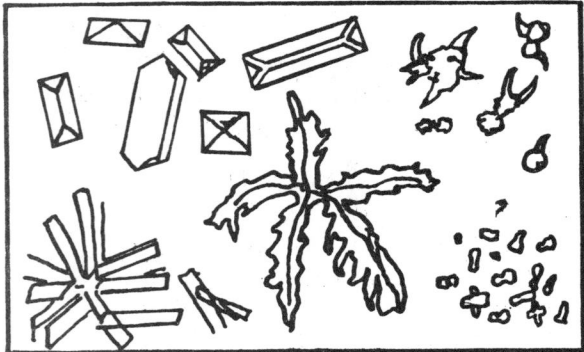

Fig. 40 Deposit in alkaline urine

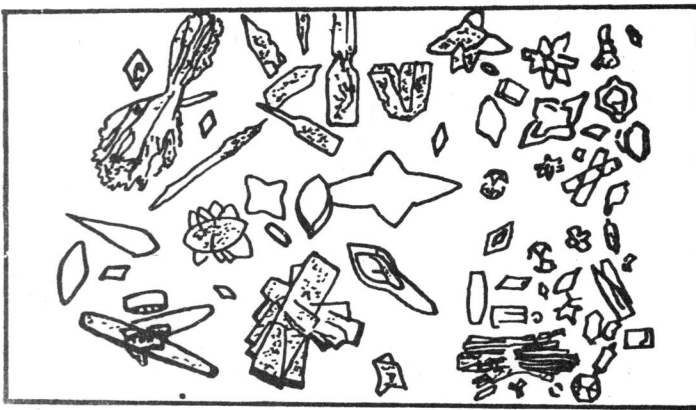

Fig. 41 Uric acid.

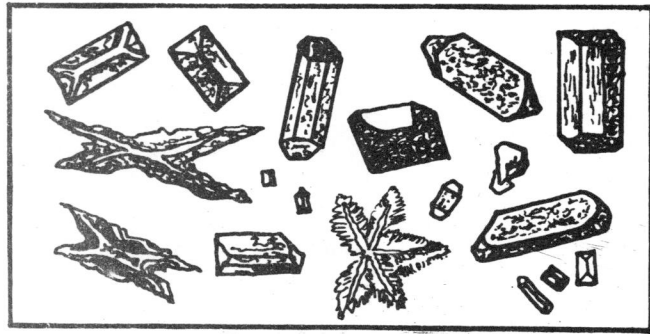

Fig. 42 Triple phosphates.

The quantity of fluid ultimately reaching the bladder under normal conditions is 1,200 to 1,500 ml during the 24-hour period and has the approximate composition given in Table 22. This composition is not constant, even in normal health, but varies with diet and fluid intake.

All three primary functions of the nephron can be measured by various tests, and in fact renal function tests are conveniently grouped into these three general classes — those testing (1) renal blood flow, (2) glomerular filtration, and (3) renal tubular activity.

Tests of Renal Blood Flow

Renal blood or plasma flow is measured by means of substances which are completely cleared from the plasma, both by glomerular filtration and tubular secretion, in its passage through the kidney. Phenolsulfonphthalein lends itself to a simple, convenient, rapid, semiquantitative test. p-Aminohippurate (PAII) is utilized in an accurate, more complicated quantitative method. The normal value for renal plasma flow is approximately 650 ml per minute with a range from 500 to 800 ml per minute.

Tests of Glomerular Filtration

Three clearance tests — urea, inulin, and creatinine — often are used to examine for impairment of glomerular filtration. Urea and creatinine are more commonly employed in clinical evaluation and inulin clearance for more meticulous experimental studies.

Determination of Urea Clearance

Principle

The urea clearance is calculated upon the basis of the blood urea concentration, urine urea concentration and rate of urine excretion.

Preparation of Subject

No special preparation of the subject is necessary other than giving two glasses of water one-half hour before beginning of the test and one at the end of the first hour to promote free flow of urine.

Procedure

1. Have the patient empty his bladder completely. This specimen is discarded. Accurately record the time of completion of urination.
2. At the end of approximately 1 hour have the patient void completely and again note accurately the time of voiding. Save this specimen.
3. Have the patient drink a glass of water. Collect a blood specimen for urea determination.
4. At approximately the end of the second hour have patient void completely and accurately record the time of voiding. Save this specimen.
5. Measure accurately (within 1 per cent) the volume of urine in each specimen by using the smallest graduate cylinder that will completely contain the specimen. Calculate the per minute excretion of urine for each specimen by dividing the total number of milliliters by the number of minutes lapsed between voidings.
6. Determine the blood urea concentration and the urine urea concentration for each separate urine specimen.

Calculation

If the per minute excretion of urine is 2 ml or more, use the formula:

$$\frac{U}{B} \times V = C_m \text{ (maximum clearance)}$$

If the per minute excretion of urine is under 2 ml, use the formula:

$$\frac{U}{B} \times \sqrt{V} = C_s \text{ (standard clearance)}$$

U = Urine urea mg per cent
B = Blood urea mg per cent
V = Volume of urine excreted as ml per minute

$\frac{C_m}{75} \times 100$ or $\frac{C_s}{54} \times 100$ = per cent of normal clearance

Creatinine Clearance

Creatinine is also useful for measuring the glomerular filtration rate and, as little is transferred across tubular cells, its clearance rate is much higher than that of urea and approaches that of inulin. Measurement of the 24-hour excretion of endogenous creatinine is convenient. This longer collection period minimizes timing errors.

Procedure

1. An accurate 24-hour urine specimen is collected ending at 7.00 a.m. and its total volume is measured.
2. Collect a blood sample for serum creatinine determination.
3. Determine serum and urine creatinine concentrations.

Calculation

$C_{Creatinine} = (U/P) \times V$
U = Urine creatinine concentration in gm per liter
P = Serum creatinine concentration in mg per cent $\div 100$
V = 24-hour urine volume in ml $\div 1,000$

The average normal 24-hour endogenous creatinine clearance is 170 litres.

Interpretation:

Normal values for men and women corrected to 1.73 sqm body surface area range from 140–180 litres/24 hours (100–150 ml/minute). To correct clearance to standard 1.73 sqm body surface area.

Clearance observed $\times \dfrac{1.73 \text{ sqm}}{\text{Estimated surface area}}$
= Corrected clearane.
(This test is superior to urea clearance).

Creatinine clearance test
Normal range: 110–150 ml/min (males)
105–132 ml/min (females)

Effect of age on normal function

Ages 50–75, subtract 5 ml for each 5-yr interval. Age 75 and above, subtract 8 ml for each 5 yr interval.

Artifacts that lower calculated figure

— Incomplete urine collection.
— Bacterial multiplication in collecting vessel.
— Ketones, barbiturates, PSP in urine at higher levels than is plasma.

Causes for reduced creatinine clearance

Acute: Shock, hypovolemia, nephrotoxic chemicals, acute glomerulonephritis, malignant hypertension, eclampsia.

Chronic: Glomerulonephritis, pyelonephritis, hypertensive nephrosclerosis, polycystic kidneys.

Since shock, severe dehydration, circulatory failure, and obstruction in the lower urinary tract diminish clearance, these conditions must be properly evaluated before low clearance values can be accepted as evidence of primary renal disease.

Glomerular filtration rate (GFR)

Inulin, a polysaccharide is eliminated exclusively through the glomeruli, is neither excreted nor absorbed by the tubules. Inulin clearance is therefore a measure of the glomerular filtration rate. Other radio-active labelled substances can be used. Normal in adults is 100–130 ml/minute per 1.73 sqm of body surface.

Table 22. *Renal function tests*

Determination		Normal values
Phenolsulfonphthlein (PSP, Phenol red)	1 m I/V	15 min 35% (28–51) 30 min 17%(13–24) 60 min 12%(9–17) 120 min 6%(3–10) } 55–60%
Clearance tests	Glomerular	Corrected to 1.73 sq m SA
Inulin clearance	filtration rate	Male 110–150 ml/min
Iothalamate	— do —	Female 105–132 ml/min
Endogenous creatinine clearance	— do —	
Iodohippurate ^{131}IPAH clearance	Renal Plasma flow	Male 560–830 ml/min Female 490–700 ml/min
Filtration fraction	FF=GFR/RPF	Male 17–21% Female 17–23%
Urea clearance (C₄)		Standard 40–65 ml/min Maximal 60–100 ml/min
Maximal glucose reabsorptive capacity	TmG	Male 300–450 mg/min Female 250–350 mg/min
Maximal iodopyracet capacity	TmD	Male 43–59 mg/min Female 33–51 mg/min
Maximal PAH excretory capacity	Tm PAH	80–90 mg/min

Tests of Tubular Function

Concentration Tests

A number of tests have been devised to examine for impairment of the important function of water reabsorption. They are all based on the ability of the kidney (nephron) to concentrate urine. These tests measuring the tubular reabsorption (concentration) function of the nephron have been called, as a group, the specific gravity tests. They are extremely important, for the ability to concentrate urine is an early kidney activity to show significant impairment in nephritis.

Dilution and Concentration Test

The healthy kidney can excrete variable quantities of fluid or water through the mechanism of reabsorption under the control of the anti-diuretic hormone of the pituitary. This power to do osmotic work can be roughly gauged by measuring the specific gravity of the urine. These tests are a challenge to the physiological function of absorption of water by the tubular epithelium.

Procedure: The patient should be on a diet containing reasonable amounts of water, salt and proteins before the test. At least an interval of 24 hours should elapse between the dilution and the concentration test.

Dilution Test: The test is done in the morning after a 12-hour fast. The patient is made to empty the bladder and then he drinks 1,200 ml of water in half an hour. Thereafter the bladder is emptied every hour for 4 hours. The total volume of the urine excreted in 4 hours should be 80 to 120 per cent of the water ingested and in at least one of the four samples the specific gravity should be 1003 or lower. If the amount of albumin in the urine is more than 1 + the specific gravity figures have to be corrected by subtracting 0.003 for each gram of albumin per 100 ml of urine.

Concentration Test: All fluids are restricted after breakfast until the following morning; the usual diet is allowed omitting foods containing free fluid. On retiring the patient empties the bladder; this sample is discarded. The following morning the bladder is emptied & the sample saved. Two additional samples are collected at hourly intervals. At least in one of the three samples the specific gravity should be 1025 or higher. The test is contra-indicated in old persons, in patients with heart diseases or those with incipient renal failure.

The dilution and the concentration tests are simple and can be done at the bed side without special equipment. They are sensitive tests, the concentration test being positive even in the case of compensated renal damage. The tests are not reliable in oedematous patients, in pregnancy, in patients with chronic liver disease and in patients with adrenocortical insufficiency. Further they do not distinguish primary renal dysfunction from that due to external causes.

Tests of Tubular Excretion and Reabsorption

The reserve function of secretion of foreign nonendogenous materials by the tubular epithelium is most conveniently test for by the use of certain dyes and measuring their rate of excretion.

Indigo-Carmine Test: The patient is given 100 mg of the dye intravenously. Normally the blue dye appears at the ureteric opening in the bladder 15 minutes after the injection. Late appearance or failure to appear indicates dysfunction on that side.

Phenolsulfonphthalein (PSP) Test: PSP is a dye which, when injected intravenously, is excreted mainly by the kidney (both glomerules and tubules); about 15–25 per cent is excreted by the liver, the amount increasing with liver disease. The urinary concentration is determined after alkalinising the urine (when the dye appears red) by colorimetry. By ureteric catheterisation the excretion by each kidney can be estimated seperately.

Procedure: The patient empties the bladder. He is given about 600 ml of water to drink to promote the urine flow. After 30 minutes 1 ml of the dye (6 mg) is injected intravenously. The dye should appear in the urine within 10 minutes normally. Beginning after 10 minutes of the injection samples of the urine are collected at 1 hour and 2 hours. The volume of the urine and the concentration of the dye are measured. If the kidneys are healthy, about 40 to 60 per cent of the dye is excreted in the 1st hour and 20 to 25 per cent in the next. A fall in the exeretion of the dye below 50 per cent in 2 hours indicates renal impairment.

Choice of Renal Function Tests

The selection of a renal function test for use in any instance is influenced by three primary considerations — the type of information desired, the nature and severity of the kidney lesion under investigation, and the scope of laboratory facilities available. If a quick, rough estimate of severe functional impairment is desired as in the case of known urinary tract obstruction or in the presence of clinical symptoms suggesting uremia, determination of the blood urea nitrogen, nonprotein nitrogen or serum creatinine is often sufficient. However, it is usually desirable to have a more accurate evaluation of the degree of reduction of renal function. Adequate assessment of kidney function requires consideration of the renal blood flow, glomerular filtration rate and tubular cell activity.

Under conditions where inadequate laboratory facilities prevent the use of tests requiring chemical determinations on blood and urine, entirely satisfactory results may be obtained by employing the specific gravity and the 15-minute phthalein excretion tests. These utilize simple equipment and procedure within the scope of any laboratory or physician's office. They test the reabsorptive and excretory abilities of the renal tubular cells and also the adequacy of renal blood flow. Combined with the examination of the urine they afford a fair appraisal of the functional and structural state of the kidneys. The picutre of the functional state will be more complete with some measure of glomerular filtration rate, such as urea or creatinine clearance. Further clarification of the structural state may require needle biopsy of the kidney.

If accurate information of kidney functional is needed for diagnostic or prognostic purposes, the rate of renal blood flow and maximal tubular reabsorptive capacity should be determined.

Renal Biopsy: Needle biopsy of the kidneys has been introduced recently. The technique, though safe in experienced hands, is much more difficult than that of liver biopsy. The tissue bit removed is submitted for histological examination. If positive, it gives the exact information of the nature of the lesion.

CHAPTER 11

Cerebrospinal and Other Body Fluids

CEREBROSPINAL FLUID (C.S.F.)

Examination of Cerebrospinal Fluid

Whenever there is clinical evidence of central nevous system disease, examination of C.S.F. is indicated. Removal of spinal fluid is also indicated for relief of abnormal pressure and for the drainage of blood or exudates, for injection of drugs, for spinal anaesthesia, etc. In certain conditions, however, extra caution is required. These are (1) a brain tumour at the cerebellopontine angle or in the region of the 3rd ventricle associated with papilloedema, (2) a recent intracranial haemorrhage, (3) a brain abscess, (4) septicaemias and acute exanthemata, (5) a state of convulsion, and (6) advanced diseases of the heart and arteries.

Normal values for lumbar C.S.F. in adults

Pressure	70–150 mm of water column (patient lying on side)
Volume	90–150 ml
Specific gravity	1.006–1.008
Total solids	0.85–1.70 gm%
Cells	0–8 lymphocytes/cu mm
	Neutrophils and erythrocytes absent

Protein		20–50 mg%
Of this		
albumin is		50–70%
α_1 globulin is		3–9%
α_2 globulin is		4–10%
β globulin is		10–18%
γ globulin is		3–9%
fibrinogen is		Absent
Sodium		144–154 mEq/L
Potassium		2.0–3.5 mEq/L
Chloride		118–132 mEq/L
pH		7.30–7.40
Creatinine		0.5–1.2 mg%
Cholesterol		0.2–0.5 mg%
Glucose		50–80 mg%
Glutamine		6–16 mg%
Iron		1–2 mg%
Thyroxine		0.1–0.2 mg%
Urea		6–16 mg%
Uric acid		0.5–4.5 mg%

Normal Physiology: The cerebro spinal fluid (C.S.F.), is formed by a process of selective dialysis of plasma by the choroid plexuses of the ventricles of the brain. It then passes through the foramina in the fourth ventricle into sub-arachnoidal cysterns at the base of the brain and travels over surfaces of the cerebral hemispheres. It is eventually asborbed into the blood in the cerebral veins and dural sinuses through arachnoidal villi and pachionian granulations. Thus it fills ventricles of the brain and subarchnoid spaces of the brain and the spinal cord. The total quantity is about 150 to 200 ml, but the daily turnover is probably to the tune of about 1000 ml The normal pressure is 80 to 180 mm of water. The functions of the C.S.F. are: (1) to serve as a fluid buffer, as a water jacket for the brain and the spinal cord; (2) to act as a reservoir to regulate contents of the cranium; and (3) to serve as a medium for the exchange of substances especially removal of waste-products — between the blood and the brain. The normal composition is shown in the table at the end.

The C.S.F. is very poor in colloids so that it does not clot on standing. Compared to the plasma it has less sugar. calcium and non-protein nitrogen; it contains very little cholestrol and no bilirubin at all.

Collection of Cerebro spinal Fluid

The C.S.F. is obtained by puncturing the subarachnoidal space in the interspace between the 3rd and 5th lumbar vertebrae. The puncture is done with all aspetic and under local anaesthesia. A special lumb ar puncture needle is used.

Routine examination of C.S.F. includes:

(1) Pressure
(2) Physical examination
(3) Chemical examination
(4) Cytological examination
(5) Bacteriological examination
(6) Serological examiantion

Pressure

C.S.F. under normal pressure flows from the needle at a rate varying from 20 to 60 drops per minute. True evaluation of the pressure is attained by the use of a manometer.

The normal adult pressure in the horizontal position is from 100 to 200 mm of water or 7 to 15 mm of mercury. Pressure above 250 mm or under 50 mm are pathological. In children the pressure is slightly lower.

Physical Examination

1. *Appearance and Colour* The pathological changes in appearance may consist of cloudiness or opalescence to frank turbidity. Opalescence and turbidity are due to the presence of cells in the fluid. In meningitis, therefore the C.S.F. will show these changes. When the C.S.F. is frankly yellow, the change is described as "xanthochromia"; it is caused by (1) haemorrhage in the subarachnoid space with conversion of haemoglobin into bilirubin; (2) severe jaundice of the obstructive (regurgitation) type; and (3) in Froin's syndrome in which xanthochromia is associated with a rise in proteins of the fluid (above 500 mg) but not in the cell count. Froin's syndrome is seen in obstruction in the subarachnoid space produced by a spinal tumour or by chronic meningitis. Another change in colour is reddish discoloration ("erythrochromasia") due

to blood in the C.S.F. If blood has appeared from accidental puncture of vein during the lumbar puncture, it is seen most in the first portion (first tube) of the C.S.F. during collection. If such a sample of the C.S.F. is centrifuged, the upper portion is clear. On the other hand, a spontaneous haemorrhage in the subarachnoid space will produce a uniformly bloody fluid in all the successive tubes and, if it has been of some standing, on centrifugation of supernatant is xanthochromic. Frank blood in the C.S.F., not produced by the puncture of a vein, may be due to a cerebral haemorrhage (intraventricular or elsewhere with rupture into the subarachnoid space), spontaneous subarachnoid haemorrhage or due to a vascular tumour. A third type of discoloration is the greenish discoloration seen in a tubria fluid; this occur in pneumococcal meningitis.

(2). *Formation of a clot*: This occurs in meningitis. In tuberculous meningitis, on standing for a few hours (especially in a refrigerator), the C.S.F. shows a fine coagulum or pellicle described as a "cobweb". Such a cobweb is used for the demonstration of Myco. Tuberculosis which gets caught in it. In purulent meningitis the clot is formed quickly and is of a coarse type. Cobweb and clot are due to the appearance of fibrinogen in the fluid.

Chemical Examination

1. *Estimation of total proteins:* This is done by taking 1 ml. of the C.S.F. in a tube and adding 3 ml of 3% sulphosalicylic acid. Mix and allow to stand for 5 minutes, and compare the turbidity with that of the standard protein tubes, or in a photo-electric colorimeter.

2. *Qualitative tests for increase in globulin*: (1) In Pandy's test 1 ml of the reagent (10% carbolic acid) is taken in a Kahn or Wassermann tube and to it is added one drop of the C.S.F. Normal fluid does not produce any change. If globulins are increased, a bluish ring or a cloud develops immediately. (2) In the Nonne-Apelt test 1 ml of saturated ammonium sulphate solution is taken in a small tube and 1 ml of the C.S.F. is layered on it. Allow to stand for 3 minutes and compare with the rest of C.S.F. Normal fluid produces just a faint opalescence at the junction; if globulins are increased, a distinct ring develops at the junction of the two fluids.

Obviously, if the C.S.F. is contaminated with blood, the tests for proteins and globulins will give false reactions. Heavy bacterial contamination of the C.S.F. (due to improper collection and storage) will also falsify the results. In all the conditions, mentioned in the table 23, the rise in the cell count (pleocytosis) is seen. Some entities are characterised by a rise in proteins without pleocytosis; these are cerebral thrombosis, subdural haematoma, brain tumours and polyneuritis.

Quantitative Protein estimation

Principle: There are 2 types of methods.
1. Protein is precipitated by using 3% sulphosalicylic acid. The resultant turbidity is proportional to the amount of protein present.
2. Proteins are simultaneously precipitated & dyed by a trichloracetic acid (ponceau S regeant). The protein bound dye is dissolved in alkali, and its absorbance compared with that derived from similarly treated protein standard.

Method 1

1. Take 0.5 ml of C.S.F. in a small test tube.

2. Add 1.5 ml of 3% sulphosalicyclic acid, shake and keep the tube for 10 mins.
3. Compare the tube with the turbidity standard which are marked in mg of protein per 100 ml of fluid.

Method II

1. Determine approximate range of protein level in C.S.F. by albustix.
   Reading 100, use 0.2 ml for assay
   Reading between 100–300 use 0.1 ml
   300–1000 use 0.02 ml
2. Set up following tubes

	Test	Std.
(a) Std. (80mg/dl).	—	0.2 ml
(b) Test serum	0.2 ml	—
(c) working trichloracetic acid (centrifuge and decant)	1.0 ml	1.0 ml
(d) NaOH (0.2m)	2.5 ml	2.5 ml

(Read absorbance at 560 nm setting 0 with water)
CSF protein (mg/dl) = T/S × 0.32 × 100/0.2
$$= T/S \times 160 \text{ mg/dl}.$$

Interpretation: Total protein content of CSF is 10–40 mg/dl. Upon electrophoresis it contains albumin, pre-albumin, β_1, β_2 & globulins with an A:G ratio of 2:1. Total proteins in CSF may increase in: 1. Meningitis (inflammations) 2. Gullian Barre syndrome (infective polyneuritis) 3. Encephalitis 4. Cerebral malignancies etc. 5. Froins syndrome (A block in spinal canal)

3. *Test for sugar and quantitative estimation*: (a) Qualitative test: In a test tube take 0.5 ml of Benedict's qualitative reagent and add to it 4.5 ml of distilled water. Heat to boil and add 1 ml of the C.S.F. Boil for 2 minutes and allow to cool. A change of color to turbid greenish yellow is the normal reaction. Absence of any change in the color indicates diminished sugar content. (b) The quantitative estimation is done by Folin and Wu technique. Tests for sugar should be always done on fresh samples.

Interpretation: Glucose in CSF is characteristically reduced in pyogenic and tuberculosis meningitis and the reduction is the result of the metabolic requirement of the infecting organisms. CSF glucose is also reduced in disseminated leptomeningeal malignancies. In viral infections glucose may be normal or even raised. Whenever CSF sugar is being estimated, a sample of blood should be taken at the same time for glucose determination because CSF sugar is always judged in relation to blood glucose.

Determination of chloride in CSF

This is an outmoded investigation of no clincal value but only of historical interest.

Cell Counts

A. *Diluting the fluid:*
1. Draw Unna's polychrone methylene blue to the '1' mark in a RBC pipette and fill pipette to '101' mark with spinal fluid. This colors white cells blue and red cells yellow.
2. Turbid fluid: when many cells are present (as in turbid or purulent fluid), better counts are obtained with a WBC pipette and WBC diluting fluid.

3. Bloody fluid: when significant number of red cells are present in the fluid, the possibility of traumatic bleeding should be considered. Fresh RBC's are intact with a smooth round margin. Older cells have crenated appearance.

B. *Count:* Count 9 large squares in the counting chamber for both RBC's and WBC's. The total multiplied by 1.1 gives the number of cells per cubic mm.

Differential count: Centrifuge the CSF and make smears from the sediment. Stain and count as for a blood smear.

Bacteriologic Examination

Smears and cultures for bacteria should be made of all fluids when indicated.

Smears: Make smears directly if fluid is very turbid, otherwise from sediment of centrifuged CSF. All smears should be stained with Gram's stain. If no characteristic bacteria are found, do an acid fast stain (Zeihl Neelsen stain) and search for mycobacteria. AFB stain should also be done if a pellicle forms on standing. An India ink preparation is required for cryptococcus. Immunofluorescent stains can be used for Hemophillus influenzae and some other organisms.

Cultures: Cloudy fluid should be streaked on chocolate agar, Sabouraud's agar, and agar plates and inoculated into blood broth and thioglycollate medium. All media are incubated at 37°C, some in candle jars (for CO_2 atmosphere). Sediment of centrifuged fluid should be cultured on special media for tuberculous bacilli and fungi and inoculated into guinea pigs. Mice should be inoculated intraperitoneally if coccidioidomycosis is suspected.

Virus isolation : This is possible only in very sophisticated laboratories and is helpful in aseptic meningitis and arthropod borne encephalitis.

Serological Examination: These are undertaken when neurosyphilis (meningo-vascular syphilis, tabes dorsalis or general paralysis of the insane) is suspected. The Wassermann reaction (complement fixation test) is considered the most dependable of various serlogical tests available. A test on the C.S.F. is warranted because tests on the blood may be negative in neurosyphilis.

Lange's Colloidal Gold test: About 5 to 7 ml of very fresh fluid collected in scrupulously clean; sterile tubes are required. The fluid must not be contaminated with blood.

Lange's test is an empirical non-specific test depending upon the alterations in the total proteins and the albumin-globulin fractions in the C.S.F. In some diseases serial dilutions of the fluid when added to colloidal gold chloride solution (brilliant orang-red colour) brings about a somewhat characterstic pattern of colour changes with precipitation, the normal fluid has no effect.

The utility of the test is very limited. Compared to the labour involved the information given is hardly conclusive. The test is, therefore, falling into background.

One can do — VDRL using CSF in syphilis. —Latex agglutination and complement fixation tests in cryptococcal meningitis.

Form of Reporting on a Specimen of Cerebro spinal Fluid

A. Physical Examination : Colour
Transparency
Coagulum or cobweb

B. Chemical Examination : Proteins
Tests for globulins, Sugar — Qualitative — Quantitative
Chlorides

C. Cytological Examination : Total cell count
Predominant cell

D. Staining : Ziehl-Neelsen, Gram

GASTRIC ANALYSIS

Digestion in the stomach consists of the action of pepsin on proteins in the presence of hydrochloric acid and of the curding of milk by rennin. Lipase of the gastric juice has very little activity except on previously emulsified fats, such as those of milk and egg yolk.

Gastric analysis denotes an examination of the gastric contents at various phases of digestion. Yet, the results of such analysis are influenced by many intragastric factors, and need to be interpreted only in the light of the clinical findings.

Although the gastric juice is secreted continuously quantities sufficiently large for examination are better obtained after administration of a suitable food. Different foods stimulate secretion to different degrees, hence for the sake of uniform results certain standard test meals have been adopted.

The chief constituents of gastric juice are
1. Hydrochloric acid, secreted by parietal cells.
2. Pepsinogen secreted by chief cells. (It is activated to pepsin by acid which also provides acid medium in which pepsin acts.
3. Renin which clots milk by converting milk casein into caseinogen.
4. Intrinsic factor which binds Vit B_{12} and aids its absorption in the intestine.
5. Mucous.

Gastric secretion is secreted in response to varied stimulants important among which are.
(i) Psychic factors such as sight, taste, smell of food, mediated by vagus nerve.
(ii) Gastrin (a hormone secreted by gastric mucosa in response to food present in the stomach).
(iii) Presence of digested products in the intestine.

Other stimutants include
1. Insulin
2. Histamine and
3. Alcohol

Various gastric function tests can be broadly put under 2 headings.

(A) Test of Resting Gastric Function
These include
1. Test of acid in gastric juice
2. Test for bile in gastric juice
3. Test for blood in gastric juice
4. Test for digestive enzymes

(B) Test of Gastric Secretion after Stimulation
1. Fractional test meal
2. Augmented histamine test
3. Insulin test (Hollander's test)

Gastric analysis can be of 2 types
1. Tube gastric analysis — gastric contents are collected by means of a double lumen tube
2. Tubeless gastric analysis

Table 23 *The CSF In Differential Diagnosis*

Disease	Initial pressure mm H₂O column	Appearance	Cells/cu mm	Protein mg %	Glucose mg%	Remarks
Normal	70–150	crystal clear	0–8, lympho's	20–50	50–80	In fasting afebrile individuals.
Acute purulent meningitis	↑	Opalescent to purulent clot	500–20,000 mostly poly's	50–1000 +	0–45	Organism in sediment or clot, culture positive.
Tuberculous meningitis	↑	Opalescent fibrin web, pellicle	10–500 mostly lympho's	45–500 +	0–45	Sugar and chloride values falling progressively.
Early, acute syphilitic meningitis	↑	Clear to turbid, occasional clot	25–2000 mostly lympho's	45–400 +	15–75	+ve (often serologic test in CSF & blood).
Late CNS syphilis	↑	Normal	Normal or ↑	Normal or ↑	Normal	Often +ve serologic test in CSF.
Aseptic meningeal reaction (brain or extradural abscess, thrombosis etc)	Usually normal	Clear or turbid, often xanthochromic	↑	Normal or ↑	Normal	CSF culture negative.
Acute poliomyelitis	Usually normal	Usually clear and colourless	↑	↑	45–100	
Viral encephalitis (arthropod borne)	Normal or ↑	Normal	0–100 mostly lympho's	Normal or increased	45–100	Proved by serologic tests.
Viral mening-oencephalitis	Normal or ↑	Normal	0–2000 + mostly lympho's	Normal or ↑	Normal	Proved by virus isolation and serologic tests.
Post-infectious encephalitis	Usually ↑	Normal	Slightly ↑	Normal or increased	Increased	
Traumatic (bloody) tap	Normal	Bloody	Many fresh RBC's	↑	Normal	Most blood in Ist tube, least blood in last tube.
Cerebral hemorrhage ventricular, subarachnoid	Slightly ↑	Bloody, supernatant yellow	Many RBC's crenated or fresh	↑	Variable	Blood present in all specimens equally.
Subdural hematoma	Usually ↑	Clear/yellow	Normal	Normal or ↑	Variable	
Brain tumor	Usually ↑	Clear/xanthochromic	Normal or increased	Usually ↑	Normal or increased	If papilledema is present lumbar puncture is contraindicated.
Spinal cord tumor (Subarachnoid block)	Normal or low	Often xanthochromic	Normal or ↑	Usually ↑	Normal or increased ↑	Little fluid obtained.
Multiple sclerosis	Low	Normal	Normal or increased	Normal or increased	Normal	50% cases have normal CSF.
Uremia	Usually ↑	Normal	Normal or ↓	Normal or ↑	Normal or ↑	CSF NPN is high.
Diabetic coma	Low	Normal	Normal or ↑	Normal	Increased	May have spasticity, weakness, convulsions.

Withdrawal of gastric contents: The gastric fluid is obtained by aspiration through a tube. There are many tubes on the market, of which 'Sawyer tube', 'Levin tube', 'Rehfuss tube', or a 'Ryle's tube may be used (Fig. 43).

If the patient is neurotic or has marked pharyngeal hyperaesthesia, spray the fauces and the nostrils with a 2 per cent solution of cocaine hydrochloride. The patient should be seated with the head tilted slightly forward and the clothing protected with towels. Place the tip of the tube on the tongue held well out and pass it back to the throat or introduce the tube along the floor of the nose until it is felt that the top turns down into the phanynx. Then the patient is encouraged to swallow quickly until the tube is passed to the desired length.

Examination of Resting contents: The tube is passed after a night's fast (no food or drink) and the stomach contents removed.

Following things have to be checked
1. Colour
2. Volume
3. Any specific odour
4. Detection of acid

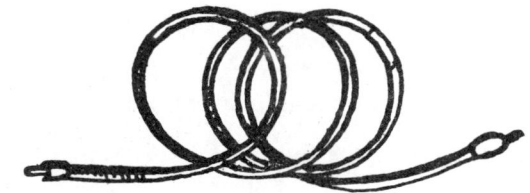

Fig. 43 Ryle's stomach tube

5. Presence of mucus (normal or excessive)
6. Detection blood
7. Detection of Bile
8. Detection for digestive enzymes
   each of these will be discussed in detail in the text.

Colour: Normal gastric juice is a colorless fluid of low specific gravity.

Volume: In most normal cases after a night fast only a small quantity (20–50 ml) of resting contents is obtained volumes above 100–200 ml may be considered abnormal.

Odour: Fermentation which gives rise to lactic acid and other organic acids may produce a rather characteristic smell with which the dealing persons soon become familiar.

Mucous: Presence of excessive amounts of mucus implies mixture of excessive amounts of saliva in the gastric juice.

Detection of Blood: Blood should not normally be present. A small amount of fresh red blood may be present and usually signifies trauma and is easily distinguished macroscopically from that arising due to any pathological condition; since blood which has been in the stomach for some time is usually brown or reddish brown in color, because of formation of acid haematin (Coffee ground) various chemical tests for detection of blood include.
1. Ortho toulidine test
2. Guaiac test
3. Benzidine test
All these have been discussed in detail under the chapter of stool.

Interpretation: The blood may be
1. Swallowed
2. from stomach itself in various conditions like-
   Gastritis
   Gastric ulcer
   Gastric carcinoma

Detection of Bile: Bile may be found occasionally but may not be of any particular significance. A small amount may regurgitate into the stomach during intubation.

Various tests for detection of bile include:
1. Iodine test
2. Gmelin's nitric acid test
3. Fouchet's test
4. Hunter-diazo test
5. Ictotest
(All have been discussed in the chapter on urine)

Some pathophysiologists believe that bile is important in the pathogenesis of gastric ulcers. Therefore detection of bile may be important and significant in some patients of gastric ulcer.

Detection and estimation of Gastric Acid: Total acid of gastric juice is devided into 2 parts:
1. Free hydrochloric acid (free acid)
2. Combined acid, this includes organic acids and HCl found in combinations with proteins or more appropriately acid that is not free for first titration with NaOH.

Testing for free & Total Acid

Take 1.0 ml of gastric juice in a test tube and to it add 2–4 drops of Topfer's reagent. If there is an initial yellow color on adding the indicator, no free acid is present, than only titrate for total acid.

If initially red color appears, titrate with 0.1N sodium hydroxide (NaOH) until unitial red colour becomes yellow.

Note down the volume of NaOH used.

Now add 2–4 drops of phenolphtalein. Again titrate with 0.1N NaOH until pink color reappears and note down the total NaOH used up for titration.

Vol. of free acid = Vol. of NaOH used for first titration × 10
Total acid = Total Vol. of NaOH used for both titrations × 10

(Topfer's reagent-p-dimethylamino azobenzene 1 gm in 100 ml. of 95% ethyl alchohol. 0.1% methylorange can be used in its place)

Thymol blue can be used as the only indicator in test for free and total acid because it has 2 color changes, one at pH 1.2–2.8 and the second at pH 8.0 to 9.5.

Interpretation: There is only a small amount of free HCl, normally present in gastric juice. This is 0–30 mEq/l. Upto 50 mEq/l may be taken to be normal. Concentrations above this point to hyperacidity. Lactic acid is the most important, among the organic acids found. All these are formed by action of micro-organisms on food which is favoured by achlorhydria associated with prolonged retention of food.

Tests for Lactic Acid

1. **Ferric chloride test:** 2ml of filtered gestric contents + 1–3 drops of $FeCl_3$ (10%; solution) in a test tube
   A yellow colour that remains on dilution with water points to presence of lactic acid.
2. **Maclean's test:** (Maclean's soln — 100 ml saturated $HgCl_2$ + 1.5 ml HCl in which 5 gms $FeCl_3$ is dissolved)
   5 ml filtered gastric contents + few drops of Maclean's solution Reddish color points to lactic acid
   It can be quantitized colorimetrically with a blank of normal gastic contents.

Tests for HCl

(Gunzberg's reagent — 2 gm phloroglucinol + 1 gm Vanillin in 100 ml of 95% ethanol)
1–2 drops gastric contents + 1–2 drops of Gunzberg's reagent in a petridish
Evaporate to dryness in a waterbath.
Reddish color signifies HCl.
(This test is positive for all mineral acids and HCl is the only mineral acid expected in gastric contents)

Fractional test meal (Fig. 44): This test has now lost its importance and is not of much use in the diagnosis of gastric disceases.
1. Begin the test after overnight fasting. Analyze the fasting contents as discussed earlier.
2. Now give the patient a meal. Various types of meals that have been used include.
   (a) 50 ml of 7% ethyl alchohol solution.
   (b) 2 spoonfulls of oat meal to ½ a glass of water.
   (c) Tea/Coffee
3. After the meal samples are drawn at interval of 15 minutes for 2 hrs. At least 10 ml of sample should be drawn.
4. Analyze for free & total acid as discussed earlier.

Interpretation: 1. Normal: After the meal free acid is found after about 45 mins. to 1 hr. It rises steadily to reach maximum at about 1½ hrs after which concentration starts decreasing. Maximum level is 15–45 mEq/litre of free acid
25–55 m Eq/l of total acid.

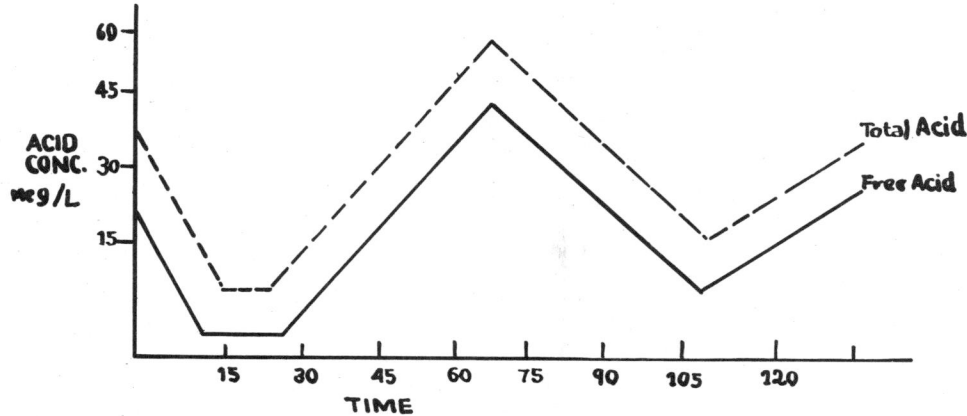

Fig. 44. Shows free and total acid concentration with time relation.

2. Hyperchlorhydria: Occurs when max. free acidity exceeds 45 mEq/l. Combined acidity is same as for normal persons. It is typically seen in 1. Duodenal ulcer, 2. Zollinger Ellison syndrome, 3. Gastric ulcer (50% cases).

3. Achlorhydria: This term is used when no HCL is secreted by gastric mucosa. Seen in (a) Tuberculosis, (b) Atrophic gastritis, (c) Late stages of gastric malignancies, (d) Microcytic hypochronic anemia due to iron deficiency.

Defined as inability of stomach to produce juice with a $pH < 7.1$ even after maximal stimulation.

Histamine test (Pentagastrin test)

Only useful test for diagnostic purposes.

Histamine or Pentagastrin is used for stimulating gastric acid secreton.

1. After overnight fasting, collect the resting contents.
2. Collect gastric contents for one hr by aspirating at 15 min intervals. At 30 mins point give 1 amp avil intramuscular.
3. At the end of first hour give the dose of Histamin. It is given in doses of 0.25 mg by S.C. injection (Pentagastrin in doses of 6 mg/kg can be given instead, S/c or i/m — Infact this is now preferred over histamine.)
4. Specimens are again collected for the next 1 hr at 15 minute intervals.
5. Now titrate for presence of acid both free and total.

Interpretation   m Eq/l/hr

	Basal acid output	Maximal output
Normal	3–4	18.5
Gastric ulcer	2	14.6
Duodenal ulcer	0	37.5
Anastomotic ulcer	2.7	31
Zollinger Ellison syndrome	22	50–100 or even more

Hollander test (Insulin test)

It is of value postoperatively to verify completeness of vagal section.

To a fasting patient give 20 unit/10 kg body weight by I/V injection and perform serial 15 min aspirations for 4 hrs (Blood sugar should fall below 35 mg/dl).

Early response: Rise in concentration of acid 20 mmol/l above basal level within 1st hr suggests incomplete vagotomy.

Delayed response: Rise in concentration of acid between 1–4 hrs suggests less than complete vagotomy.

Negative response: No increase in gastric acid concentration suggests complete vagotomy.

Tubeless Gastric Analysis

In 1950–53 Segal et all published a series of papers in which a new method for determining the production of free acid by stomach was put forward.

Principle: When a quininium — resin indicator is given by mouth, hydrogen ions from HCl in stomach can liberate quinine ions (the Q H cation). At pH values less than 3 quinine HCl is formed, is absorbed in the intestine and begins to be excreted in the urine. The quinine can be extracted from the urine and determined by measuring its fluorescence in U-V light.

Procedure: This test is marketed as a ready made kit in foreign countries.

It is called [Gastro test marked by ortho pharmacenticals
       Diagnex Test marketed by Squibb Ltd.]

It contains the reagent Diagnex Blue (Azure A-3 amino 7 dimethyl amino-phenazath onium Cl).

Tablets for this test are available. Each test unit contains (2), 250 mg tablets of caffeine sodium benzoate.

1. Do not break fast in the morning.
2. Empty the bladder on rising and discard the urine.
3. Take the tablets of caffeine sodium benzoate with a glass of water.
4. Empty the bladder 2 hrs later. This is the test urine
5. Azure A may be excreted in blue form or colorless form which may be converted to blue form by acidification boiling & standing for 2 hrs.
6. It is measured by a visual type of colored comparator.

PERICARDIAL, PLEURAL, PERITONEAL, AMNIOTIC AND SYNOVIAL FLUIDS

Examination of these fluids is useful in the diagnosis of disease of organs adjoining the body cavities which accommodate the fluids. The specimen for examination are collected by puncturing the cavities with a suitable needle. Two specimens are necessary: (1) in a plain sterile test (about 10 to 20 ml) and (2) in a tube containing sodium citrate as an anticogulant (in the proportion of 1 ml of sodium citrate 2.5 per cent solution to 10 ml of the fluid). Cytological and bacteriological examinations require fresh fluid.

Routine Examination: The pattern of examination runs like the one for the cerebro-spinal fluid. The first step is, however, to decide whether the fluid is a transudate or an exudate. Transudates are filterates generally due to mechanical causes, while exudates are inflammatory fluids. The following table summarises the differences between the two kinds of fluids.

Table 24: *Differences between transudates and Exudates*

	Transudate	Exudate
Appearance	Clear, Usually straw-colored	Cloudy or frankly purulent
Spontaneous coagulation	Absent	Frenquently present
Specific gravity	Usually under 1018	Usually over 1018
Proteins	Usually under 2 g/100 ml	Usually over 2 g/100 ml
Cells	Red cells, endotheilal cells and few lymphocytes. Bacteria absent.	Red cells, neutrophilis & lymphocytes in large numbers. Bacteria may be present

The distinction, however, is not always clearcut.

Physical Examination: The appearance (clear or turbid), the color, the presence of blood and the presence of clot are noted. In the absence of trauma a haemorrhagic fluid is suggestive of a malignant tumour. A "chylous" fluid-milky due to mixture of chyle with the effusion also indicates the same. Glandular carcinomas produce a mucinous fluid.

Chemical Examination: Proteins: Qualitative tests: To 3ml of the fluid are added 4 drops of 5 per cent (tricholracetic acid). Transudates show no change or a slight opalescene. Exudates become turbid. In the quantitative test proteins are estimated by one of the methods used in the determination of serumproteins (see the specific gravity method).

Cytological Examination:

1. *A Differential Cell Count:* A total cell count does not give any information. The differential count done by staining a smear of the centrifuged deposit by Giemsa or Leishman stain) is useful in distinguishing between transudates and exudates. Further plenty of neutrophils in the fluid suggest an exudate produced by phogenic infections: lymphocytes, as predominant cells, indicates chronic infection, tuberculosis, or an old collection of fluid. Mesothelial (endothelial) cells predominate in transudates; these are large cells with abundant cytoplasm and one or more vesicular nuclei, and frequently occur in clumps.

2. *Cytological examination for tumour cells:* This is a valuable procedure. Smears made from fresh fluid are fixed immediately (while wet) in ether-alcohol and stained by papanicoloau stain; haematoxylin and eosin stain also can be used. Alternatively, the clot or the packed sediment is fixed in formalin-saline and treated as a tissuebit for cutting sections. A cancer which has produced an effusion in the adjoining serous sac is one which is well advanced, possibly beyond treatment.

Bacteriological Examination:

1. Smears made from the sediment are stained by Gram and Zeihl-Neel-sen stains.
2. Cultures are done on suitable media.
3. Animal inoculation can also be done in case of fluids suspected to be tuberculous.
4. Fluids obtained from "cysts" are examined for scolices and hooklets to establish the diagnosis of E. Granulosus infection.

AMNIOTIC FLUID: It is the fluid contained in the amniotic sao. At term (40 weeks of gestation), the sac contains 5 to 8.5 litres of fluid. The source of the fluid is unknown. The amniotic fluid is in dynamic equilibrium with both fetal and maternal plasma and reflects the physiologic state of the mother and the fetus. Normal amniotic fluid is similar to water in appearance. Its specific gravity and viscocity are slightly greater than water. It consists of 98 to 99 per cent water with 1 to 2 per cent solids. About half of the solids are organic and half of this material is proteins. It also contains fetal cells squamous and RBC.

Following are some of the objectives where examination of amniotic fluid obtained by amniocentesis is necessary.

1. RH isoimmunization syndrome: (Erythroblastosis fetalis). Rh isoimmunization leads to haemolysis in the fetus. This causes an increase in the unconjugated bilirubin in the fetus as well as in the amniotic fluid. Increase in the amniotic fluid bilirubin can be estimated by spectrophometry and accordingly the time for indicated interruption of pregnancy or intrauterine transfusion is selected.

2. Sex determination of the fetus and ABO blood group determination is also done by cytological examination of the amniotic fluid cells-squamous and red blood cells.

3. Hereditary diseases-chromosomal or genetic (inborn errors of metabolisms) can be diagnosed from the examination of amniotic fluid. Karyotypic studies of amniotic fluid cells can be used to detect chromosomal abnormalities like Down's syndrome; whereas determination of certain substances like protein bound iodine can help in diagnosis of genetic abnormality as in hypothyroidism.

4. Foetal Lung Maturity: Phospholipids (lecithin and sphingomyelin) contents of amniotic fluid reflect those in the lungs of the growing fetus. The determination of lecithin and sphingomyelin amniotic fluid predicts fetal lung maturity and is determined by thin-layer chromatography. Lecithin-Sphingomyelin ratio increases with fetal lung maturity and thus with duration of pregnancy. This is the single most accurate test for fetal maturity.

Immature lung (upto 30th week L/S ratio is less than 1 of gestation)

Mature lungs (35th week ofL/S ratio is more than 2 gestation)

Postmature lungs   Abundant lecithin with trace or no sphinogomyclin.

The determination of foetal maturity is indicated to predict development of the respiratory distress syndrome and to determine when it is safe to interrupt gestation because of threat to fetus.

Synovial Fluid (SF)

Normally about 1 ml of SF is present in each large joint: knee, ankle, hip, elbow, wrist, and shoulder.

Table 25 *Synovianalysis in Arthritis*

	Appearance	Viscoslty	White Cells	Mucin clot	Protein (Avg-gm%) Total	Globulin	Remarks
Normal	Straw-coloured clear, cloudy	High	200–600 25% poly's	Good	1.36	0.05	
Traumatic	Yellow to bloody	High	±2000 30% poly's	Good	4.27		
Osteo-arthritis	Yellow, clear	High	±1000 20% poly's	Good	3.08	0.75	Cartilage fibrils
Rheumatic fever	Yellow, slightly cloudy	Low	±10,000 50% poly's	Good	3.74	1.07	
Systemic lupus erythematosus	Straw-coloured, slightly cloudy	High	±5000 10% poly's	Good			
Gout	Yellow to milky cloudy	Low	±12,000 60% poly's	Fragile	4.18	1.54	Urate crystals
Tuberculous arthritis	Yellow, cloudy	Low	±25,000 50–60% poly's	Fragile	5.3	2.0	Tubercle bacilli bacilli
Septic arthritis	Grayish or bloody, turbid	Low	±80,000 90% poly's	Fragile	5.64	2.45	Bacteria
Rheumatoid thritis	Yellow to greenish, cloudy	Low	±15,000, 65% poly's	Fragile	4.74	1.79	Rheumatoid factor*

Viscosity: When normal fluid drips from a syringe, a tenacious 'string' at least 4 cm long forms with each drop. This provides an estimate of whether viscosity is normal, decreased (string less than 4 cm in length), or markedly decreased (string less than 1 cm in length).

Another method for evaluating viscosity is to see how far a drop of fluid can be stretched between the thumb and index finger before breaking. Fluids with very low viscosity will behave like water. Decreased viscosity reflects decreased hyaluronate in the synovial fluid.

Mucin clot test (Ropes' Test): This is done by adding 1 ml of synovial fluid to 20 ml of 5% (v/v) acetic acid in a small beaker. Normally a compact large clot will form, surrounded by clear solution; this is graded as 'good'. If a soft clot forms in a turbid solution, this is graded as fair. A friable clot with cloudy surrounding fluid is graded as 'poor' or 'fragile'. No clot formation, with flakes in a cloudy suspension, is graded as 'very poor'. Good clots do not break up when agitated, while poor clots break up into small shreds. This procedure actually is an estimate of synovial hyaluronate and not mucin, which is absent in joint fluid.

Microscopic Examination: Total and differential counts as for CSF. But the usual leucocyte with 1% glacial acetic acid precipitates synovial fluid hyaluronate and is unsatisfactory, instead methylene blue in saline can be used. If the fluid is very turbid, use saline dilution or digestion with hyaluronidase (2 ml SF incubated with 150 IU hyaluronidase for 1 hr ar 37°C) may be helpful. Differential count can be done from EDTA sample (sediment) that has been centrifuged, a film made and stained as for peripheral blood.

LE cells are frequently seen in stained SF from patients with Systemic Lupus Erythematosus. Sometimes they can be seen in cases of rhematoid arthritis. Large phagocytes containing neutrophils may be found in SF and are called 'Reiter cells'; they are non-specific and may be present in effusions of varying etiology. RA cells or 'Ragocytes' are neutrophils containing 0.5 to 1.5 μ inclusions better seen with phase microscopy. They are seen in 94% cases of rheumatoid joint fluids but are non-specific for they can also be found in septic arthritis, gout, etc. (Table 25).

Examination of Seminal Fluid: Semen is formed by the testes as well as accessary male reproductive organs. It consists of spermatozoa suspended in seminal plasma. The seminal plasma provides medium for the spermatozoa. Examination of seminal fluid is usually performed as part of infertility investigation involving both partners of a barren marriage. It is a relatively simple examination and hence, is often done before the more complicated and expensive examination of the female partner. The results of the semen analysis must be interpreted in the light of the detailed history and thorough medical examination of the male and female partners. Indeed, it has been suggested that for the purpose of infertility investigation the male and female involved should be considered not as individuals but as a reproductive unit. In case of an abnormal result on first examination it is recommended that the test be repeated one or more times. It is required in forensic studies to examine vaginal secretions or clothing stains for the presence of semen in alleged or suspected rape. Semen examination is also requested to investigate the effectiveness of vasectomy, of recanalization operation and; it also supports or disproves a denial of paternity on the grounds of sterility.

The semen sample is collected in a clean, dry container preferably in the pathology laboratory. It is recommended that the sample be collected following a three-day period of abstinence. Freshly ejaculated semen is highly viscid, opaque, white or gray-white or grey-white coagulum that may have a distinct musty or acrid ordor. After 10–20 minutes it liquifies spontanously to form a translucent, turbid viscous fluid which is mildly alkaline (pH 7.7). The normal semen volume averages 3.5 ml with a range of 1.5 to 5.0 ml.

Microscopic Examination

Quantity: Measure the volume of semen in a small graduated cylinder. There is quite a variation in amount in different samples from one donor, depending on the period of continence preceding the examination. The average lies between 3 to 4 ml.

Viscosity: Freshly ejaculated semen is highly viscous. Self-liquefaction takes places and should be completed in 15 to 30 minutes. The absence of liquefaction may inhibit the movements of spermatozoa, thereby interfering with fertilization.

Color: The normal semen is whitish with the typical seminal smell. Frank hæmorrhage in the vesicles may color the fluid red, and suppurative infection imparts a yellow color and a foul smell.

Reaction: It is always found to be on the alkaline side (pH 7.2 to 8.0).

Motility of spermatozoa: Make a hanging drop preparation using a well slide. Ring the well with vaseline. Place a large drop of seminal fluid on a cover-glass, invert it over the well and press it down gently to make an airtight seal. Motility can then be observed:

(i) Absence of spermatozoa (*Azoospermia*), which should be confirmed after centrifugation of the specimen.

(ii) Only a few motile spermatozoa found (*Oligozoospermia*)

(iii) Spermatozoa are present but immobile (*Necrozoospermia*)

(iv) When motile spermatozoa are present, the proportion of motile to immobile cells should be noted. The microscopic field is made very small by fitting in the eyepiece of the microscope a disc of black paper with a central slit. Immobile spermatozoa are counted after motile ones.

(v) If the motility is very low, the specimen is incubated at 37°C, which may restore motility. Ten to fifteen per cent of immobile spermatozoa are encountered in fertile samples.

Duration of motility is one essential to fecundation. For stydying the duration, a thick smear covered with a coverglass is prepared and the preparation is sealed with vaseline. Hour to hour examination should be made for studying the motility. A normal specimen shows little cessation of motility at the third hour after emission, and considerable cellular activity is noted at the fifth or sixth hour. Complete or considerable subsidence of motility within this limitation should be regarded as an index of deficiency.

Microscopic Examination of Semen :

It is done as seen as possible after liquification of the semen has taken places ie within 15–30 minutes of collection.

1) **Sperm count:** Mix the semen sample thoroughly and draw the sample to the 0.5 mark on a white blood cell pipette (WBC pipette). Dilute to the mark with the semen diluting fluid.

Semen diluting fluid;

Sodium bicarbonate	— 5 gms
Formalin (neutral) or Phenol	— 1 ml
Distilled water	— 100 ml

Charge the improved Neubauer counting chamber. Allow the semen to settle (for 2 mins) and then count the sperm in the four corner squares as in a WBC count. The formula for calculation is similar to the WBC counting formula except that we report sperm count per c.c. or ml. instead of per cu mm, so an additional multiplication factor of 1000 is added.

Sperm/ml $= (N \times 10 \times 20 \times 1000)/4$

The total number of sperms is multipled by 50,000

Normal sperm count is between 60 to 150 million/ml. Even if the count is below 60 million/ml (Oligospermia), the patient may still be fertile. Total absence of sperm is known as azo-spermia and is associated with sterility.

2) **Motility:** Active motility is necessary for the sperms to penetrate the cervical mucous and subsequently migrate to fertilize the ovum in the fallopian tube. Motility can be assessed by placing a small drop of liquified semen on a microscopic slide. It is covered by coverslip which is ringed by vaseline to prevent drying. The preparation is scanned under the high dry objective of a microscope until at least a total of 200 sperms are observed. Normally about 80 per cent of the spermatozoa are actively motile and about 20 per cent are sluggishly motile or non motile. Decreased sperm motility is associated with infertility.

3. **Morphological Examination of Spermatozoa:** Stained smears are employed for the purpose.

A thin smear of semen on a clean glass slide is dried in air, and fixed by heat. Add one per cent chloramine for several minutes to remove excess of mucus. Wash by blotting on filter paper. Stain for 2 to 5 minutes with the following:—

Ziehl-Neelsen's carbol fuchsin	....	2 parts
Conc. alcoholic sol. of eosin	....	1 part
Alcohol 95 per cent	....	1 part

Wash with water and counterstain with Loeffler's methylene blue for a few seconds. Wash, dry and examine under oil immersion. The heads of the spermatozoa are stained purplish, while the tail and middle piece are red.

Count the number of spermatozoa in a microscopic field. The same field is searched for immature forms of spermatozoa. The different developmental stages may be encountered in pathological semen but rare in fertile specimens.

Examine 100 to 500 spermatozoa for the following abnormalities:— (Fig. 45).

(i) Heads — too small or too large, pointed, ragged edges, atypical distribution of chromatin, presence of acidophilic vacuoles, double heads.

(ii) Middle pieces — absent, swollen, bifurcated, etc.

(iii) Tails — double, curled, rudimentary or absent.

Semen containing upto 20 per cent, abnormal spermatozoa is still considered fertile.

4. **Other Cells:** RBCS, epithelial, cells, polymorphonuclear cells, immature germ cells and numerous granules and globules are observed during the microscopic examination of the semen. Presence of trichomonas is also looked for.

Investigations: Other tests performed on seminal fluid:— post coital (Sims Huhner) test, determination of antibodies to spermatozoa etc. are some additional elaborate tests carried out in the infertility investigations.

Form for reporting routine semen examination:

A) Microscopic or Physical examination: 1. Volume, 2. Viscosity, 3. Color and 4. Reaction.

B) Microscopic examination: 1. Count of sperm, 2. Motility of sperm, 3. Morphology or abnormal forms and 4. Other cells.

EXAMINATION OF SPUTUM:

The sputum is the material coughed up from the lungs, the bronchi, the trachea and the larynx, and consists of mucus secreted by the respiratory mucosa, products of tissue disintegration due to disease, exudate from lesions and materials from near-by structures that might have established communication with the respiratory tract. Expectoration of the sputum is the body's attempt to rid itself of material irritating the respiratory mucosa. The amount of mucus secreted in health is so small that normally there is no expectoration. Lesions in the lungs will produce sputum provided they are communicating with the bronchi and provided the material to be coughed out is fluid enough.

Examination of the sputum is a valuable means of investigating diseases of the respiratory tract.

Collection of Specimen: The patient is instructed to rinse the mouth with water to avoid contamination by food residues. He is further explained that the material required is expectoration

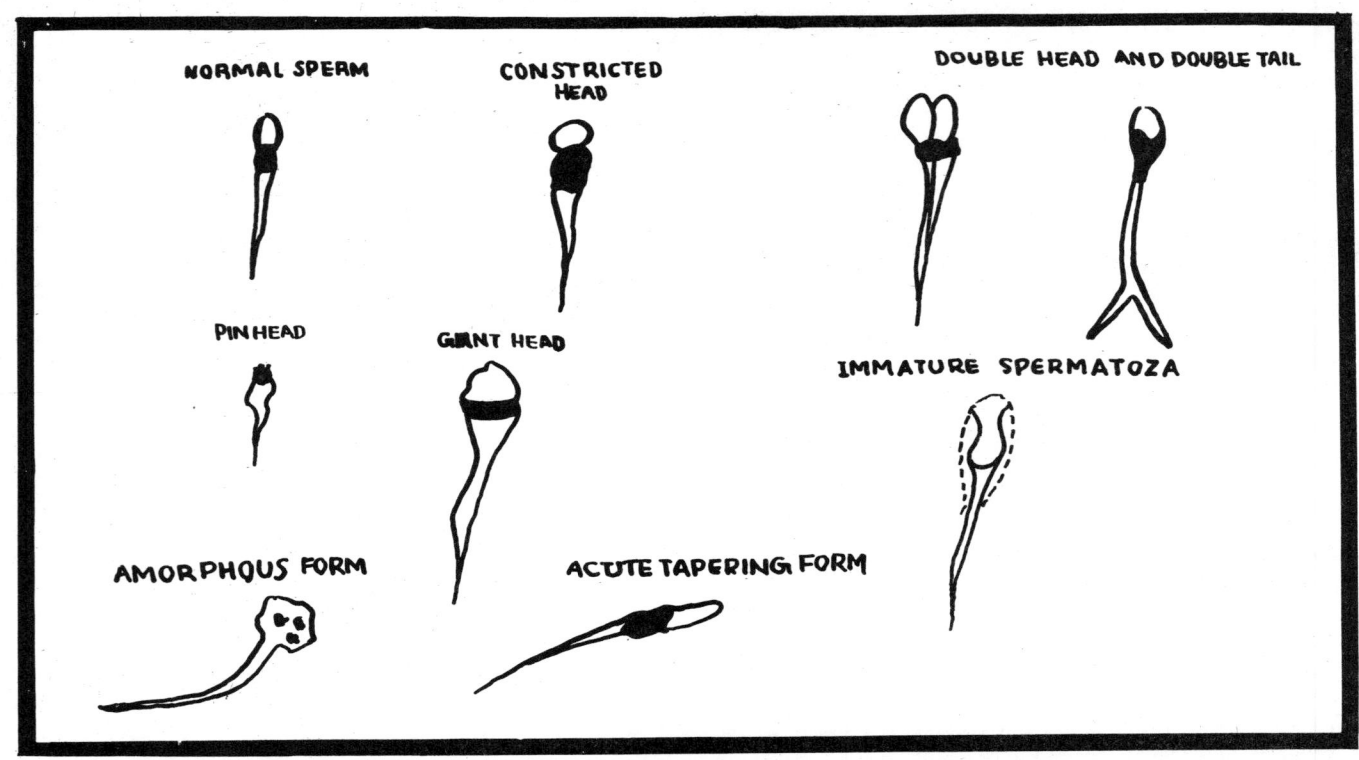

Fig. 45 Shows normal and abnormal sperms

brought out after a fit of coughing and not saliva. The sputum is collected directly into the container. Conveniently the container can be clean, widemouthed bottle (capacity 30 to 60 ml) with a tight-fitting screw-cap. The most common examination of the sputum is the detection of tubercle bacilli and for this, the early morning specimen (consisting of the material collected overnight in the bronchi) is preferred. If this specimen proves negative, a specimen collected over a period of 24 hrs is the next step. When a cultural examination for pyogenic organisms or fungi is to be done, the sputum should be collected in a sterile Petri dish and examined immediately; in the case of the cultural examination for the tubercle bacillus a 24 hrs sample in a clean bottle is sufficient. Cultural examination of any kind should, however, be done before antibiotics or chemotherapeutic drugs have been given. After the specimen has been examined the remnants should be destroyed by heat or a chemical disinfectant (strong lysol).

Procedure for Routine Examination

1. **Physical examination:** Quantity: Large amount of sputum (over 100 ml per day) are produced in bronchietasis and lung abscess.

Appearance and Consistency: Sputum is described as mucoid, mucopurulent serous (watery) and blood-stained. The characterstic appearance are; watery, frothy sputum in pulmonary oedema; tenacious rusty (blood-stained) sputum in lobar pneumonia; purulent sputum in lung abscess; and thin sputum separating into layer on standing in bronchietasis. Frank blood may be seen in the sputum in pulmonary tuberculosis, pneumonias, congestive cardiac failure from mitral stenosis, pulmonary infarction and malignant tumours of the bronchi and the lungs. Rupture of an amoebic abscess of the liver into the lung produces sputum with the appearance of "anchovy sauce".

Odour: A foul odour is seen in abscess of the lung and in an empyema that has ruptured into the lung. The sputum of bronchiectasis has usually a sweet smell.

2. **Microscopic examination:** (a) A wet or coverslip preparation: Suspicious portions of the sputum, as judged by the physical examination after pouring the sputum in a Petri dish, are selected. A small portion is put on a glass slide; add saline, if necessary to thin and put a coverslip. Examine under the low and the high power.

Elastic Fibres: Appear as slender, curled, highly refrectile fibres; they are seen in any destructive lesion of the lung-tuberculosis, abscess, bronchiectasis or carcinoma. Curschman's spirals are spirally twisted, mucoid strands closing epithelial cells and leucocytes (chiefly eosinophils). Curschman's spirals are seen in bronchial asthma.

Charcot-Leyden crystals are either colorless, painted hexagones, or needle-like. They are supposed to be derived from disintegration of eosinophils. They are encountered in bronchial asthma or parasitic infection of lung.

Fungi: These may take the form of yeast-like cells, non branching or branching double-contoured filaments or as tangled masses of filaments with "clubbed" ends (ray fungus). Fungi may occur in the sputum as contaminants from the mucous membrane of the upper respiratory tract and have no significance. That they come from bronchi or lungs is proved by demonstrating their presence repeatedly in the sputum raised by deep coughing or in specimens obtained by bronchoscopy. Fungi can also be demonstrated by special staining methods and cultural examinations.

Animal Parasites: On rare occasions parasites may be found in the sputum. E. histolytica may be discovered in the sputum if any amoebic liver abscess has ruptured into the lung. In the case of hydatid disease of the lung the sputum may show the laminar membrane and the germinal layers or scolices containing groups of minute hooklets. Other parasites found are trichomonas hominis, ova of P. westermani and larvae of S. sterocoralis and hookworms.

Cells: A coverslip preparation may show red cells, puscells and haemosiderin-containing macrophages ("heart-failure cells"). The last type seen in congestive cardiac failure, must be distinguished from macrophages containing carbon pigment, a common findings in the sputum city-dwellers.

(b) Stained Smears: The suspicious portion is selected and, with a pointed match-stick or a platinum loop, a thin smear is made on a clean glass slide. The smear meant for bacteriological examination is fixed by passing it slowly through the flame three to four times.

Leishman or Giemsa Stained Smear for Cytological Study: This smear is not to be fixed by heat. It is handled exactly like the blood smear. In bacterial infections the sputum will show a large number of polymorphs, Monocytes (macrophages) are seen in chronic infections macrophages with vacuolated cytoplasm (due to fat) may be seen in lipoid pneumonias. However, the only significant fingding is the presence of a large number of eosinophils in bronchial asthma and tropical eosinophilia.

Smears Stained by Gram Stain:The sputum is always contaminated by organisms contained in the upper respiratory tract and the mouth. A mixture of organisms is the usual findings. None carry a diagnostic significance. The different type of cells, referred to above, can be identified with a little experience in the smears stained by gram's stain also.

Smear Stained by Ziehl-Neelsen Method: This is by far the most important step in the routine examination of the sputum because it shows the presence of mycobacterium tuberculosis. The technique of Ziehl-Neelsen staining is given below:

1. Fix the smears by passing through the flame 3–4 times.
2. Cover the smear with carbol fuchsin.
3. Warm the slide until steam rises from the staining solution; this is done twice. Do not boil the staining solution. Allow the heated stain to act for 5 minutes.
4. Wash the smear with water.
5. Decolorise the smear with 20% (by volume) sulphuric acid.
6. Now counterstain with Lowffler's methylene blue for 1 minute.
7. Wash with water. Dry the smear in air. Examine with the oil-immersion lens.

Mycobacterium tuberculosis is an acid-fast bacillus and appears as a redstained rod with beaded appearance. To detect mycobacterim tuberculosis by this in the sputum-estimated to be about 50,000 per cu mm. A negative result does not, therefore, exclude pulmonary tuberculosis. At least three different specimens of sputum should be examined before the negative report is accepted. When direct microscopy is negative, further procedures are available to detect mycobacterim tuberculosis in the sputum. These are described separately below.

Special Methods for Detection of Myco tuberculosis

(a) **Fluorescence Microscopy:** This is a simple and efficient method but requires special equipment. The bacilli in the sputum are stained with a fluorescent dye, Auramin O. The stained bacilli when irradiated with ultraviolet light and observed with the fluorescent microscope, appear as brilliant yellow rods against a black background, and can be easily spotted out. The yield of positives by this method in trained hands is better than with smears stained by Ziehl-Neelsen method.

(b) **Concentration Method for Mycobacterim tuberculosis:** Many techniques are available. The principle under all is the same; destroy the extraneous matter like mucus, cells and the contaminating organism by means of chemical digestion so that only live tubercle bacilli are preserved and concentrated in a small amount of the deposit obtained from the original volume of the sputum. The most commonly used method for concentration is that of Petroff. This is as follows:

A 24 hours collection of the sputum is made. The sputum is mixed with an equal volume of 4 per cent NaOH and placed in the incubator at 37°C for 30 minutes; the container is shaken every few minutes. The mixture or digest is now centrifuged at 3000 rpm for 30 minutes and the supernatant discarded. The deposit is neutralised with 8 per cent HCl; the acid is added, drop by drop, using phenol red as an indicator. The neutralised deposit is the concentrated material ready for examination. Three kinds of examinations can be done on the deposit:

1. Smears can be prepared and stained by Ziehl-Neelsen stain.
2. The deposit can be cultured on special media; the most commonly used media are Lowenstein-Jensen medium and Dorsett's egg medium.
3. Guineaping inoculation. About 1 to 2 ml of the deposit from the concentrated material is injected subcutaneously (in the flank) or intramuscularly (in the thigh). A nodule appears at the site of injection in 7 to 21 days. The neighbouring lymph nodes are also affected and later lymph nodes in other parts of the body; they become enlarged and caseous. The animal loses weight and dies within 6 weeks to 3 months. At the autopsy it will show tubercles in the liver and the spleen in large numbers; the lungs may show a few tubercles. In the living animal mycobactrim tuberculosis is demonstrated in smears made from enlarged regional node at the autopsy. The organism is present in smears from different lesions.

In the diagnosis of pulmonary tuberculosis examination of gastric contents or of post-pharyngeal or larynegeal swabs for Myco. tuberculosis are available alternatives, especially in children.

Exfoliative Cytology on Sputum: This is a useful method for the diagnosis of bronchial and lung carcinomas. Smears of the fresh material are fixed immediately (while wet) in ether-alcohol and stained by papanicolaou stain. The diagnosis depends upon the identification of cancer cells by their special features (cytological diagnosis of cancer). The bronchial secretion obtained by bronchoscopy gives even better results.

Form of reporting a sputum specimen:

A. Physical Examination: Quantity, Colour, Odour, Mucus, Pus, Blood and Miscellaneous findings.

B. Microscopic Examination: (i) Wet unstained preparation, (ii) Stained preparation, Ziehl-Neelsen, Gram and Leishman.

CHAPTER 12

STOOL EXAMINATION

IMPORTANCE OF STOOL EXAMINATION

Most clinicians consider examinatin of faeces as being limited to a search for intestinal parasites or thier ova, or for pathogenic bacteria. Much, of clinical value, may be learned, however, by physical, chemical and detailed microscopic examinations of the stool. Examination of stool may therefore be,

1. **Physical** —
   1. Amount
   2. Form & Consistency
   3. Colour
   4. Odour
   5. Reaction &
   6. Mucous.

2. **Chemical** —
   1. Occult blood
   2. Bilirubin
   3. Urobilin (stercobilin)
   4. Urobilinogen
   5. Fats &
   6. Nitrogen

3. **Microscopic** —
   1. Intestinal parasites/ova/cyst
   2. Pathogenic bacteria
   3. Remnants of food
   4. Cellular exudates &
   5. Erythrocytes

NORMAL APPEARANCE & COMPOSITION

Stool/faeces is the end product of the digestive system of the body. The faeces are normally composed of food residues, materials secreted through the wall of the intestines & in the bile, leukocytes, desquamated epithelial cells & bacteria.

The contents of jejunum & terminal ileum are liquid and about 400 gms in weight per 24 hrs. As they pass through caecum and colon, most of the water is absorbed converting the contents to a soft but formed mass, about 150–200 gms in weight. Normal characteristics of stool are as follows:

MACROSCOPIC

1. No. of evacuations/day — usually 2 (2–4)
2. Weight in gms/day — 150–200
3. Form & consistency — Soft but formed
4. Colour — Light to dark brown due to stercobilin
5. Odour — Aromatic
6. Reaction — 6.9–7.2
7. Mucous — Scanty, intimately mixed with stool.

MICROSCOPIC

1. Undigested and indigestible remnants of food — details to be discussed under text.
2. Desquamated epithelial cells.
3. Bacteria — commensals of alimentary tract.
4. Protozoa — Commensals in intenstines.

COLLECTION OF SPECIMENS FOR STOOL EXAMINATION

In this we will mention not only collection of stool specimens for routine examination but also discuss something about the other techniques which improve the chances of finding ova/cyst etc.

Collection of Faeces

1. The faeces to be examined, should be passed into a clean vessel without admixture of urine and antibiotics.
2. A small portion of stool sample is sufficient for routine examination, collected in a wide mouth glass container it should be sent to the laboratory within a few hrs owing to changes caused by decomposition.
3. The stool should not be sent in a match box or wrapped in a paper as it is unhygienic & decomposition takes place quickly.
4. The patient should not usually be given any purgative before the stool is collected, oils should especially be avoided.
5. For benzidine test for occult blood it is advised that patient be given a diet free from meat & green vegetable for 3 days to avoid a false positive test.
6. In case of delay, stool may be collected in a suitable transport medium & may be sent within 4–5 hrs or even 24 hrs; various transport media in use include.
   i. For vibrios — Alkaline peptone water & Venkat-Ramakrishan (VR) fluid.
   ii. For other enteropathogens — Cary & Blair medium.
   iii. For all parasite/Ova/cyst-stool should be collected in a 30 ml bottle containing 15 ml of 10% formaldehyde solution.
   iv. Hanks Soln (salt, 0.4% bovine albumin, pencillin & streptomycin) especially useful for preserving rectal swabs.

Rectal Swab: Sterile swabs are dipped in sterile buffered glycerol. Separate the buttocks before introducing the swab in the rectum to avoid contamination with the perianal skin. The swab is inserted either in a sterile glass container or in a preservative medium like V R fluid or Cary & Blair's medium. Rectal swabs are taken when stool samples are not available.

NIH Swab: This consists of a wooden applicator to which a piece of cellophane tape is attached. Early in the morning without washing, sticky face of the applicator is applied against perianal skin. Immediately transfer to a microslide. Wash away the glue with xylol and examine immdiately under microscope. This swab is especially useful for identifying the ova of enterobius vermiculares (Pinworms).

PHYSICAL EXAMINATION

In the complete routine examination of faeces, attention should be paid to the physical characterstics. Much information of clinical value may be derived in relation to amount, form & consistency, color, odor, mucous, concretions and animal parasites.

Physical examinations are especially indicated in most patients with suspected gastrointestinal diseases & should be rarely omitted in cases of diarrhoea, constipation, jaundice, anaemia or in infants with feeding problem.

AMOUNT: The amount is commonly characteristically increased in states producing:
  (i) Steatorrhoea — due to an increase in faecal lipids eg. obstructive jaundice.
  (ii) Indigestion of carbohydrates — e.g. sprue when stools are foamy.

Form & consistency

  (i) Excessively hard faeces, sometimes called scybala are commonly observed in habitual constipation & indicate atony of muscular coat of colon.
  (ii) In spastic constipation the faeces are characterized by numberous hard, ball like masses.
  (iii) Flattened, ribbon like stools may result from taking mineral oil but otherwise indicate obstruction of rectum, generally a structure from a healed ulcer (most frequently syphillis or LGV).
  (iv) In dysentry, stools are invariably small, numerous & composed largely of mucus & blood with very small amount of fecal material.

  Color: of faeces may depend a lot on diet, any drugs taken or disease.

  (i) Diet: Milk diet — light yellow faeces.
  Cocoa chocolate — dark grey faeces
  Fruits — reddish black faeces
  Spinach & other chlorophyllic vegetables — green faeces
  Beetroot — red colored faeces
  Rhubarb — yellow colored faeces.
  (ii) Drugs: Calomet — green stools due to biliverdin,
  Iron — dark brown or black stools
  Neoprontasil — red stools
  Santonin/senna — yellow stools
  BaSO₄ — clay colored stools.
  (iii) Diseases — *Obstructive jaundice* — clay colored stools
  Haemorrhage in upper GIT — black tarry stools (Malena)
  Diarrhoea due to chromogenic bacteria — green colored stools.

  Odor: Variations of odor may occur
  (i) Sour rancid odour — increased faecal fat.
  (ii) Putrid odour — in severe diarrhoeas
  (iii) A foul stench — ulcerative/gangrenous lesions.

  Blood & Mucus: Obvious pus, blood & mucus in faeces indicate the presence of ulcerative lesions or infections of the lower bowel. Blood (bright red) coating surface of stools may be due to haemorrhoids, fissure in and or ulceration in the rectum.

  In the so called mucous colitis, shreds & ribbons of mucous, sometimes representing complete casts of portions of colon, are passed especially after an enema. This mucous does not contain pus cells.

  Reaction: Various methods may be used to test pH of stool.
  (i) Thoroughly mix the stool & test with red and blue litmus paper, red paper turns blue with alkali.
  (ii) Test with Congo red paper
  (iii) To a watery suspension of faeces, add a few drops of 1% alcoholic solution of phenolphthalein. It turns pink if alkaline.

CHEMICAL EXAMINATION

Blood in Faeces

  Quite often blood in the stool is not visible grossly and may be revealed only by specific tests (Occult blood).

  Principles: Haem compounds catalyze the oxidation of organic substances such as benzidine, orthotolidine by H_2O_2 (hydrogen peroxide). The tests are made specific by boiling the faeces, which destroys true peroxidases, leaving only haem compounds that are thermostable.

Precautions:

1. To avoid false positive reactions patients should be on a meat free diet for 72 hrs before collection of specimen.
2. Faeces should be mixed thoroughly before testing.
3. Cross check results by 2 methods.
4. Exclude aspirin & related drugs.
5. Exclude lettuce, apples & oranges from diets.

(1) Benzidine Test:

1. Prepare a thin emulsion of faeces with water in a test tube.
2. Prepare the benzidine reagent by dissolving a knife point of benzidine HCl crystals in 5 ml of glacial acetic acid and adding an equal volume of 10 Vol% H_2O_2 (Alternatively prepare a saturated solution of benzidine in glacial acetic acid and store away in a brown bottle in a dark place).
3. Now add 5 ml of boiled faecal emulsion to the reagent. (Alternatively haem compounds can be extracted from faeces using 3% v/v acetic acid).
4. A deep green color indicates a positive test for occult blood.

(2) Orthotolidine Test:

1. Prepare the reagent by dissoving 4 gm of 0-tolidine in 100 ml glacial acetic acid. Keep in a brown bottle and prepare at monthly intervals.
2. To a 1 ml of water suspension of faeces add 1 ml of reagent & 1 ml of 3% H_2O_2.
3. A positive reaction is indicated by development of a bluish/bluish green color within 30–60 secs.

(3) Alvarez & Wright's Modification of Gregersen Test:

1. Dissolve 225 mg of a mixture of 8 parts barium peroxide (200 mg) 1 part benzidine (25 mg) in 5 ml of a 50% solution of acetic acid. Prepare a fresh before use.
2. Rub a small portion of faeces into a few drops of water on a porcelein plate. Add few drops of the above solution. Interpret results according to Gregersen scale mentioned below:
  Deep blue in 3 seconds — + + +
  Distinct blue in 15 secs — + +
  Blue green in 30–60 secs — Doubtful positive ±

(4) Guaiac Test:

1. Prepare reagent by dissolving 2 gm of powdered guaiac in 10 ml of 95% ethyl alcochol.
2. Prepare a smear of faeces on a filter paper.
3. Add 10 drops of reagent followed by 1–2 drops of glacial acetic acid & 1–2 drops of H_2O_2.
4. Development of blue/dark color within 30 seconds constitute a positive reaction.

Test for Reducing Substances

Benedicts qualitative test is used in a way similar to urine except that a faecal suspension is used instead of urine.

Test for Bile Acids

1. Extract a small amount of faeces with alcohol & filter. Evaporate the filtrate in a dish over a water bath.
2. Dissolve the residue in water made slightly alkaline with KOH solution
3. Add 0.3 ml of a 5% sucrose solution.
4. Transfer to a test tube & carefully run down the sides about 3 ml of concentration H_2SO_4. Cool in running water.
   A red ring at the point of contact is a positive reaction.

Test for urobilin

The test depends on formation of urobilin mercury with production of red color.

1. Rub a small amount of faeces in a mortar with a saturated solution of $HgCl_2$.
2. Transfer to a shallow white dish & let stand for 24 hrs.

Presence of urobilin is indicated by a deep color imparted to particles of faeces. If unaltered bilirubin is present, a green color is produced through its oxidation to biliverdin.

Urobilin is absent to greatly reduced in obstructive jaundice & its return to faeces often the first sign of relief.

MICROSCOPIC EXAMINATION

(a) Preparation:

1. **Saline Preparation:** A minute portion of faeces is diluted with normal saline (0.9%) and a drop taken on a clean glass slide. A coverslip is gently put over it so as to spread the emulsion into a thin, uniform & transparent layer.
2. **Iodine Preparation:** Lugol's iodine solution is prepared as follows:

Powdered iodine crystals	— 5 gms
Potassium iodine	— 10 gms
Distilled water	— 100 ml

Potassium iodine is dissolved in distilled water, iodine crystals slowly added while shaking. Filter & store in an amber colored bottle. One drop of saline emulsion is taken on a glass slide. Add 1 drop of lugol's iodine and place a coverslip over it.

(b) Examination:

Both unstained and stained preparations are first examined under low power objective starting from one end of the cover slip, the whole slide is examined. Any suspicious object is focussed under high power objective for detailed diagnosis.

CONCENTRATION TECHNIQUES

1. Concentrated Saline Floatation:

(a) Preparation of Saline Soln.
1. Add NaCl in hot water & continuously stir until excess salt added does not dissolve.
2. Check the Sp. gravity and adjust to 1020.
3. Filter the solution before use
(b) Technique:
1. Take a vial 1″ in diameter & 2–2½″ long of 20 ml capacity.
2. Fill up 1/4 of vial with saline solution.
3. Add faeces of a small marable, and mix thoroughly.
4. Fill the vial to the brim with solution and superimpose a grease free microscopic slide so that it is in contact with the suspension.
5. Allow to stand for 10–60 minutes and lift the slide straight up without tipping.
6. Invert the slide carefully without allowing the drop to slide off & examine under microscope, imediately.

2. Formal Ether Concentration:

1. Take a stool sample of the size of a marble in a mortar. Mix & suspend with 10 cc distilled water to destroy blastocysts.
2. Strain about 10 cc of suspension through a funnel having gauze of 40 meshes/inch & centrifuge at 2500 rpm for 2 mins. Decant supernatant: If it is much larger or smaller, adjust the proper quantity by resuspending & pouring out some fluid or adding more faecal suspension & repeating the process (centrifugation & decantation).
3. Add 7 ml of 10% formalin to the sediment, make it a suspension by thorough mixing. Add 3 ml of ether, stopper the tube with a stopper, shake vigorously in an inverted position for 30 sec Remove the stopper with care.
4. Centrifuge at 2500 rpm for 1–2 mins when 4 layers will be formed. Loose the plug of debris by a pricking needle, & quickly & carefully pour off the upper 3 layers leaving sediment undistrubed. Keeping the tube horizontal, remove the debris adhering to wall of tube by cotton swab.
5. Mix the sediment with the small amount of fluid drained back from the wall by a pipette & prepare iodine stained & saline mount & examine under microscope.

The bulk of stool consists of granular debris. Among the recognizable microscopic structures encountered in normal and diseased conditions are:

1. **Remnants of Food:** (Fig. 52)
(a) **Vegetable fibres:** Spiral structure with pits, dots or reticulate marking.
(b) **Vegetable cells:** Show double contours & sometimes chlorophyll bodies.
(c) **Vegetable hairs:** Are homogenous, elongated, tube like structures with highly refractile wall.
(d) **Starch granules:** Best identified by adding drop of lugol's iodine which stains them blue.
(e) **Muscle Fibres:** Usually appear as short, transversely striated cylinders.
(f) **Fats:** May appear as:
   1. Neutral fats (droplets).
   2. Fatty acids (Needle like crystals).
   3. Soap (Yellow masses or coarse crystals).
(g) **Elastic fibres and connective tissue:** Appear as colorless/yellowish threads, rendered more distinct by acetic acid.
2. **PUS Cells:** Present in ulcerative conditions of the intestine. In amebic dysentry, their presence indicates superadded infection.
3. **Macrophages:** are sometimes present and are liable to be mistaken as E. histolytica. They are most common in bacillary dysentry.
4. **Epithelial Cells:** A few cells are always present. Increase number of epithelial cells occur in catarrhal condition of the colon.
5. **Red Blood Cells:** Unaltered erythrocytes are seen in diseases of colon, rectum or anus. In amebic dysentry RBCs are present in clumps and are redish yellow, while in bacillary dysentry, they are bright, discrete or in rouleaux.

6. **Crystals:** Various crystals may occur
  (i) **Triple Phosphates:** More likely in a vegetable diet
  (ii) **Calcium Oxalate:** More likely in a vegetable diet.
  (iii) **Charcot Leyden Crystals:** Particularly common in ulcerative conditions of colon, especially amebic dysentry. Absent in bacillary dysentry. These crystals are colorless, pointed, often needle like, hexagonal on cross section & variable size.
  (iv) **Hematoidin Crystals:** Yellowish brown needle like or rhombic crystals. They may occur after haemorrhages within gastro intestinal tract.
  (v) **Bismuth Suboxide Crystals:** Seen after administration of Bismuth.
  (vi) **Cholesterin Crystals:** Especially found in cases of Chole Lithiasis.
  (vii) **Calcium Bilirubiate:** Same as above
7. **Bacteria:** A study of bacteria in a saline or iodine preparation of stool is usually unnecessary.
8. **Yeasts & Moulds:** Yeast cells are present in large nomber in cases of intestinal fermentation. The cells show buds and form short chains. Moulds if present are commonly contamination from unclean vessels or air.
9. **Protozoa:** Amongst the protozoa, a medical lab. has to mainly identify Entamoeba histolytica and Giardia intestinalis. In fresh stool, trophozoites are seen, whereas cysts should be identified in iodine preparations, preferably after concentration. The cyst may be present in carriers. This is the infective form and carriers are public health hazards.

(i) **Giardia Intestinalis**

Trophozoites are not usually seen in stool.

Cysts Oval in shape, 12 micron × 7 micron axostyles diagonally split the cyst into two. Four nuclei, clustered at one end or paired at opposite poles (Fig. 47).

Trophozoite is pear shaped, 12–20 microns in length. Has a depression on one side of the blunt and 3 pairs of flagellae around the depression and one at the pointed end. 2 nuclei seen.

(ii) **E. Histolytica:** has to be differentiated from the Endolimax-nana and Entamaeba Coli by the undermentioned characteristics.

Table 26

(iii) **Chilomastix Mesnili**

Pear shaped, 13–24 microns long with 3 anterior flagella & no undulating membrane. Contains a large round nucleus and a large, elongated cystostome anteriorly. Posterior end is projected into a narrow tail like process (Fig. 49).

Cyst is pear shaped to oval 7.5–8.5 microns in length.

(iv) **Balantiduim Coli**

Oval shaped, 60–100 microns long & 50–70 microns wide. It is covered with cilia. It contains a bean shaped mactronucleus, a globular microns nucleus, contractile vacuoles and various sizes granules. At anterior end is a funnel shapped mouth. It is actively motile (Fig. 48).

10. **Helminthic ova:** (Fig. 50)

The ova which may be encountered in faeces of man are:

(i) **Ascaris lumbricoides**

a) **Fertilised egg**

Round or oval in shape (60–75 microns in length by 40 to 50 microns in breadth).
— Always bile stained and brownish (golden brown) in color.
— Surrounded by a thick smooth translucent shell with an outer albuminous coat which is thrown into rugosities or mamillations, this outer layer is sometimes lost (decortacated egg).
— Contains a very large conspicuous, unsegmented ovum (the nucleus is concealed by a larger amount of coarse yolk granules there is a clean crescentric space at the each pole.
— Floats in saturated solution of common salt.

(b) **Unfertilised egg**

— Narrower, longer (80 microns by 55 microns and more elliptical).
— Brownish in color (Bile stained).
— Has a thinner shell with an irregular coating of albumin.
— Contains small atrophied ovum with a mass of unorganised highly refractile granules of various sizes.
— Do not float in salt solution (heaviest of all helminthic eggs).

Morphology	E. Histolytica	E. Coli	E. Nana
Trophozoite			
(Fresh unstained) size	20–30 microns	20–40 microns	8 microns
Motility	Actively motile	Sluggish	Sluggish
Nucleus	Not visible	Visible	Visible
Cytoplasmic inclusions	Red cells, leycocytes tissue debris present bacteria absent	Bacteria & other materials present,	red cells never found
Cytoplasm	Clearly defined into ectoplasm & endoplasm.	No clear division	No clear division.
(Iodine stained) nuclear character	Central Karyosome, fine chromatin granules line nuclear membrane	Eccentric Karyosome coarse, chromatin granules line nuclear membrane	Large, irregular & eccentric karyosome, no chromatin granules.
Cyst (stained with Iodine)			
1. Size	6–15 Microns	15–20 microns	8–9 microns
2. Nucleus	1–4 Central karyosome	1–8 Eccentric karyosome	1–4 Karyosome may be central or eccentric
3. Glycogen mass	Rounded bars Chromatoid bars	Filamentous with square or pointed ends	Not seen

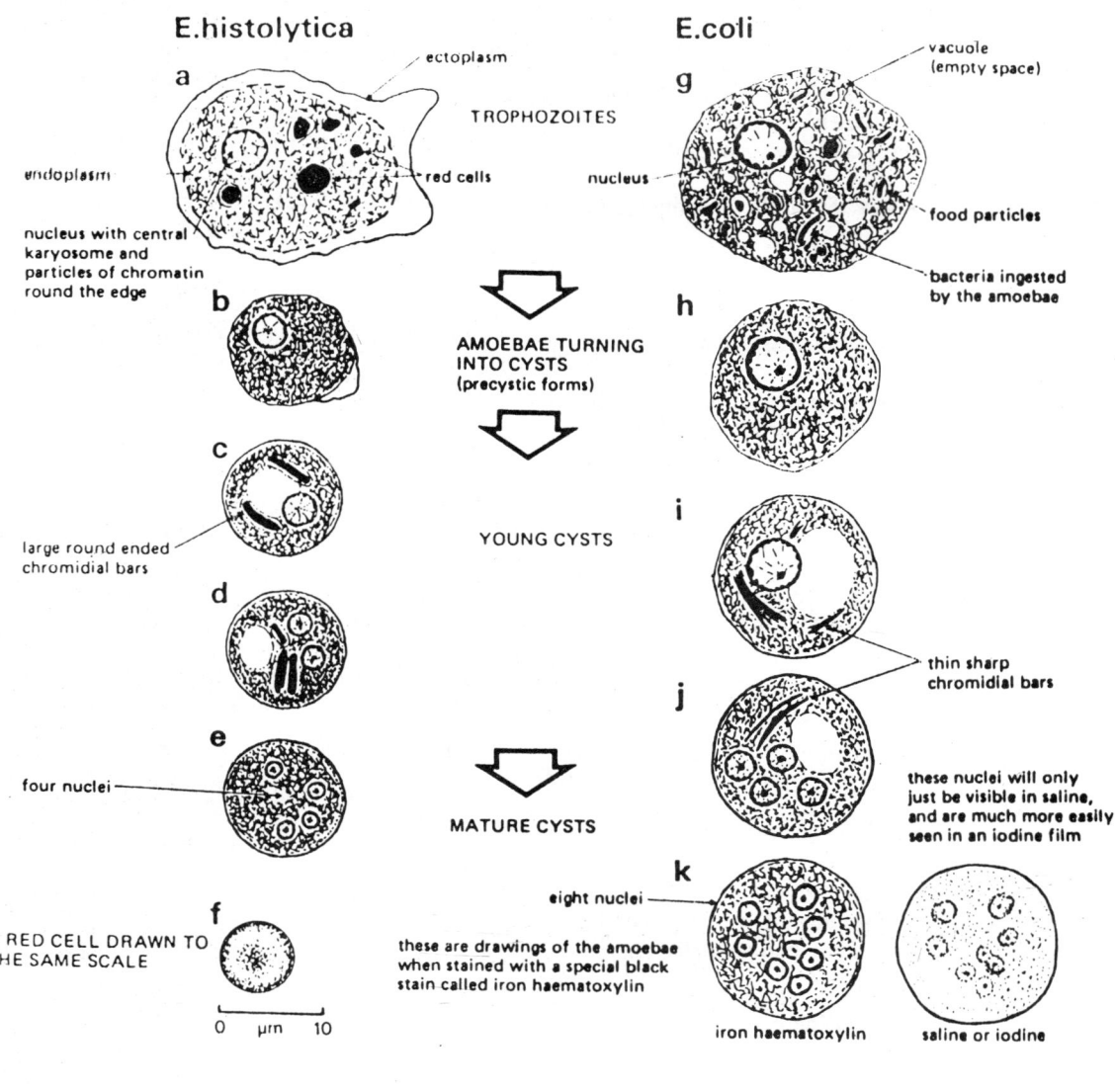

E.histolytica

a ectoplasm

TROPHOZOITES

endoplasm — red cells

nucleus with central karyosome and particles of chromatin round the edge

b

AMOEBAE TURNING INTO CYSTS (precystic forms)

c

large round ended chromidial bars

YOUNG CYSTS

d

e

four nuclei

MATURE CYSTS

f

A RED CELL DRAWN TO THE SAME SCALE

0 μm 10

E.coli

g vacuole (empty space)

nucleus

food particles

bacteria ingested by the amoebae

h

i

thin sharp chromidial bars

j

these nuclei will only just be visible in saline, and are much more easily seen in an iodine film

eight nuclei

k

these are drawings of the amoebae when stained with a special black stain called iron haematoxylin

iron haematoxylin   saline or iodine

DIFFERENT SPECIES OF AMOEBAE HAVE DIFFERENT NUCLEI

to see these details, make an iodine preparation, seal it with vaseline and wax, and use an oil immersion objective

these are diagrams and are not to the same scale as the figure above

Don't worry about identifying these species, the important thing about them is that they are not Entamoeba histolytica

fine chromatin round the edge

coarse chromatin round the edge

Plate 88

fine central karyosome

coarse non-central karyosome

Entamoeba histolytica   Entamoeba coli   Endolimax nana   Iodamoeba butschlii   Dientamoeba fragilis

Fig. 46 *Entamoeba histolytica* and *Entamoeba coli*

74

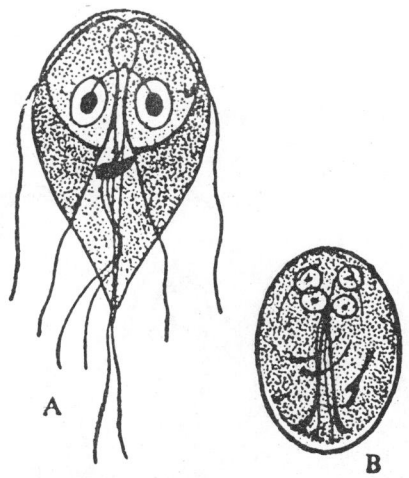

Fig. 47. *Giardia intestinalis.*
A. — Trophozoite. B.— Cyst

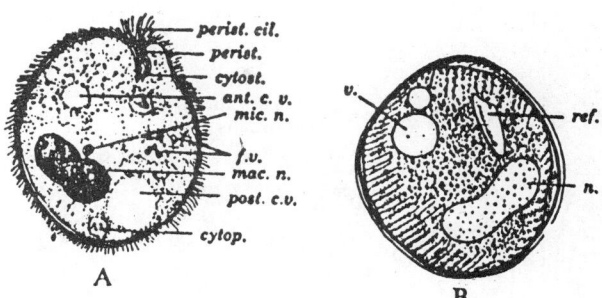

Fig. 48. *Balantidium coli.* A. — Trophozoite, B. — Cyst, *c.v.* — Anterior countractile vacuole, *Cystost.* — Cystostome, *Cystop.* — Cytophyge, *f.v.* — Food vacuoles, *mac. n.* — Macro-nucleus, *perist. cil.* — Peristoneal cilia, *post c.v.* — Posterior contractile vacuoles, *mic. n.* — Micronucleus. *ref. b.* — Refractile vacuole, *n.* — Vacuole

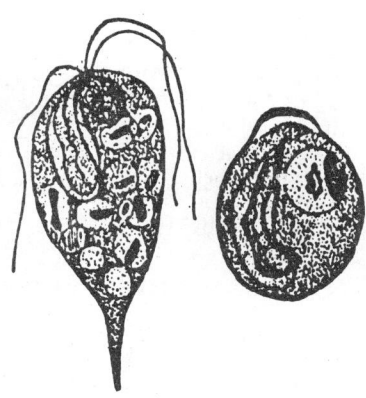

Fig. 49. *Chilamastix mesnili,* Trophozoite and cyst.

(ii) **Trichuris trichura**

— Size about 50 to 25 microns.
— Color brown (Bile stained). It has a double shell, outer one being bile stained.
— Barrel shaped with a mucous plug at each pole.
— Contains an unsegmented ovum when the egg leaves the human host.
— Floats in saturated solution of common salt.

(iii) **Ankylostoma duodenale**

— Oval or elliptical in shape 65 microns by 40 microns.
— Colorless (not bile stained).
— Surrounded by a transparent hyaline shell.
— Contains a segmented ovum usually with 4 blastomeres; has a clear space between the egg shell and segmented ovum.
— Floats in saturated solution of common salt.

(iv) **Enterobius vermicularis**

— Colorless (not bile stained).
— Asymmetrical in shape being planoconvex i.e. flattened on one side and convex on the other side.

— Measures 50 to 60 microns by 30 microns.
— Surrounded by a transport shell.
— Contains a coiled tadpole like larva.
— Floats in saturated solution of common salt.

(v) **Hymenolepis nana**

— Spherical or oval in shape measuring 30 to 45 microns in diameter. (not bile stained).
— There are two distinct membranes (a) the outer membrane is thin and colorless and (b) the inner embryophore encloses an oncosphere with three pairs of lancet shaped hooklets.
— The space between the two membranes is filled with yolk granules and polar filaments emanating from little knobs at either end of embryo phore.
— Floats in saturated solution of common salt.

(vi) **Taenia soluium/saginata/echinococcus granulosus** (Fig. 51).

— Spherical and brown in color (bile stained).
— Measures 30 to 43 microns in diameter.
— Thin, outer transparent shell. When present, represents the

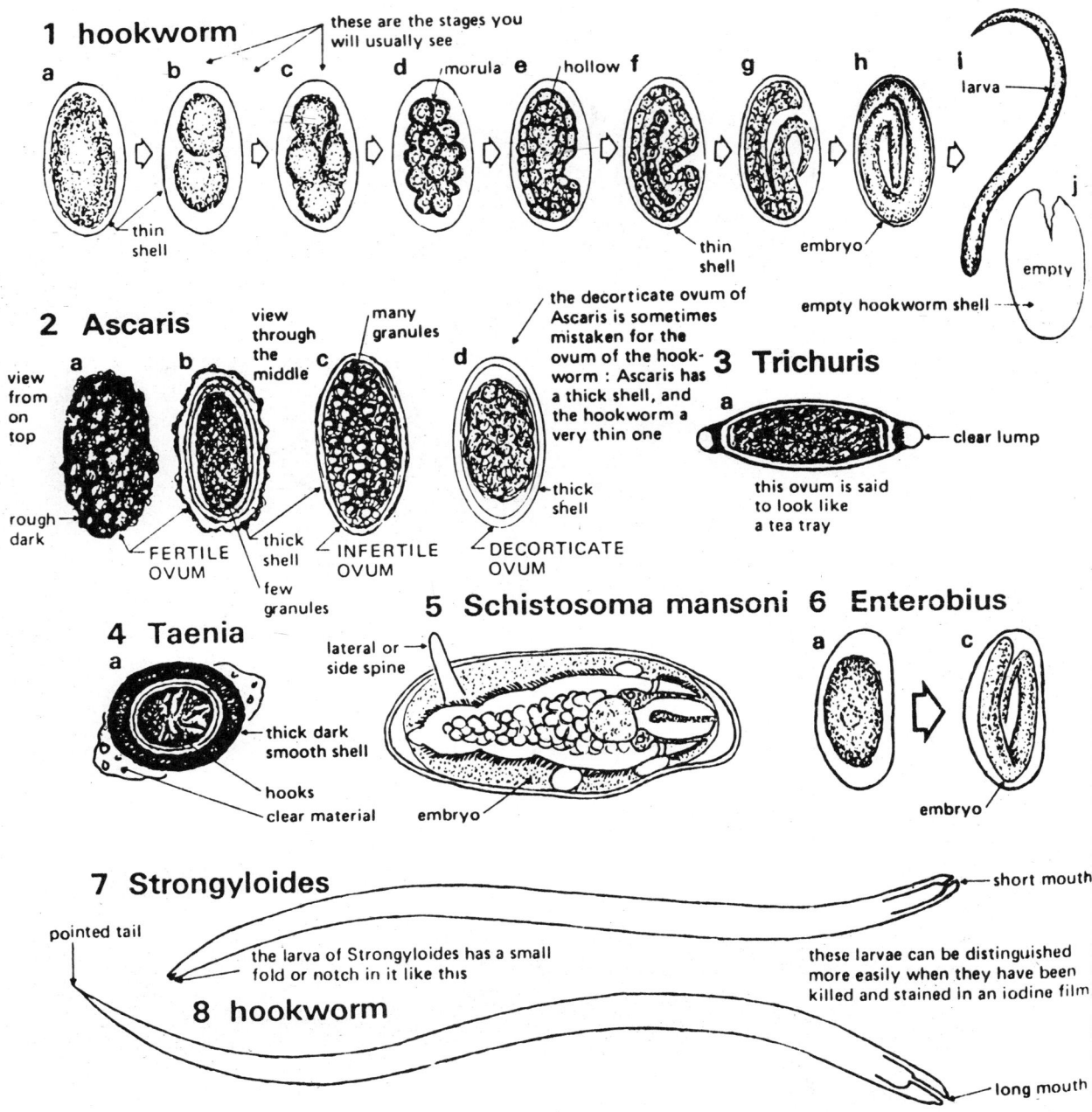

1 hookworm

these are the stages you will usually see

a b c d morula e hollow f g h i larva

thin shell

thin shell

embryo

j empty

empty hookworm shell

2 Ascaris

view through the middle

many granules

the decorticate ovum of Ascaris is sometimes mistaken for the ovum of the hookworm : Ascaris has a thick shell, and the hookworm a very thin one

view from on top

a b c d

rough dark

FERTILE OVUM

thick shell

INFERTILE OVUM

few granules

thick shell

DECORTICATE OVUM

3 Trichuris

a

clear lump

this ovum is said to look like a tea tray

4 Taenia

a

thick dark smooth shell

hooks

clear material

5 Schistosoma mansoni

lateral or side spine

embryo

6 Enterobius

a c

embryo

7 Strongyloides

short mouth

pointed tail

the larva of Strongyloides has a small fold or notch in it like this

these larvae can be distinguished more easily when they have been killed and stained in an iodine film

8 hookworm

long mouth

hookworm larva in Picture 1i above drawn much larger so that it can be compared with the larva of Strongyloides

Fig. 50. *Some common ova — a diagram*

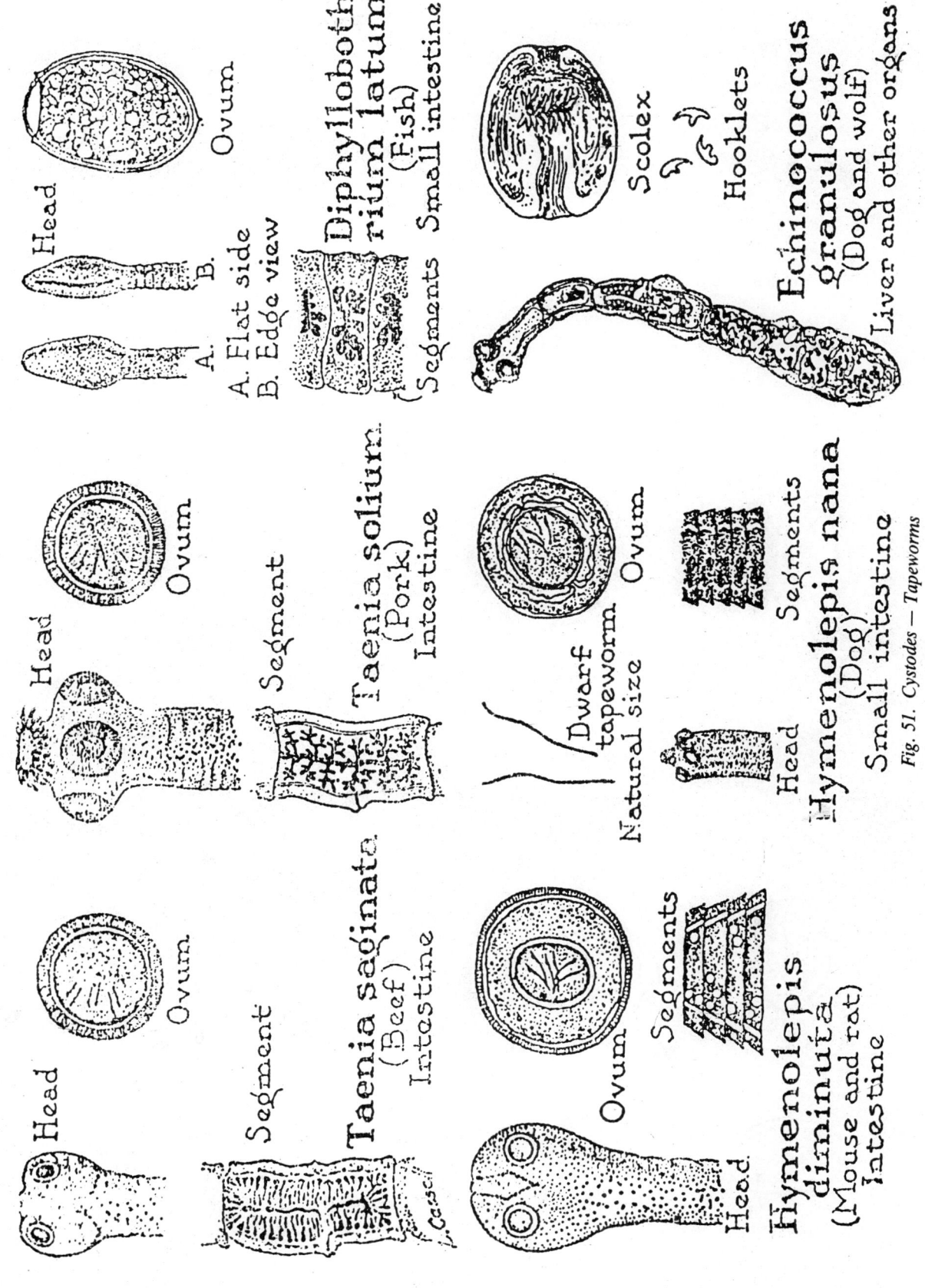

Head
Ovum
A.
B.
A. Flat side
B. Edge view
Segments
Diphyllobothrium latum
(Fish)
Small intestine

Scolex
Hooklets
Echinococcus granulosus
(Dog and wolf)
Liver and other organs

Head
Ovum
Segment
Taenia solium
(Pork)
Intestine

Dwarf tapeworm
Natural size
Ovum
Segments
Head
Hymenolepis nana
(Dog)
Small intestine

Fig. 51. Cystodes — Tapeworms

Head
Ovum
Segment
Taenia saginata
(Beef)
Intestine

Cases

Ovum
Segments
Head
Hymenolepis diminuta
(Mouse and rat)
intestine

77

Objects in Faeces Mistaken for Protozoan cysts & Helminthic Ova.

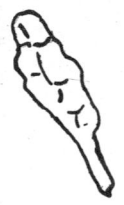

1. Alternaria spore

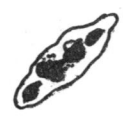

2. Acrothecium spore

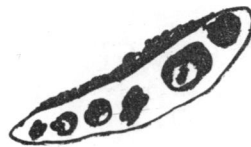

3. Helminthosporium spore

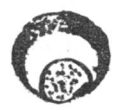

4. Blastocystics hominis

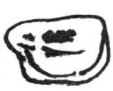

5. Hemp-pollen

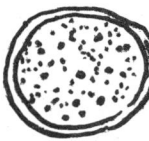

6. Drashard grass pollen

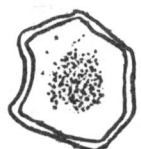

7. Timothy pollen

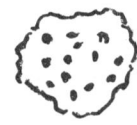

8. Ragweed pollen

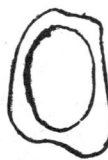

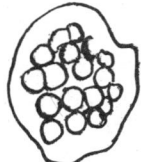

—————— 9., 10., 11., 12., Vegetable cells ——————

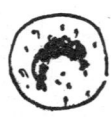

13. Leucocyte

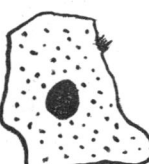

14. Squamous epithelial cells

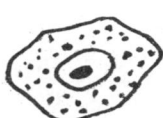

15. Epithelial cell

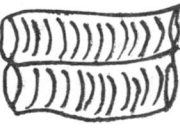

16. Muscle fibre

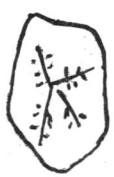

17. Corn starch

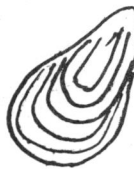

18. Potato starch

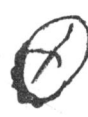

19. Rice starch

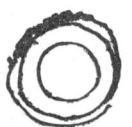

20. Oil globule

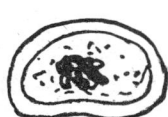
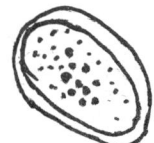
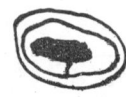
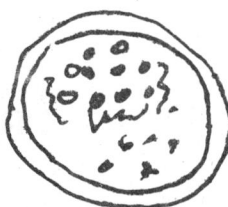

——————— 21., 22., 23., 24., Cellophene bodies ———————

Fig. 52. (1 to 24)

remnant of the yolk mass; it causes the eggs to clump together.
— The inner embryophore is brown, thick walled and radially striated (Bile stained).
— Contains an oncosphere (14 to 20 microns in diameter) with 3 pairs of hooklets.
— Does not float in saturated solution of common salt.

(vii) Schistosoma (General)

Eggs are non-operculated and when laid are fully embrynated (containing a ciliated embryo, miracidium).

S. Haematobium — 150 microns by 50 microns, terminal spine.
S. Mansoni — 150 microns by 60 microns, lateral spine.
S. Japonicum — 100 microns by 65 microns, lateral knob.

(viii) Fas-ciola hepatica/Fasciolopsis buski

— Large operculated, brownish yellow (Bile stained).
— Size 140 microns by 80 microns.
— Contains a large unsegmented ovum in a mass of yolk cells.
— Does not float in saturated salt solution.

(ix) Clonorchis sinensis

— Large operculated, brewnish yellow (Bile stained) flask shaped and operculated.
— Possesses a terminal hook like spine (Resembling an electric-bulb).
— Small in size, measuring 35 microns by 20 microns.
— When oviposited, contains a ciliated embryo (Miracidium).
— Does not float in saturated salt solution.

(x) Diphyllobothrium latum (Fig. 51)

— Oval and brown in color (Bile stained).
— Measures 70 microns by 45 microns.
— Contains abundant yolk granules and an unsegmented ovum.
— There is an inconspicuous operculum at one end with a small knob at the other end. Does not float in saturated solution of common salt.

(xi) Paragonimus westermani

— Golden brown in color (Bile stained).
— Oval in shape.
— Flattened operculca.
— Measure 80 microns by 55 microns.
— Contains an unsegmented ovum surrounded by yolk cells.

(xii) Strongyloides stercoralis

As soon as the eggs of the stronglyoides sterconalis are laid, the rhabditiform larvae start hatching and move their way out, into the lumen from where they are passed in the faeces. Hence it is the larvae, not the eggs which are found in the faeces. Two types of larvae are found.

(a) Rhabditiform larvae measure 200 to 250 microns in length by 16 microns in breadth, they have short mouth and double bulb esophagus.

(b) Filariform larvae are longer, more slender. They have short mouths and cylindrical esophagus.

SECTION III
PARASITOLOGY

CHAPTER — 13

PROTOZOA

CLASSIFICATION

Without going into details of zoological classification, a simplified classification of protozoa of medical importance has been designed mentioning the the diseases caused by them.

Organism	Disease
I. Flagellates	
1. Leishmania	Leishmaniasis or Kala Azar
2. Trypanosoma	Sleeping Sickness
3. Giardia	Giardiasis
4. Trichomonas	Vaginitis
5. Naegleria	
6. Choilomaslix	
7. Enteromonas	
II. Amoebae	
1. Entoamoeba	Amoebic dysentry
	Amoebic abscess
2. Dientamoeba	
3. Iodamoeba	
4. Hartmanella	
III. Sporozoa	
1. Plasmodium	Malaria
2. Toxoplasma	Toxoplasmosis
3. Babesia	Babesosis
4. Pneumocystis	Pneumonitis
5. Sarcocystis	
IV. Ciliates	
1. Balantidium	

Further in the text, all the organisms mentioned above have been discussed in relavant details in the order of their medical importance.

MALARIAL PARASITE

Introduction

Malaria is a very important disease for two prime reasons:
1. Nearly 15–20 million people all over the world are affected by malaria every year, especially in Africa, Asia and South America where it is an important cause of morbidity & mortality.
2. It is potentially eradicable, but is still rampant for a number of reasons. We say it is eradicable because there is i) A single

reservoir of injection — humans ii) A single vector responsible — Female anopheline mosquito

It has not been eradicated due to numerous medical and administrative problems and also the extent of disease.

Malaria is caused by genus *Plasmodium*, which is transmitted to man by female of the anopheles species of mosquito. (Details will be discussed under life cycle). Four species of plasmodium are of importance to man.
1. Plasmodium falciparum (by far the most dangerous)
2. Plasmodium vivax (by far the commonest)
3. Plasmodium malarie (rare in India).
4. Plasmodium ovale (not found on the Indian subcontinent).

Clinical importance and features (Fig. 53)

As discussed above in the life cycle, merozoites are released in the blood in cycles repeated every 48–72 hrs, depending upon the infecting species. On basis of the periodicity of these cycles, malaria has been classified into
I. Tertian — cycle is repeated after 36–48 hrs
   A. Benign — caused by plasmodium vivax
   B. Malignant — caused by plasmodium falciparum.
II. Quartan — cycle is repeated after 72 hrs caused by *P. malariae*.

Occasionally Quotidian (Cycles of 24 hrs) malaria may be seen with a double infection — some parasites maturing on days 1, 3, 5, and some on days 2, 4 & 6. Also now a days most of the cases of malaria do not follow any of the above, fixed courses. In fact it may present as irregular or even continuous features.

Typical attack of malaria

After an incubation period of 1–2 weeks depending on the infecting species, a typical attacks of malaria follows 4 labelled phases.

1. **Prodromal phase:** Characterized by nonspecific malaise and prostration accompanied by bodyaches and headache. There may be a chilly sensation . Lasts for 2–3 days.

2. **Stage of heat:** Most prominent feature of an acute malarial attack characterized by shaking chills and rigors; following which the temperature mounts steadily to reach upto as much as 40°C. (104°F) or more, Lasts for few hrs.

3. **Stage of lysis:** Characterized by profound sweating and decline of temperature to normal or even subnormal. May be accompanied by vomitting.

4. **Stage of recovery:** Patient is afebrile but is markedly prostrated. He feels extremely weak.

LIFE CYCLE OF PLASMODIUM

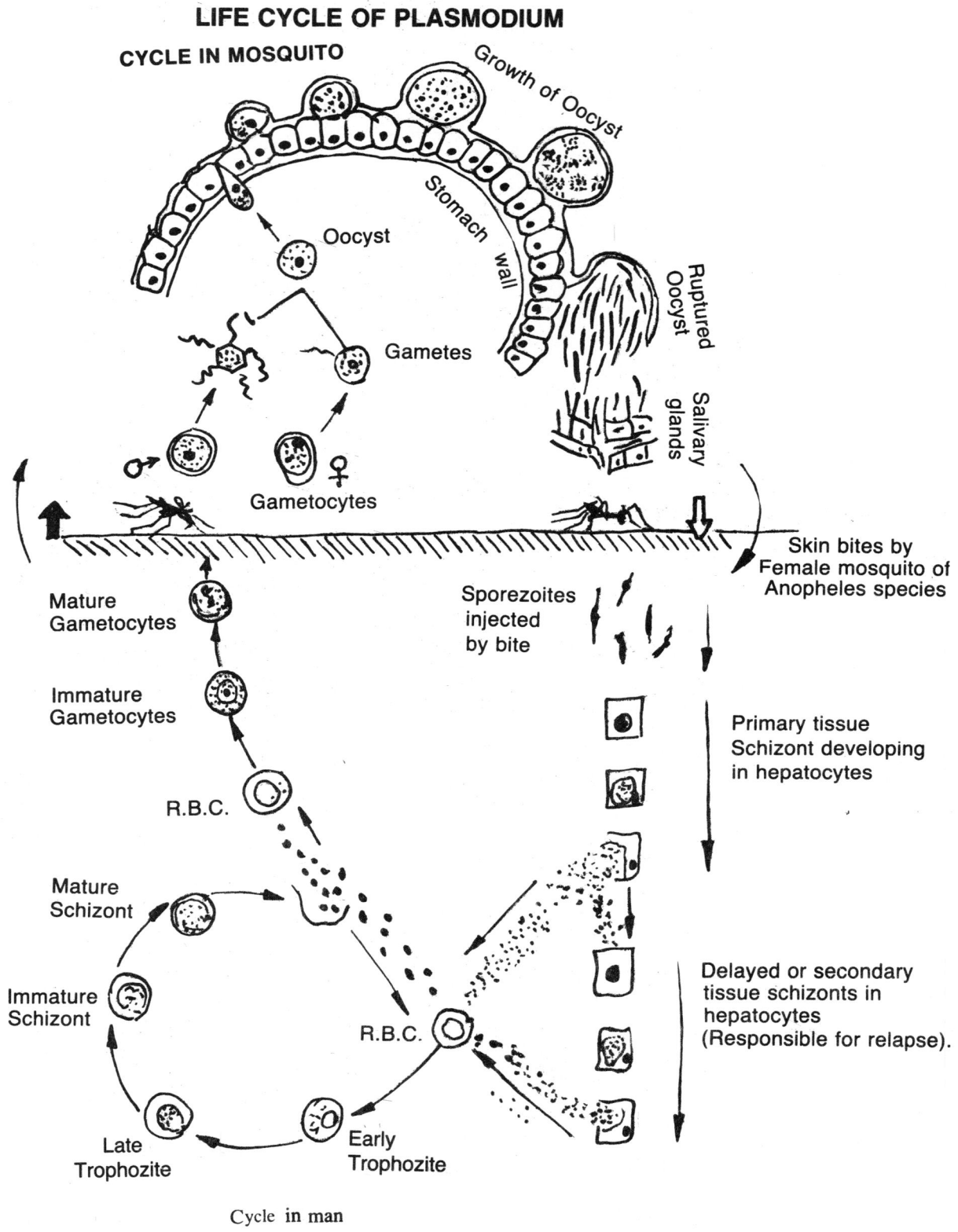

Fig. 53 Life Cycle of Plasmodium

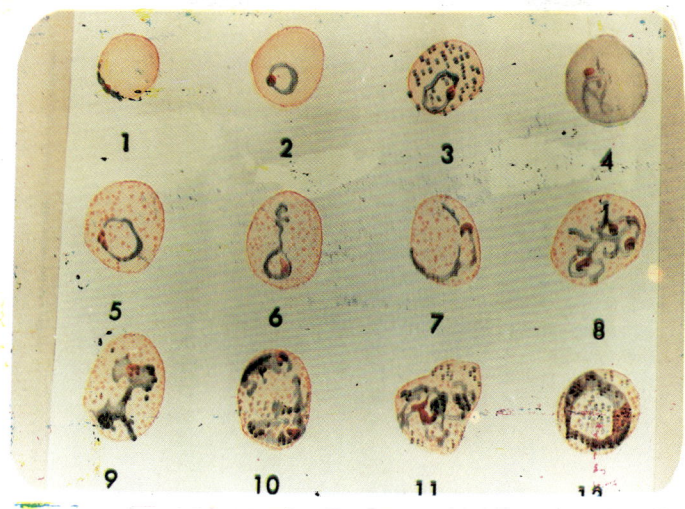

Fig. 54: Showing 1 to 12 development stages of plasmodium vivax

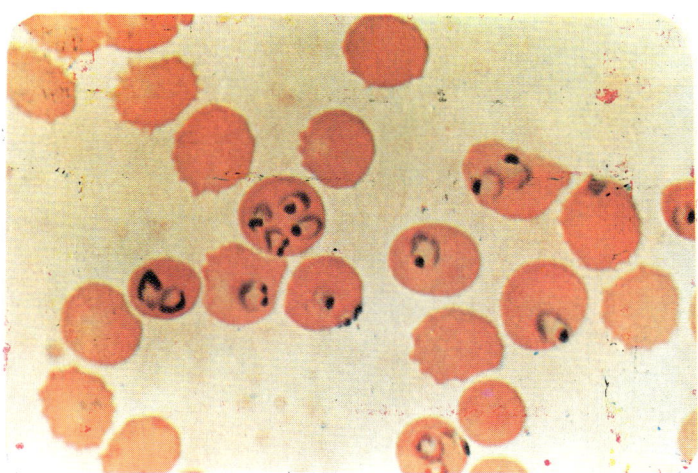

Fig. 55: Blood smear showing ring stage plasmodium falciparum

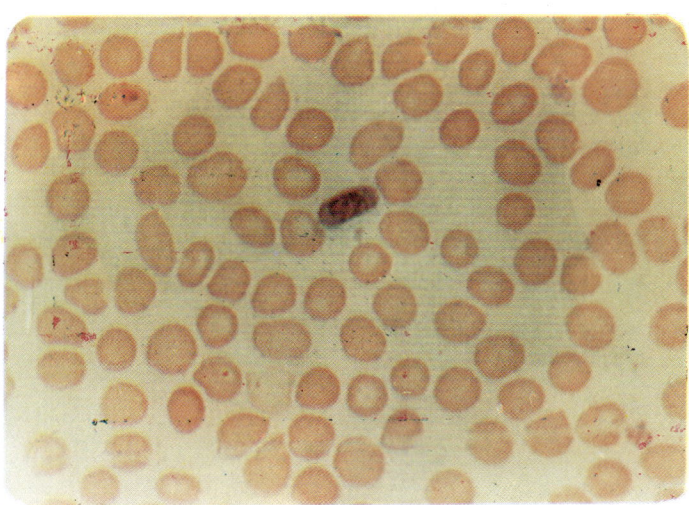

Fig. 56: Blood smear showing gametocyte (male) plasmodium falciparum

Clinical Signs

May consist inconsistantly of the following:
1. Mild to moderate pallor
2. Mild icterus
3. Fever
4. Hepato &/or splenomegaly
5. Lymphadenopathy.

Complicated Malaria

This generally occurs with plasmodium falciparum and is the fatal form of malaria, which can kill a non-immune person within no time. Here we will be discussing primarily 4 conditions.

1. **Pernicious malaria:** Pernicious malaria carries high number of parasites in the peripheral blood (1,00,000 parasites/mm$_3$). It may result in death rates of 20% or more.

2. **Cerebral malaria:** It is a severe form of pernicious malaria characterized by:
1. Hyperpyrexia (41.6°C or 107°F)
2. Infection of $\geq$ 5% erythrocytes
3. Delirium and coma which may come on very early in disease
4. Behavioural changes
5. Convulsions (epileptiform)
CSF is under pressure, with increased lymphocytes and proteins.

3. **Algid malaria:** It results from an overwhelming infection, with collapse and peripheral vascular failure, possibly resulting from acute adrenal failure. Patient is hypothermic and hypotensive and coma supervenes very fast.

4. **Blackwater fever** (Malarial haemoglobinuria): Characterized by sudden, extensive intravascular haemolysis, which results in:
1. Haemoglobinuria
2. Icterus
3. Hepatosplenomegaly
4. Epigastric pain
5. Vomiting & diarrhoea
All the 4 conditions listed above are potentially life threatening and early diagnosis and immediate treatment is absolutely indispensable.

Diagnosis of Malaria

Diagnosis depends primarily on demonstration of malarial parasite in peripheral blood. Ideally blood should be taken in the stage of heat (i.e. when patient is febrile)

Demonstration of Malarial Parasite in Blood

This consists in staining peripheral smears and identifying malarial parasite in erythrocytes. 2 types of methods are used for making blood films.

1. Thin films: These are made as any other blood smear and stained with Romanowasky stains.

2. Thick films: This has the advantage of having increased volume of blood on the slide, the probability of positive diagnosis increases. However it is difficult to identify the infecting species in thick smears.
Thick smears are prepared as follows:—
Place a good sized drop of blood on a clean slide & spread it with a glass rod until it covers an area of approximately 2 cm diameter. Ideal thick smears are ones through which newspaper print can be just read.

For staining the smears various stains are used. Some of these are:
1. Giemsa stain
2. Leishman's stain
3. Field's stain
4. J.S.B. stain
   (i) **Giemsa stain:** Fix smear by dipping it in acetone free methyl alchohol for a few seconds. Air dry and cover it for 10–20 minutes with 5% Giemsa stain. Wash with distilled water and air dry. Used both for thin and thick films.
   (ii) **Leishman's stain:** Fix smear as above. With slide on a level bench, add 7–8 drops of leishman's stain. Leave for 20 seconds. Add 12–15 drops (double the amount of stain) of

Identification of various plasmodium species (Fig. 54–56)
(Both clinical and laboratory features)

No.		P. vivax	P. malariae	P. falciparum
1.	Incubation period	12–17 days	½ to 1 month	9–14 days
2.	Exo-erythrocytic phase	+	+	−
3.	Merozoites in tissue schizont	>10,000	2000	≥40,000
4.	Erythrocytic cycle	48 hrs	72 hrs	36-48 hrs
5.	Parasitemia (no. of parasites/cu mm)	20–30,000	6000–20,000	20,000–50,000
6.	Primary attack severity	Mild to severe	Mild	Severe
7.	Relapses	+ + +	+	−
8.	Febrile paroxysm (duration — hrs)	8–12	8–10	16–36 or even more.
9.	Infected erythrocyte	larger than normal & slightly distorted Schuffner's Dots present. Infection usually single	Normal in size or smaller Ziemman's granules seen. Infection always single.	Normal in size multiple infection common Maurer's Dots seen.
10.	Trophozoite (Ring stage)	Irregular cytoplasm which scatters away chromatin bead	Regular compact deep blue cytoplasm around single bead	Not common in peripheral blood, Regular rings, broken rings & comma shapes seen.
11.	Mature schizont	12–24 merozoits, relatively large, pigment granular & clumped.	6–12 merozoites, pigment compact clump of granules.	12–24 or more merozoites, pigment a single dark mass.
12.	Gametocyte.	Round or oval, relatively large with uniform cytoplasm frayed at edges	Rounded, compact with abundant peripheral pigment in round granules	Distinct crescenteric shape with central pigment & chromatin

distilled water (pH 7.2). Leave for 20 minutes. Wash with distilled water and air dry. Used for both thin & thick films.

(iii) **Field's stain:** Field's stain consists of 2 solutions, solution 1 & 2. Used only for thick films. Immerse dried, unfixed film for 1–3 seconds in solution 1. Remove & rinse immediately for about 5 seconds in clean tap water. Immerse in solution 2 for 2 seconds. Rinse for 2–3 seconds in clean tap water. Allow to air dry.

(iv) **J.S.B. staining (Jasbir Singh-Bhattacharya stain):** It can be used for both thin and thick films JSB stain also consists of 2 solns. JSB I & II (It is a modified Romanowsky's stain). Take the smear, dip it in, JSB-I, leave for 2–3 mins. Then dip in methanol. Take out immediately. Dip in JSB-II and take out immediately. Wash it with running water and dry in air.

Basic difference between thin and thick films staining is that thin films have to be fixed before staining while there is no need to fix thick films.

2. Leishmania (Kala — Azar)

Introduation

In this section we are mainly concerned with 3 species namely
1. Leishmania donovani — causes Kala Azar
2. Leishmania tropica — causes oriental sore
3. Leishmania braziliensis — causes Espundia

Genus leishmania was created by Ross in 1903. In 1900 Sir William Leishman discovered the parasite in spleen smears of a soldier who died in Calcutta. In same year Charles Donovan found the same parasite in a spleen biopsy in Madras. The parasite has 2 forms.
1. Aflagellate or Amastigote
2. Flagellate or Promastigote

As amastigote, it exists in the reticuloendothelial system, especially spleen, liver and marrow. It may also be rarely found in peripheral blood. Promastigote forms occur in the gut of sandflies (Phlebotomus) which are responsible for the transmission of disease.

Clinical importance and features

(A) Kala Azar: Caused by L. donovani. It is a disease of the reticuloendothelial system. Vectors for kala azar are sandflies (Genus-Phlebotomus). It occurs as a result of infected sandfly bite.

Reservior of infection: Though animals of canine genus do act as reservoirs. In India, the only reservoir is man. In India the disease is primarily active in Eastern belt including Eastern U.P., Bihar, Assam, West Bengal etc.

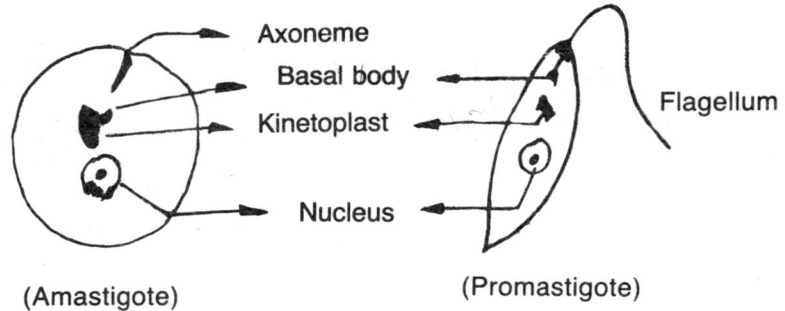

(Amastigote)   (Promastigote)

Life Cycle:

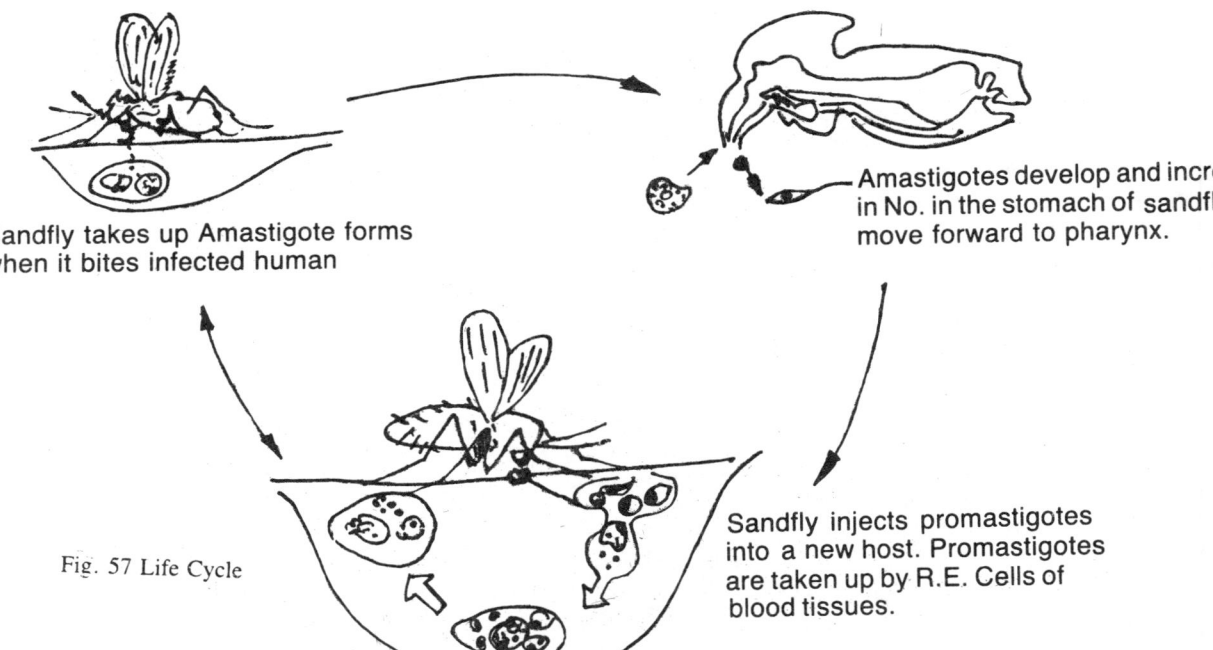

Sandfly takes up Amastigote forms when it bites infected human

Amastigotes develop and increase in No. in the stomach of sandfly and move forward to pharynx.

Fig. 57 Life Cycle

Sandfly injects promastigotes into a new host. Promastigotes are taken up by R.E. Cells of blood tissues.

Incubation Period: 2–4 months usually. Kala azar is characterized by:
1. Malaise
2. Low grade fever (occasionally fever is high grade with chills and rigors).
3. Wasting & marked emaciation
4. Anemia
5. Protrusion of abdomen
6. Edema of face and feet

Clinical signs

1. Pt. is Febrile
2. There is marked pallor, and pt. may be icteric.
3. Marked splenomegaly
4. Mild to moderate hepatomegaly
5. Lymphadenopathy may occur

Since immunity in Kala azar is markedly diminished, there is marked susceptibility to secondary infection of (1) Respiratory tract and (2) Gastro-intestinal tract.

(B) Oriental sore: Also called dermal leishmaniasis caused by Leishmania tropica Initially a small, red papule develops at the site of bite. It develops a thin crust that hides a spreading ulcer underneath. 20 or more ulcers may coalesce to form a large sore. Secondary infection may occur as

Yaws — by spirochetes
Myiasis — by maggots

If no infection occurs; the sore heals in 2 months time, leaving a depressed unpigmented scar.

(C) Espundia: It is a disease, essentially of South America and resembles oriental sore in many ways. Only difference being that espundia is characterized by secondary muco-cutaneous lesions which involve larynx, buccal cavity & lips.

Diagnosis of Kala Azar

Investigations

Direct evidence	Indirect evidence
— Peripheral blood	— Hemogram (reveals anaemia with leucopenia)
— Blood culture	
— Biopsy	— Serological tests
(i) Lymph node aspirate	1. Aldehyde test
(ii) Bone marrow (Fig. 58)	2. Complement fixation test
(iii) Liver biopsy	3. Immunoglobulin assay
(iv) Splenic puncture (surest method of diagnosis)	4. Counter immunoelectro-phoresis (CIEP)
	5. ELISA (Enzyme linked immunosorbent assay).

1. Demonstration of Amastigote Forms (Donovan Bodies) in peripheral blood.

This may practically be very difficult. Owing to small number of leishmania parasites in peripheral blood, casual examination of thin smear may often be negetive. Chances of finding L. donovani are greatly increased by adopting any one of the following procedures.
1. By making a thick film.
2. By producing a straight leucocytic edge. When a thin blood film is being drawn and before the blood is almost exhausted, spreading slide is abruptly lifted off to prevent tailing.
3. By centrifuging citrated blood. Sediment at the bottom is

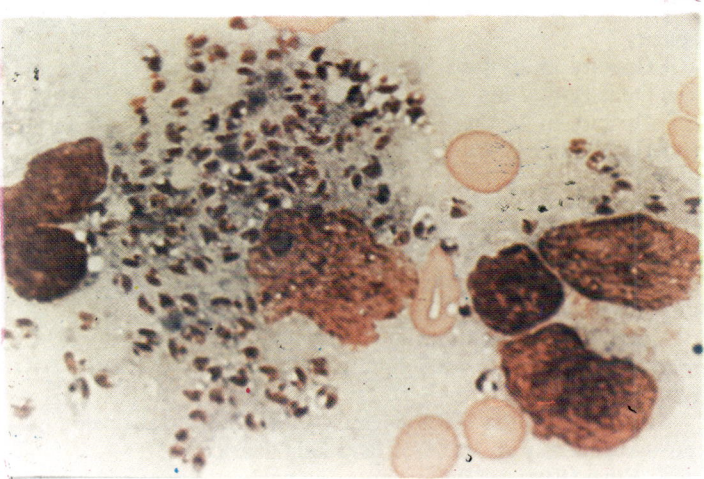

Fig. 58 Bone Marrow showing L.D. bodies

withdrawn, smeared, dried & stained with Leishman's or Giemsa's stain.

Staining procedures are same as for malarial parasite i.e. by Romanowsky stains
1. Giemsa stain
2. Leishman's stain

2. Demonstration in biopsy specimens

Biopsy specimen smears are fixed and stained. (Refer to section on histopathology).

Identification in blood & biopsies: Amastigote form appears as an ovoid or rounded body measuring 2–3 mm in length and living intracellularly in monocytes, polymorphs or endothelial cells. Cyloplasm of these stains light blue and nucleus and kinetoplast red (Fig. 59).

3. Culture of L. Donovani

Blood cutture of L. Donovani is done in the following media
1. NMN medium (Nory, Macneil, Nicolle)
2. Grace's insect tissue culture medium

1–2 ml of venous blood is mixed with 10 ml of citrated saline. Incubate at 22°C overnight. Centrifuge. Inoculate into water of condensation of N.M.N. medium. Incubate at 22–26°C for 1–4 weeks. Positive cultures may appear in 3 days or may take as long as 4–6 weeks. Promastigote forms are found in this culture.

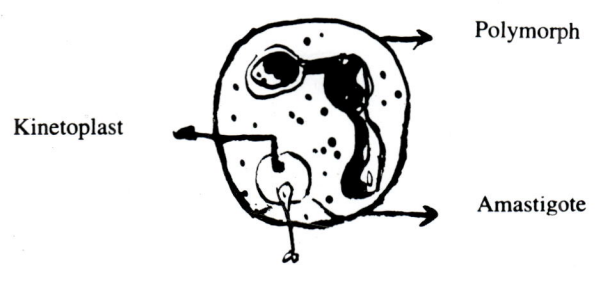

Fig. 59.

4. Serological test

1. **Aldehyde test** (Formol test): 1 drop commercial formalin solution is added to 1 ml clear serum — look for solidification and opacity.

 (i) Opacity in 20 mins $+3$
 (ii) Opacity in 2 hrs $+2$
 (iii) Opacity in 24 hrs $+1$
 (iv) No solidification $-$ve test

2. **Complement fixation test:** Antigen is prepared from Kedrowsky's acid fast bacillus. Antibodies appear during first 3 months of infection and disappear within 6 months of cure. Titres of 1/10 or more are significant. Cross reaction's occur with Chagas disease, Leprosy and T.B.

3. **Immunoglobulin assay:** Immunoglobulins, mainly IgG is markedly raised upto 4400 mg/dl. This leads to a reversal of A.G. ratio.

4. **C.I.E.P.:** It is 100% negative in non-kala-azar fevers, 80% positive in early & 100% of later kala-azar cases.

5. **Elisa (Enzyme linked immuno sorbent assay):** It is highly sensitive & more specific.

ENTAMOEBA HISTOLYTICA (AMOEBIASIS)
Introduction

Amoebiasis is an infection of the large intestine produced by Entamoeba histolytica. It is mostly asymptomatic but may cause chronic mild diarrhoea to fulminant dysentry. Among extra intestinal complications, the commonest is amoebic liver abscess. In this section, apart from entamoeba histolytica, we will also deal with certain other closely related pathogens.

Morphology

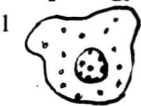 Trophozoite: 20–30μm in size, irregularly shaped, surrounded by a single layered cell membrane covered by a fuzzy layer, Cytoplasm is granular and contains a single nucleus.

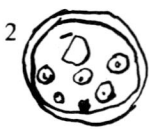 12–25μm, round in shape, cyst-wall is double in contour. It contains 2 chromatoid bars, a glycogen mass and 2–4 nuclei.

Clinical importance and features

Amoebiasis is a disease of unhealthy sanitary conditions. *Transmission* is through faeco-oral route via contaminated water, vegetables etc. Infected food handlers form a very important crosslink in transmission of disease.

Incubation period is usually 3–4 weeks. However it may be much less with a massive infection with amoebic cysts. Trophozoites are the virulent forms of entamoebae. They invade the mucosa of large intestive producing amoebic ulcers which in turn are responsible for the intestinal manifestation of the disease. In 75–80% cases ulcers are confined to rectum and sigmoid colon.

Mild amoebic diarrhoea: There is intermittent diarrhoea consisting of 1–4 foul smelling loose or watery stools daily, sometimes containing blood and mucous.

Fulminant amoebic dysentry: Onset is abrupt with high fever, between (40–40.6°C), severe abdominal cramps and profuse bloody diarrhoea with tenesmus.

On examination there is diffuse abdominal tenderness.

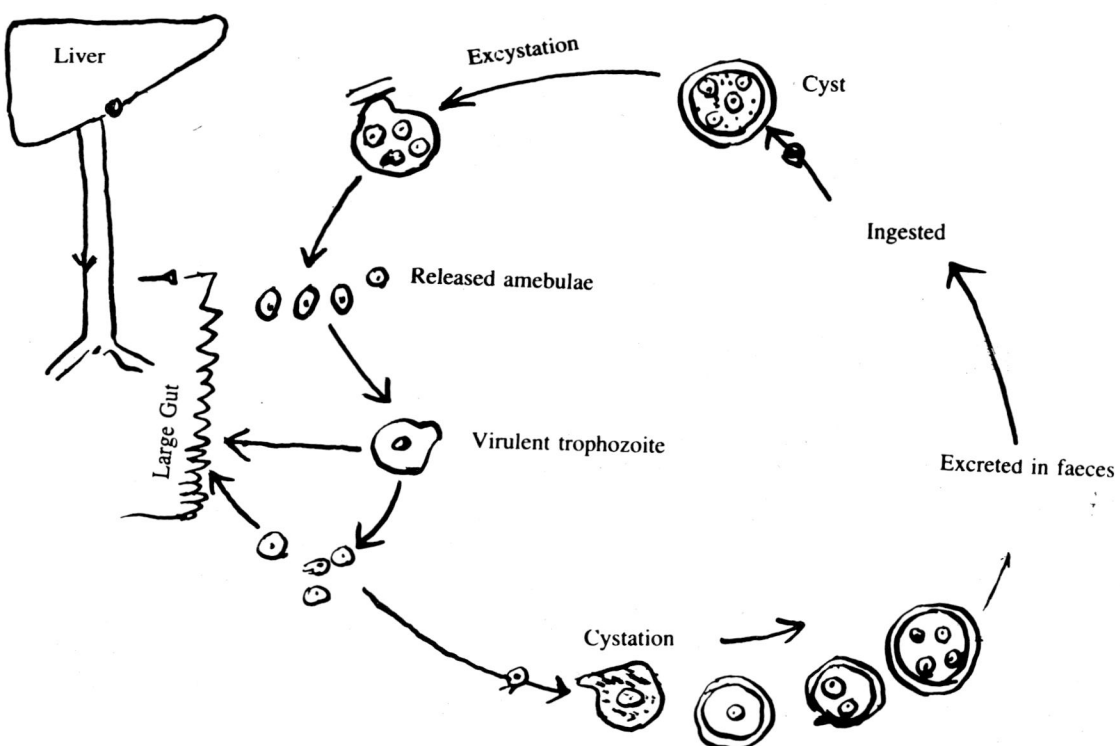

Fig: 60 Life cycle of E. histolytica

Intestinal Complications

1. Amoebic tiphlitis — amoebic infection of caecum. Characterized by pain in Rt. iliac fossa. On examination there is tenderness over caecum. It has to be distinguished from appendicitis
2. Amoebic appendicitis
3. Severe rectal haemorrhage
4. Amoeboma — A granulomatous lesion involving primarily caecum, although other parts of large intestine may also be involved.

Extraintestinal Complications

Commonest is amoebic liver abscess. It is characterized by
1. Severe pain abdomen, localized to Rt. hypochondrium
2. Vomiting
3. Fever may or may not be present.

These symptoms may or may not be accompanied by symptoms of amoebic diarrhoea. On examination there is
1. Tender hepatomegaly
2. Severe intercostal tenderness.

Table: 27. Amoebic & Bacillary (Bacterial) dysentry — A comparison

Macroscopic	Amoebic dysentry	Bacillary dysentry
1. Number of Stools/day	6–8	10
2. Amount	Copious	Small
3. Odor	Offensive	Odourless
4. Colour	Dark red	Bright red
5. Nature	Blood and mucous with faeces	Only blood and water. Mucous may be present but faecal matter is absent
6. Reaction	Acidic	Alkaline
7. Consistency	Not adherent to container	Adherent to container
Microscopic		
1. RBCs	In clumps, red to yellow in color	Discrete, bright red
2. Pus cells	Scanty	Numerous
3. Macrophages	Scanty	Abundant
4. Eosinophils	Present	Scare
5. Pyknotic bodies	Present	Nil
6. Ghost cells	Nil	Numerous
7. Parasites	Trophozoites	Nil
8. Bacteria	numerous (commensals)	Nil
9. Charcot leyden crystals	Present	Nil

Diagnosis of Amoebiasis

(1) Indentification of organism in stool

Details of the procedure have been discussed in the section on stool examination.

Collection of Faeces:

1. For the detection of trophozoites, collect fresh faecal sample and examine within 1 hr of collection.

2. For detection of cysts, stool is collected and placed in 10% formalin, and sent for examination.

Examinaiton of Faeces:

1. Place a drop of normal saline on one end of the slide and drop of iodine (2%) on the other end.
2. Pick up a very small portion of faeces with the help of a wooden applicator stick and emulsify in each solution seperately.
3. Seal the preparation with a coverslip and examine.

Concentration Techniques

Used to increase the possiblity of detection of the cysts in the stool sample. Various techniques used are basically of 2 types:
(a) Floatation procedures e.g. Concentrated saline floatation and
(b) Sedimentation procedure e.g. Formol-ether concentration.

(A) Concentrated Saline Floatation

1. Take a vial 1″ diameter and 2–2½″ long of 20 ml capacity.
2. Fill up one fourth with saline solution (saturated NaCl solution of sp. gr.1020).
3. Add faeces of size of a small marble and mix thoroughly. Fill upto brim with solution and superimpose a grease free 3″ × 2″ slide over it so that its under surface remains in contact with the suspension.
4. Invert the slide without allowing the drop to slide off and examine under microscope without a coverslip.

(b) Formal Ether Concentration

1. Take stool sample of the size of a marble in a mortar. Mix and suspend in about 10 cc of distilled water.
2. Strain the suspension through a funnel having gauze of 40 meshes inch^2 and centrifuge at 2500 r p m for 2 mins. Decant supernatant.
3. Add 7 ml of 10% formalin (buffered) to the sediment. Make a suspension by thorough mixing. Add 3 ml of ether, stopper the tube with a rubber stopper, shake vigorously in an inverted position for 30 seconds.
4. Remove stopper. Centrifuge at 2500 rpm for 1–2 minutes, when 4 layers are formed.
5. Carefully pour the 3 layers leaving the sediment undisturbed. Examine preparations of the sediment.

Morphological characteristics under microscope: It is very important to know that Entamoeba histolytica in the stool has to be distinguished from Entamoeba coli which is a normal commensal.

(2) Serological tests

Especially useful for extraintestinal complications of amoebiasis
1. Indirect haemagglutination
2. Indirect immunoflorescence
3. CIEP
4. Agar gel diffusion

4. GIARDIA

Introduction

Giardia is an organism that is cosmopolitan in distribution, but is most common in warm climates. Children are particularly susceptible. Giardia lamblia (intestinalis) resides in the duodenum and upper jejunum. It may or may not cause, symptomatic infection.

Table 28: *E. Histolytica & E. Coli — A comparison*

Morphology	E. histolytica	E. coli
Trophozoite		
1. Fresh (Unstained)		
Size	20–30 μm	20–40 μm
Motility	Actively motile	sluggish
Nucleus	Not visible	Visible
Cytoplasm	contains RBCs, tissue debris, bacteria etc.	RBCs never present
2. Iodine stained	Nucleus shows central karyosome, fine chromatin granules line the nuclear membrane	Econcentric karyosome
Cyst		
1. Iodine stained		
Size	6–15 μm	15–20 μm
Nucleus	1–4, central karyosome	1–8 eccentric karyosome with square or pointed ends

Morphology

Trophozoite —
14μm × 7μm size
Rounded at anterior end and narrow, pointed posterior end. Organism is dorsoventrally flattened with dorsal surface convex. Ventral surface bears a bilobed adhesive disk. A pair of dark colored median bodies behind the disks. There are 4 pairs of flagellae.

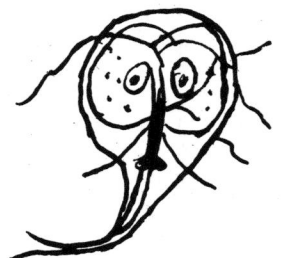

Fig. 61 Trophozoite

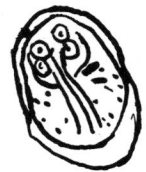

Fig. 62 Cyst

Cyst
12μm × 7μm size
Oval in shape, diagonal lie what are called false axostyles, four nuclei are distributed about these axostyles.

Life cycle

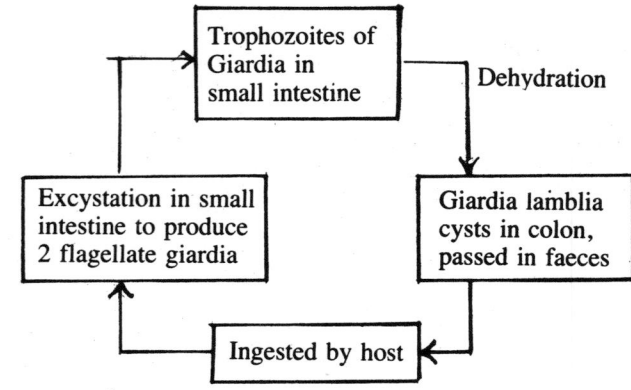

Clinical features importance

Most of the persons who harbour giardia remain asymptomatic. People who become symptomatic have varied symptoms as:
1. Vague abdominal pain
2. Diarrhoea
3. Flatulence
4. Weight loss
5. Anorexia

Diagnosis

Stool is examined as discussed earlier. Trophozoites are not usually seen in the stool. Usually only cysts are seen.

5. TRICHOMONAS

Introduction

There are 3 main species of trichomonas
1. Trichomonas vaginalis
2. Trichomonas tenax
3. Trichomonas hominis
Trichomonas vaginalis is one of the normal flora of vagina and urethra in females and prostate, seminal vesicles and urethra in males.
Trichomonas tenax is a normal commensal of oral cavity and found primarily in tartar and pyrrhoeic sockets. In females, trichomonas vaginalis causes severe vaginitis which will be discussed later.

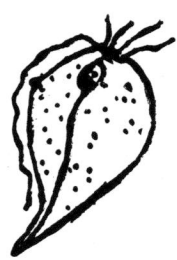

Fig. 63. Trophozoite

Morphology

1. It is 7–32 μm long and 5–15 μm wide.
2. It is oblong in shape.
3. It has 4 free anterior flagellae.
4. A fifth flagella curves back along the margin of undulating membrane & ending posterior to midline. Undulating membrane contains an extra filament.
5. A Basal body or kinetome is present anteriorly
6. A tube like axostyle extends from kinetome posteriorly to protrude from post end.
   It is a freely motile organism

Clinical features and importance

It is the cause of vaginitis in females.

It is transmitted during sexual intercourse and also by infected linen.

It causes severe itching and a copious white discharge (Acidity of vagina discourages infection but once established, it causes a shift towards alkalinity).

Diagnosis

A drop of the vaginal secretion is placed on a 3″ × 1″ glass slide. 2 drops of methylene blue are added and examined under microscope. Highly motile organisms are seen.

CHAPTER 14

HELMINTHOLOGY-I NEMATODES

CLASSIFICATION OF NEMATODES

Nematodes

Intestinal

1. Caecum & Appendix
(a) Enterobius vermicularis (pinworm)
(b) Trichuris trichuria (whipworm)

2. Small Intestine
(a) Ascaris lumbricoides (round worm)
(b) Ankylostoma duodenale (Hook-worm)
(c) Necator americanus

(d) Strongyloides stercoralis

(e) Trichinella spiralis

Somatic or Tissue

1. Lymphatic system
(a) Wuchereria bancrofti

(b) Brugia malaysi (Filariasis)

2. Subcutaneous tissue
(a) Loa Loa

(b) Onchocerca volvolus

(c) Dracunculus medinensis (guinea worm)

3. Lungs
(a) Strongyloides stercoralis

4. Mesentery
(a) Diapetalonema perstans
(b) Manzonella Ozzardi

(f) Capillaria phillipensis

5. Conjunctiva
(a) Loa Loa

6. Skeletal Msl
(a) Trichinella spiralis

In the subsequent discussion we will limit overselves to the important nematodes of the Indian subcontinent.

1. ENTERO-BIUS VERMICULARIS (PINWORMS)

Geographical distribution

It has a cosmopolitan distribution with a special affinity for temperate zones, affecting at least 500 million people in the world.

Habitat

Illeocaecal region of human intestine.

Morphology

These worms are 3–13 mm long and slender. Females are longer than the males. Both are white in color. Life span is 2–3 weeks.

Life Cycle (Pin worms)

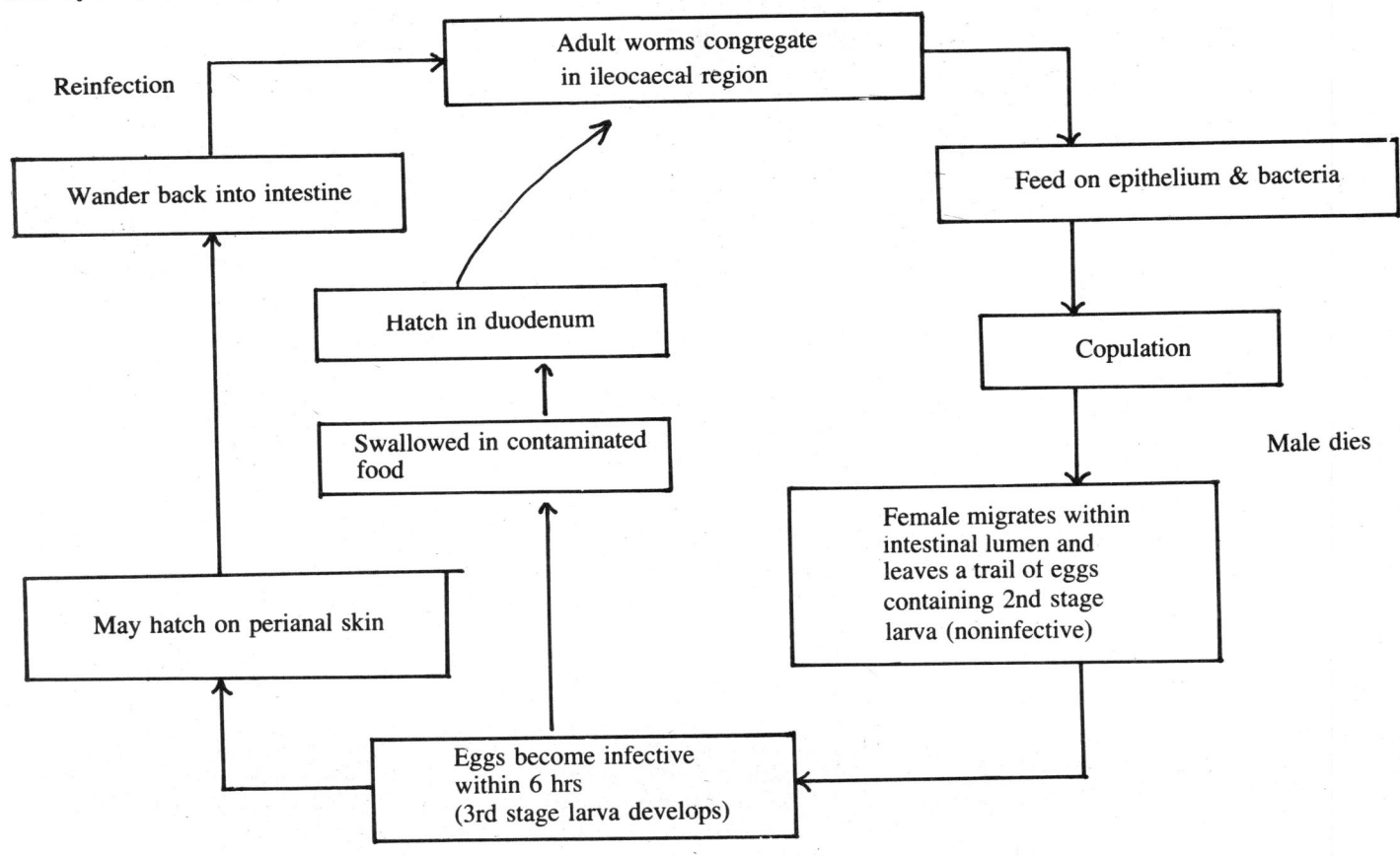

Clinical importance

Modes of infection are
1. Eating contaminated food
2. Contamination through food handlers who may be carriers of pinworms
3. Reinfection

Infection may be totally asymptomatic or cause one of the following symptoms.
1. Perianal pruritus and pain
2. Vulvo-vaginal irritation
3. Anorexia
4. Restlessness
5. Insomnia & nightmares

Diagnosis

(a) Detection of adult worms

1. Faecal examination (gross)
2. Perianal examination early in the morning
3. Discovery by patients in stool.
4. Enema

(b) Detection of eggs
(more commonly used)
1. Faecal examination
2. Perianal swab

Perianal swab:

It is the surest method of diagnosing enterobius infection. Eggs are often left behind in the perianal folds.

Swab used consists of a cellophane tape held against a wooden applicator. Early in the morning before bathing, sticky side of the swab against anoperianal junction, reversed and stuck to a microslide. Add a drop of xylene which clears away the glue.

Diagnosis depends on identification of typical eggs.
1. Nonbile stained (white colored).
2. Floats in saturated solution of saline
3. A transparent shell
4. Planoconvex in shape
5. 50–60 μm × 30 μm
6. A coiled larva is present within the egg.

2. TRICHURIS TRICHURIA (WHIPWORM)

Distribution

It is worldwide in distribution, being more common in warm, moist climates.

Habitat

Ileocaecal region of human intestines.

Morphology

They are about 30–50 mm long with males being shorter than females. A whipworm is slender, thread like throughout but abruptly becomes thick at the posterior end (reminiscent of a whip).

Life Cycle (Whip worm)

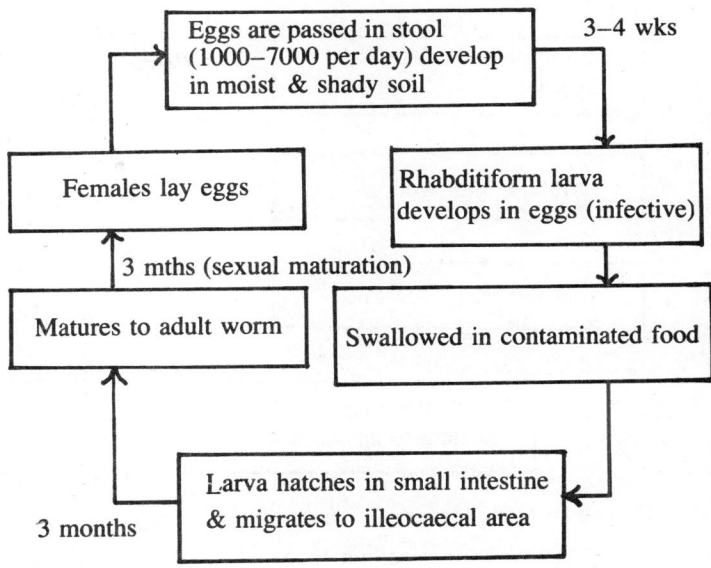

Clinical importance

Vast majority of infections are mild and cause no symptoms. In heavy infections, a patient may show
1. Wasting
2. Diarrhoea with tenesmus
3. Blood streaked stools
4. Anaemia
5. Abdominal pain & flatulence

Hyperinfection is indicated by 30,000 eggs/gm of faeces.

Diagnosis

Specific diagnosis depends on demonstrating characteristic eggs in the stool.
1. Bile stained
2. Float in saturated soution of saline
3. 50 μm × 25 μm in size
4. Barrel shaped with a mucus plug at each pole
5. Contains an unsegmented ovum.

3. ASCARIS LUMBRICOIDES (ROUND WORM)

Geographical distribution

It is most common in the tropics, though the distribution is worldwide. two populations of ascaris lumbricoides exist, one in human and one in pigs, both show a strong host specificity.

Habitat

Jejunum of man.

Morphology

Adult worms are 15–45 cm long 2–6 mm wide with females slightly longer and wider than males. Posterior ends are curved ventrally. Both sexes are brownish pink in color.

Life Cycle (Round worm)

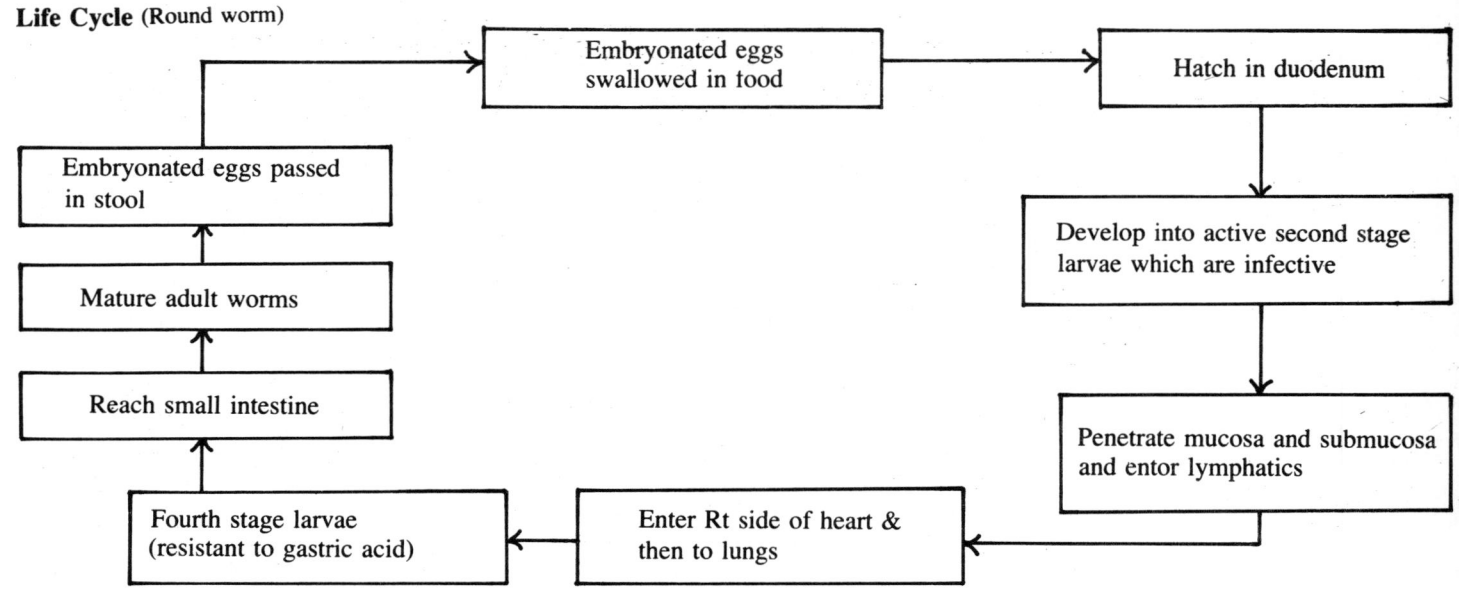

```
Embryonated eggs          →    Embryonated eggs          →    Hatch in duodenum
passed in stool                swallowed in food                    ↓
    ↑                                                        Develop into active second stage
Mature adult worms                                           larvae which are infective
    ↑                                                                ↓
Reach small intestine                                        Penetrate mucosa and submucosa
    ↑                                                        and entor lymphatics
Fourth stage larvae       ←    Enter Rt side of heart &   ←
(resistant to gastric acid)    then to lungs
```

Clinical importance

1. **Of larvae:** On reaching lung, when larvae break into the alveolar space and cause minute haemorrhages, larvae may cause.
   1. Mild chest pain
   2. Dry cough
   3. Mild rusting of sputum
   4. Breathlessness on exertion
   Superimposed bacterial infection may occur. Investigation may reveal eosinophilia

2. **Of adult worms:** May cause a variety of symptom complexes in small intestine
   (a) Malnutrition and under-development in children
   (b) Abdominal pain which may be colicky
   (c) Sensitization phenomena including
       1. Skin raskes
       2. Eye pain
       3. Breasthlessness
       4. Insomnia & restlessness
   (d) Fatal intestinal obstruction.
       Wandering worms may lead to
       1. Clogging of appendix, leading to appendicitis
       2. Anal irritation
       3. Obstructive jaundice by blockage of bile ducts
4. Nausea & vomiting on entering stomach where gastric acidity irritates them.
   5. Sudden consternation as a result of exit through nose & mouth.
   6. Extensive damage of eustachian tubes & middle ear.

Diagnosis

Direct		Indirect
Finding of adult worm	Finding of eggs	
1. In stool (by gross examination)	1. In Stool	1. Blood eosinophilia
2. In vomit	2. In duodenal aspitate (eggs may be fertilized, unfertilized or decorticated)	2. Scratch test with powdered ascaris antigen
3. X-Ray after Barium meal followthrough		

Characteristics of voa:
1. Bile stained
2. Floats in saturated saline
3. 70 μm × 45 μm
4. Thick outer shell surrounded by an albuminous coat thrown into mamillations.
5. A large unsegmented ovum containing yolk granules
6. A clear crescentric space at each end
Unfertilized egg is narrower, longer with an inconspicuous ovum and it settles down in saturated saline.

4. HOOK WORM

Two main species of hookworm known to cause infection are:
1. Ankylostoma doudenale
2. Necator americanus

Geographical distribution

Ankylostoma duodenale is abundant in Southern Europe, North Africa, India, China & S.E. Asia and in small scattered areas of United States, Carribean Islands & South America. Nector americanus is more abundant than *A. duodenale*. It was first discovered in Brazil, then Texas. Now it is indigenous in Africa, India, S.E. Asia, China & S.W. Pacific Islands.

Habitat

Small intestine of human being.

Morphology

Characteristic	A. duodenale	N. americanus
1. Size	8–13 mm long thicker (stouter)	7–11 mm long slender
2. Anterior end	Bends in direction of body curvature	Bends opposite to the body curvature
3. Buccal capsule	6 teeth, 4 hooklike on ventral surface & 2 knoblike on dorsal surface	4 chitinous plates, 2 ventral & 2 dorsal. A pair of subventral & subdorsal teeth.
4. Posterior end of female	A spine is present	No spine is present.

Life Cycle (Hook worm)

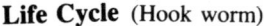

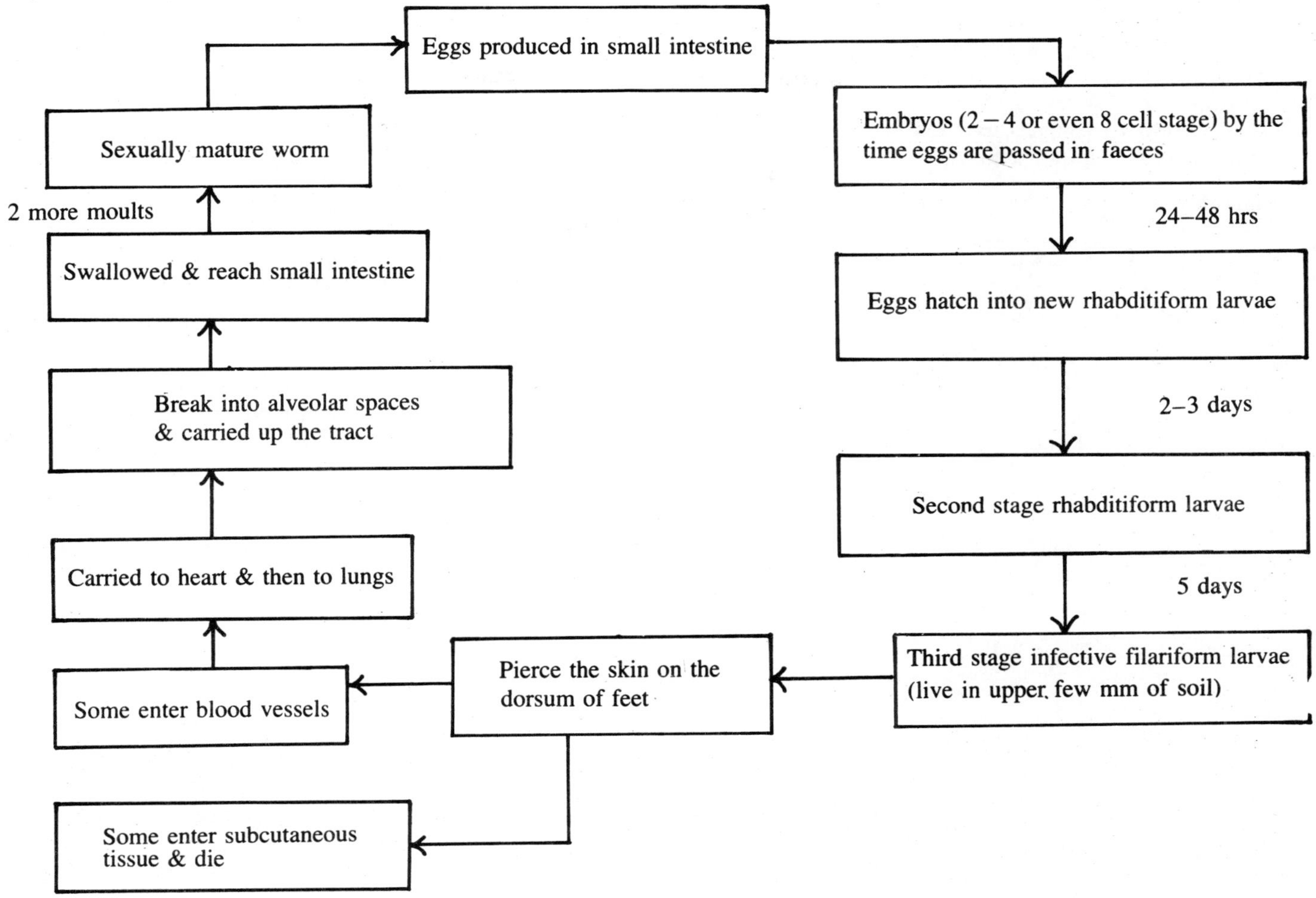

```
                          ┌─────────────────────────────┐
              ┌──────────→│ Eggs produced in small      │──────────────┐
              │           │ intestine                    │              │
              │           └─────────────────────────────┘              ↓
    ┌─────────────────────┐                        ┌─────────────────────────────────────┐
    │ Sexually mature worm│                        │ Embryos (2 – 4 or even 8 cell stage) │
    └─────────────────────┘                        │ by the time eggs are passed in faeces│
 2 more moults    ↑                                └─────────────────────────────────────┘
    ┌─────────────────────────┐                              │  24–48 hrs
    │ Swallowed & reach small │                              ↓
    │ intestine               │           ┌─────────────────────────────────────┐
    └─────────────────────────┘           │ Eggs hatch into new rhabditiform     │
              ↑                            │ larvae                               │
    ┌─────────────────────────┐           └─────────────────────────────────────┘
    │ Break into alveolar     │                              │  2–3 days
    │ spaces & carried up the │                              ↓
    │ tract                   │           ┌─────────────────────────────────────┐
    └─────────────────────────┘           │ Second stage rhabditiform larvae     │
              ↑                            └─────────────────────────────────────┘
    ┌─────────────────────────┐                              │  5 days
    │ Carried to heart & then │                              ↓
    │ to lungs                │  ┌──────────────────┐  ┌─────────────────────────────┐
    └─────────────────────────┘  │ Pierce the skin  │←─│ Third stage infective       │
              ↑                   │ on the dorsum of │  │ filariform larvae (live in  │
    ┌─────────────────────────┐  │ feet             │  │ upper few mm of soil)       │
    │ Some enter blood vessels│←─└──────────────────┘  └─────────────────────────────┘
    └─────────────────────────┘        │
    ┌─────────────────────────┐        │
    │ Some enter subcutaneous │←───────┘
    │ tissue & die            │
    └─────────────────────────┘
```

Clinical importance

Whether hookworm infestation, manifests as hookworm disease depends on 3 factors.

No. of worms present –	A. duodenale	N. americanus
5	Asymptomatic	
25	Mild symptoms	asymptomatic
25–100	Moderate symptoms	Mild symptoms
100–500		Moderate symptoms
100–1000	Severe symptoms	Severe symptoms
1000	Fatal	Fatal

Thus A. duodenale infection is in general more severe in comparison to N. americanus infection. This is because while one N. americanus sucks 0.03 ml blood/day; one A. duodenale sucks 0.15 ml blood/day i.e. 5 times more.

A. Symptoms during cutaneous phase

This phase is symptomatic only if there is secondary bacterial infection; when urticarial rash result in GROUND ITCH. One thing that must be discussed here is:

Cutaneous larva migrans or Creeping eruption: It is caused when animal invading strains or species of hookworm invade human beings (caused by A. braziliense & A. connum). After penetrating the superficial layers, they are incapable of penetrating stratum germinatum. So they begin an aimless wondering leaving a red, itchy, scaly wound that usually gets infected.

B. Symptoms during pulmonary phase:

It is usually asymptomatic, though there may be some amount of dry cough and sore throat.

C. Intestinal phase:

It is the most important clinical phase because juvenile after attaching themselves to intestinal mucosa, begin to feed on blood Upto 200 ml of blood may be lost daily in severe infections.

I. A moderate infection manifest as

1. Iron deficiency anaemia
2. Slight, intermittent abdominal pain
3. Loss of normal appetite
4. Desire to eat soil

II. Additional symptoms of heavy infection are

1. Dry skin & hair
2. Edema & potbelly in children (due to protein deficiency).
3. Mental dullness
4. Even heart failure

Hook Worm Anaemia is usually a microcytic hypochromic anaemia, severity depending on worm load & dietary iron intake.

Diagnosis

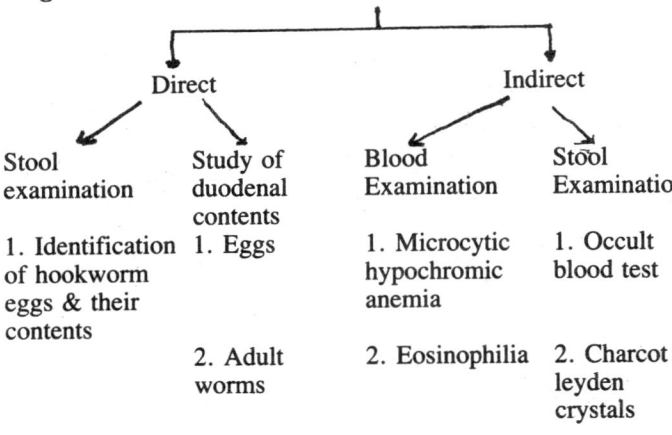

Direct
- Stool examination
  1. Identification of hookworm eggs & their contents
- Study of duodenal contents
  1. Eggs
  2. Adult worms

Indirect
- Blood Examination
  1. Microcytic hypochromic anemia
  2. Eosinophilia
- Stool Examination
  1. Occult blood test
  2. Charcot leyden crystals

Specific diagnosis depends on
1. Identification of worms
2. Identification of eggs

Characteristics of ovum:
1. Not bile stained.
2. Float in saturated saline.
3. Elliptical in shape.
4. 65–70μm × 35–40μm.
5. transparent hyaline shell membrane.
6. A 4 celled segmented ovum with a peculiar clear space between ovum & shell membrane

(Eggs of both A. duodenale & N. amerticanus are similar)

5. STRONGYLOIDES STERCORALIS

It is a curious organism capable of free living as well as living as a parasite. It has a worldwide distribution in the tropics & temperate climates. Free living forms exist mostly in the moist tropics. They are not common in India.

Morphology

Females are about 2 mm long & males about 0.7 mm in length brownish pink in color. They possess a cylindrical esophagus. Free living adults have a rhabditiform esophagus.

Life Cycle

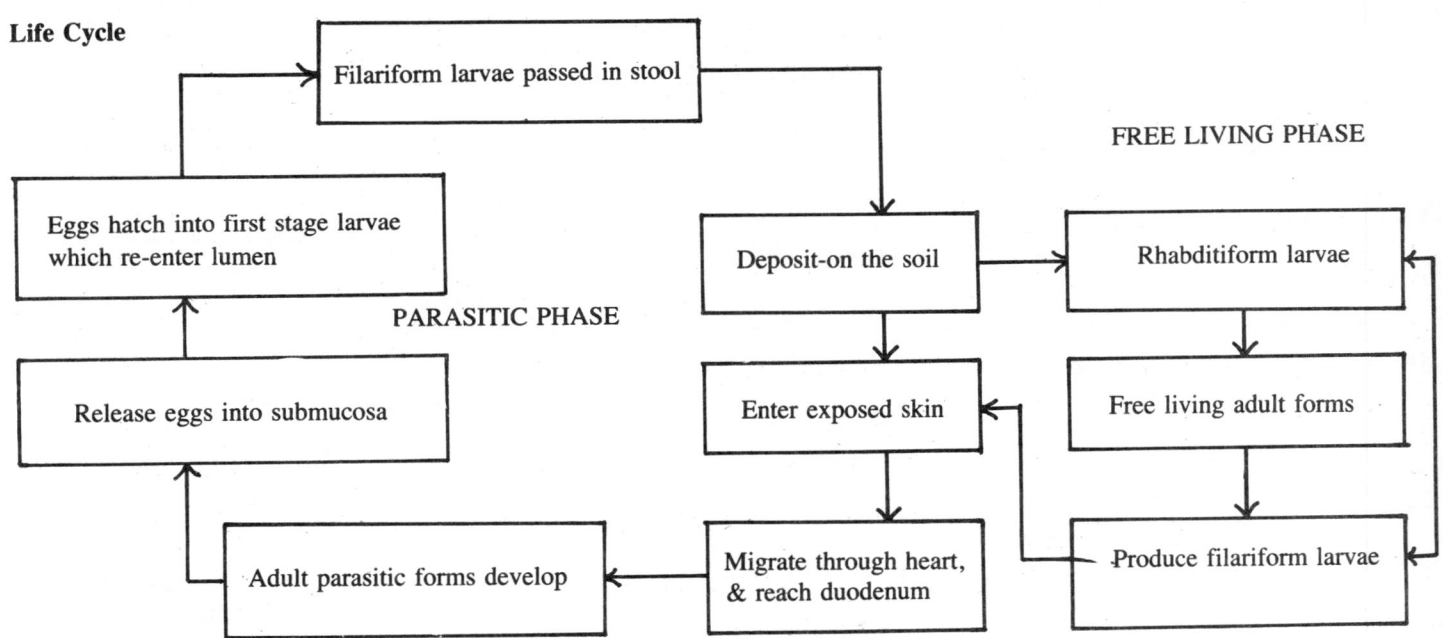

Clinical importance

Clinical manifestations of strongyloideasis are
1. Watery mucous diarrhoea (occasionally alternating with constipation)
2. Fat malabsorption cause steatorrhoea
3. Vit B_{12} deficiency
4. Eosinophilia with cough & dyspnoea
5. Skin rashes etc.

Diagnosis

Best means of diagnosis is demonstration of filariform larvae in fresh stools.

Larvae are 490–630μm long & 9μm in breadth and possess a cylindrical esophagus.

6. FILARIA

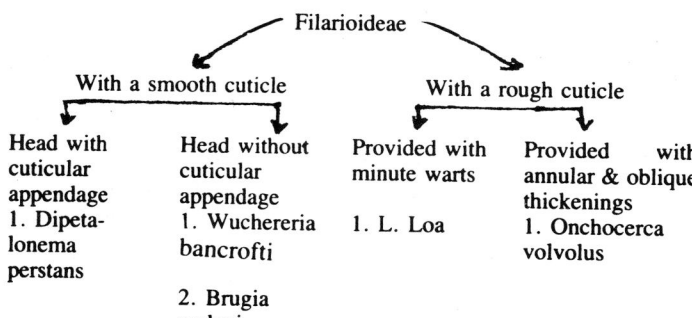

These different filaria are responsible for different disease complexes.

Wuchereria bancrofti Lymphatic filariasis (endemic in India)
Brugia malayi

Onchocerca volvulus Subcutaneous & optic infections causing river blindness (not found in India)

Dipetalonema perstans — causes illness similar to the first two but is found only in Africa & S. America

Loa Loa — causes conjunctival & corneal infection (not found in India)

Therefore we will limit our discussion to Wuchereria bankrofti and Brugia malayi.

1. Bankroftian filariasis is widespread in the world, particularly in Asia, Africa, & parts of S. America. In India, it is endemic along sea coasts and the big river systems.
2. Brugia malayi is indigenous primarily in Asia. In India it has been seen in Kerala, Orissa, Madhaya Pradesh & Assam.

Habitat

Adult worm — lymphatic system
Microfilariae — In blood

Morphology

Here we will discuss the morphology of adult worms. That of microfilaria will be discussed under the diagnosis of filariasis.

Feature	W. bancrofti	B. malayi
1. Size	Female 60–100 mm long Male 40 mm long (About 250–300 μm wide) (Both the species are cuticular)	Half the size of W. bancrofti
2. Papillae	2 circles of well defined post anal papillae	3–4 pairs of post-anal papillae.

The tail of both worms is finger like and curved ventrally. Differences are more pronounced in the microfilaria.

Life Cycle

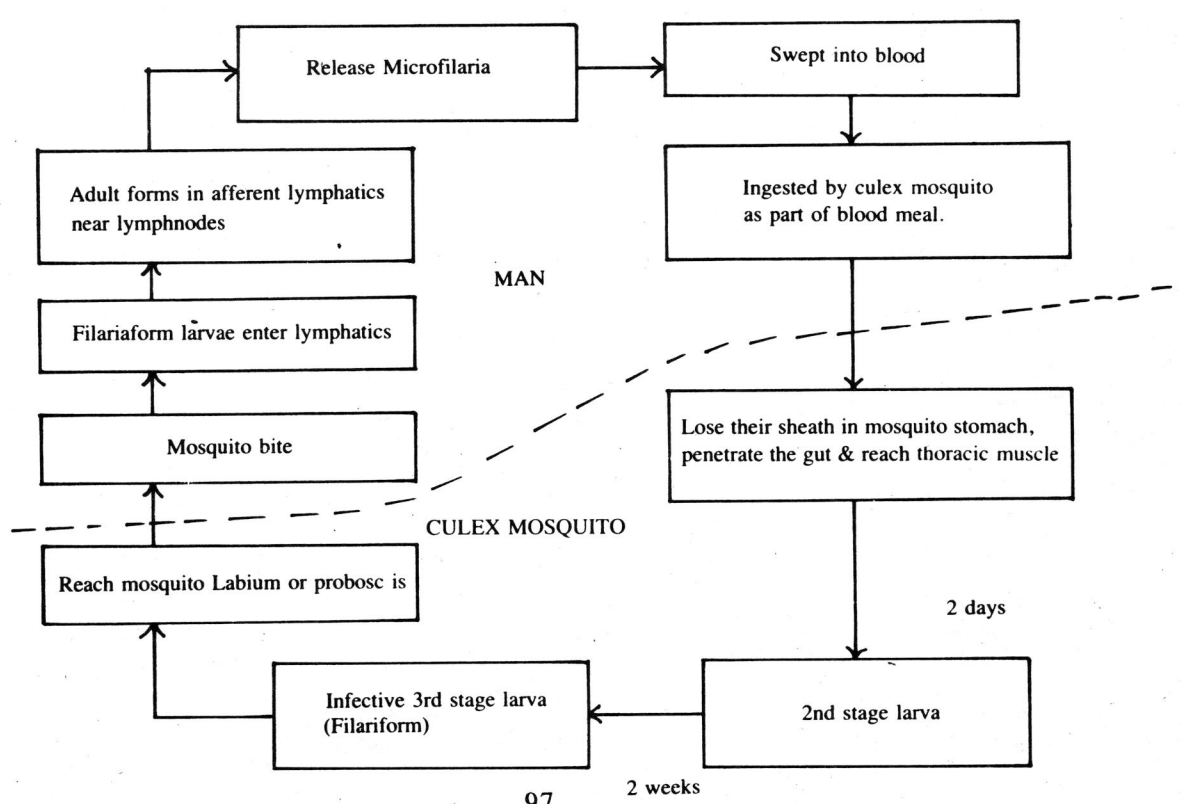

There is a marked periodicity of microfilariae in peripheral blood, that is they are seen at certain times & at other times they virtually disappear from circulation. Maximum number are found between 10 p.m. & 2 a.m.

Clinical Importance

1. Incubation Phase: Period between infection and appearance of microfilariae (mf) in the blood. It is largely asymptomatic but there may be
1. Mild fever &
2. Malaise.

2. Acute Phase: This starts when females reach maturity and start releasing microfilaria. There is intense inflammation, usually in the lower half of the body, symptoms include:
1. Chills especially at midnight
2. Fever with midnight rise
3. Tender, inflamed inguinal lymphnodes
4. There may be orchitis (testicular inflammation)
5. Epididymitis.
   Acute febrile episode of elephantoid fever recur frequently
1. Sudden onset of rigors
2. Fever (upto 104°F)
3. Sweating & lysis of fever
   It recurs periodically after few days.

3. Obstructive Phase: It is caused by obstruction of lymphatics by adult worms and are marked by chronic inflammatory reaction. It is characterized by
1. Lymphvarices
2. Chyluria
3. Hydrocele
4. Elephantiasis involving primarily scrotum and lower limbs.

Diagnosis

(a) Direct   (b) Indirect

Microfilaria detected in	Adult worms	Indirect
1. Peripheral blood	1. Lymph node biopsy	1. Eosinophilia
2. Cylous urine	2. Calcified worms by radiographs	(2) Intradermal test
3. Exudate of lymph Varix		3. Complement fixation test
4. Hydro cele fluid		

Detecting Microfilaria in blood:

Can be detected by many techniques (Fig. 64).
1. Peripheral smears taken preferably between 10 p.m. & 2 a.m. and stained with Romanowsky stains.
2. Put 0.25 ml. of fresh blood in 0.5 ml of 3% acetic acid. Then smears are made. In these preparations, microfilaria appear as transparent fibrils.
   Characteristics as seen by Romanowsky stains

	Microfilaria malayi	Mf. bancrofti
General	Minor angulations besides 4–5 major curves.	Shows 3–4 major curves with a graceful appearance.
Nucleus	Blurred and intermingled	Well defined & spaced. Quite discrete

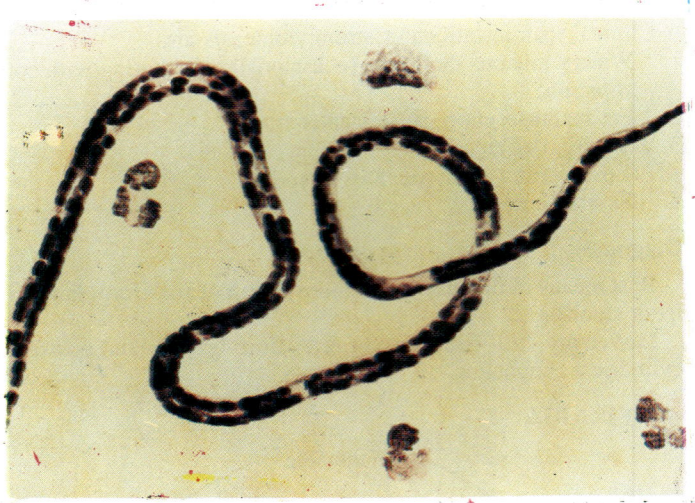

Fig. 64 Microfilaria in peripharal blood smear

Tail	Tapers to a fine point contains nuclei	Terminal portion devoid of nuclei
Cephalic space	Twice as long as broad	As long as broad
Sheath	Well stained	Hardly visible

Diethylcarbamazine Provocative test

Nocturnally periodic microfilariae may be demonstrated in the blood at any time of the day by giving 100 mg diethylcarbomazine & taking blood 45 minutes later.

(Administration of 4–6 mg/kg with examination at 30–60 mins for W. bancrofti 90 mins for B. malayi. It is of no use in sub-periodic filariasis).

7. DRACUNCULUS MEDINENSIS (GUINEA WORM)

Geographical distribution

It is widespread in India; Pakistan; Burma; S. Arabia; Iraq; Iran; East U.S.S.R.; West & Central Africa, West Indies and South America.

In India it is limited to Punjab, Rajasthan, Madhya Pradesh, Gujarat, Maharashtra & parts of South India.

Habitat

Subcutaneous tissue of especially extremities

Morphology.

It is one of the largest known nematodes.

Adult females are upto 80 cm long, males are only 1.2–4 cm long (only females are important from clinical standpoint since males die immediately after copulation). Female worm is of the thickness of a knitting needle. Body is cylindrical, white and smooth. Tail is pointed, forming a blunt hook. Head is rounded, terminating in a thickened cuticle cap or cephalic shield Mouth is triangular, small & surrounded by 6 papillae & an outer circle of 4 double papillae. Whole worms occupied by a double uterus filled with empryos.

Embryos

Measures 500–750 × 17μm. It is flattened, with a long, slender tail and a rounded head.

Life Cycle (Guinea worm)

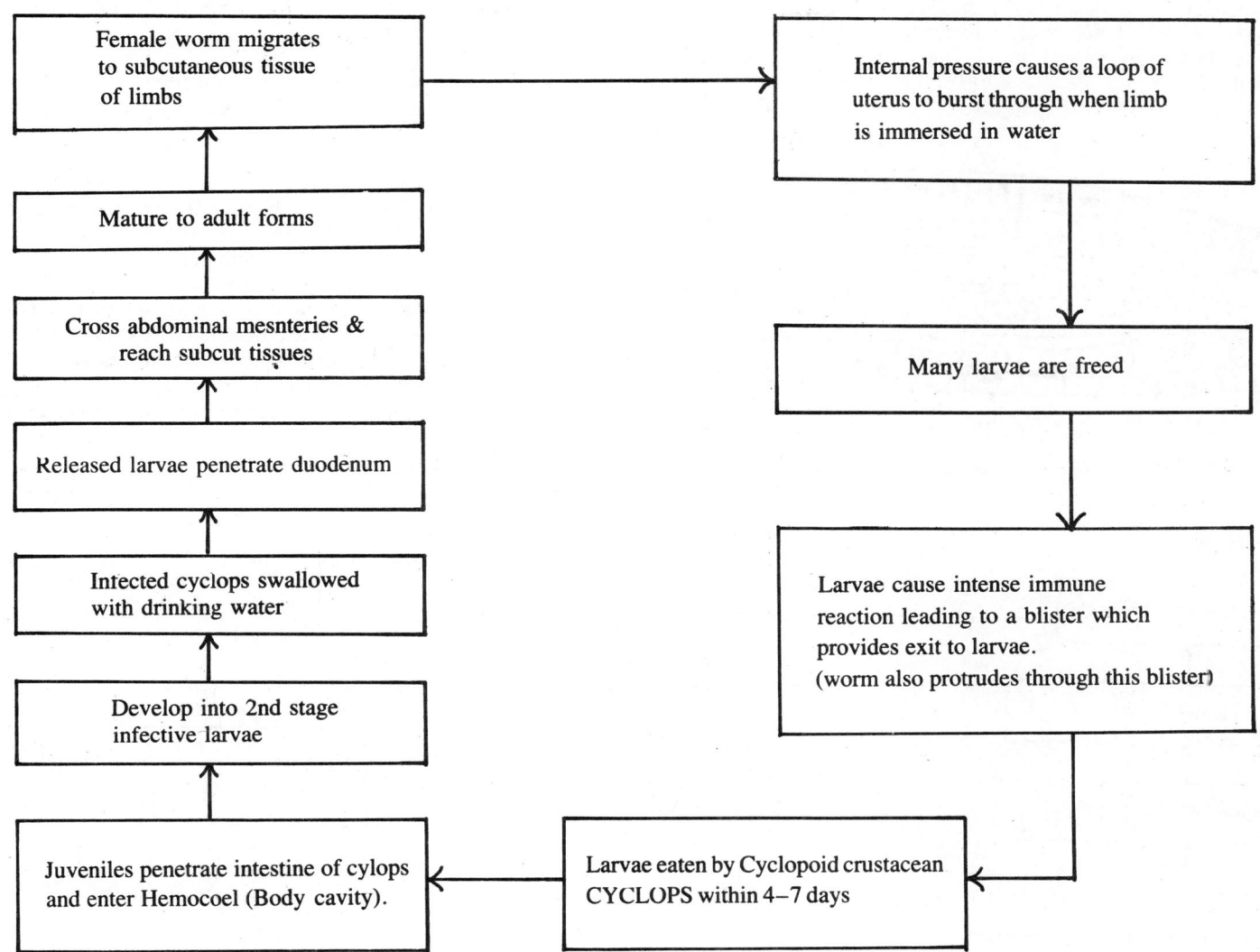

Clinical importance

At onset of migration to subcut tissue and skin of limbs, there may be an allergic reaction, characterized by
1. A rash
2. Nausea & vomiting
3. Dizziness
4. Localized oedema

Worms remain under skin for a month before a reddish papule develops. This rapidly becomes a blister. Feet and legs are the commonest site of blisters. On rupture of blister the allergic reactions subside. A tiny hole remains through which the worm protrudes; when expelled, complete healing occurs.

Secondary bacterial infection may ensue and lead to a host of complications including tetanus,, abscesses etc.

Diagnosis:

It depends on
1. **Detection** of adult worm on the skin
2. **Detection of embryos:** Bathe the affected part in water. Now mount the water on a side and observe under microscope.

3. **Intradermal test:** Inj. of dracunculus antigen, intradermally causes a wheel to appear in 24 hrs.
4. **X-Ray** may reveal calcified worms
5. **Hemogram** may reveal eosinophilia

8. TRICHINELLA SPIRALIS

It is the widespread organism in the world. It is less common in tropical regions but is well known in Mexico, S. America, Southern Asia & Middle East.

Habitat

Human skeletal muscle

Morphology

Adult worms: Males are 1.4–1.6 mm long and are more slender anteriorly than at posterior end. Anus is terminal and has a large papilla on each side.

Females are 2.6–3.4 mm long. They also taper anteriorly. Anus is nearly terminal. Vulva is located about the middle.

Larvae: Measure 100μm × 6μm. They remain encysted in

striated muscles. Inside the cysts, larve continue to grow and become 1 mm, which is the infective stage. However when encysted in human skeletal muscle, they reach a dead end and are calcified.

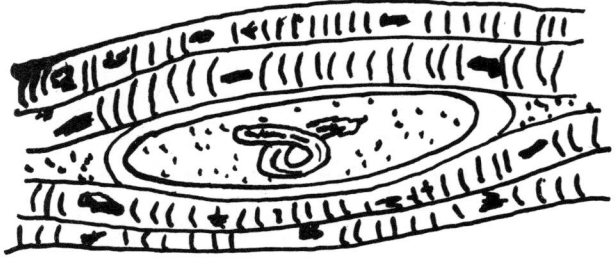

Fig 65: Larvae of To Spiralis

3. Penetration & encystment in skeltal muscle: It may cause
   1. Intense muscular pain
   2. Swelling of masseters
   3. Nervous symptoms such as hallucinations
   4. Difficulty in breathing and/or swallowing.
   5. Extreme eosinophilia

Diagnosis

1. Routine examinations of stool, blood milk etc. rarely detect larvae.
2. Haemogram shows marked eosinophilia (20–60%)
3. Trichinoscopy: Larvae can be detected in skeletal muscle by biopsy. Small samples of deltoid, biceps, gastrocnemeous & pectoralis major are obtained and digested by gastric juice for several hrs at 37°C and concentrated by centrifugation. Larvae can be detected in this specimen.
4. Xenodiagnosis: Diphragmatic or other biopsy material is fed to

Life Cycle

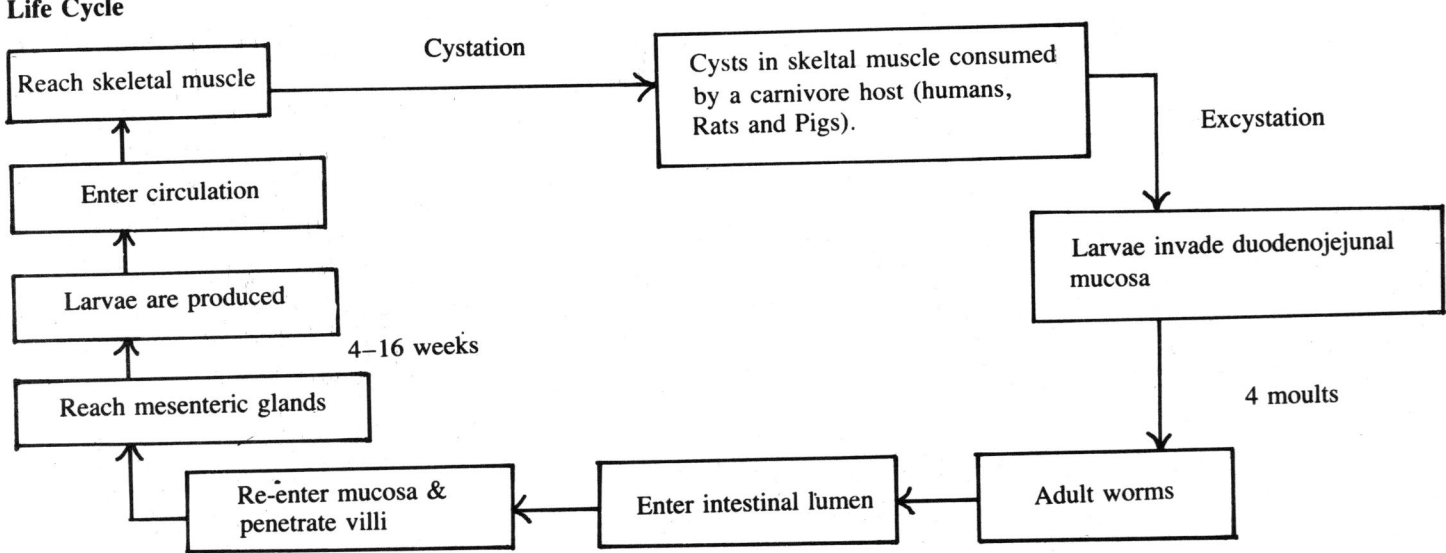

Clinical importance:

Can be studied under three headings

1. Penetration of adult females into mucosa: It results in
   1. Intestinal pain
   2. Nausea & vomiting
   3. Diarrhoea
   4. Red blotches on skin
2. Migration of larvae: Migration of larvae usually damage small blood vessels with resultant localized edema, particularly in face & hands. Wandering larvae may rarely cause any of the following.
   1. Pneumonitis
   2. Encephalitis
   3. Nephritis
   4. Eye damage (subconjunctival haemorrhage)
   5. Myocarditis
   6. Sublingual haemorrhage.

uninfected albino rats. These rats are examined one month later for encysted larvae.

5. Biochemical tests: Raised serum creatinine, creatine phosphokinase (CPK) & Lactate dehydrogenase (LDH) during acute phase.
6. X-Rays: Calcified cysts seen on X-Rays.
7. Serology: It includes
   1. Kline test — Slide agglutination test using an alkaline extract of lyophilized whole Trichinella.
   2. Bentonite & latex flocculation test — (BFT & LFT) Test of choice for diagnosis in man. Bentonite & Latex particles are added to Trichinella extract & glycerin saline solution test becomes positive on the 15th day.
   3. Charcoal agglutination test (CAT)
   4. Flourescent antibody test
   5. Complement fixation test
   6. Intradermal test (BACHMAN)

CHAPTER 15

HELMINTHOLOGY II CESTODES

CLASSIFICATION OF CESTODES
A. ORDER PSEUDOPHYLLIDEAE
   1. Diphyllobothrium latum (Fish tapeworm)
B. ORDER CYCLOPHYLLIDAE
1. Family Taenideae
   (a) Taenea solium (Pork tapeworm)
      T. Saginata (Beef tapworm)
   (b) Echinococcus granulosus (Dog tapeworm)
2. Family Hymenolepididae
   (a) Hymenolepis nana (Dwarf tapeworm) (b) H. dimunata.
   Of these D. latum is rather rare to absent in India.

1. TAENIA SAGINATA & SOLIUM (TAENIASIS)

Geographical distribution

Cosmopolitan. They occur in all parts where beef & pork are a part of the diet. T. saginata is therefore rare in Hindus who shirk eating beef while T. solium is rare in Muslims who do not eat pork.

Habitat

They live in the human jejunum and move against the peristaltic movements.

Morphology

They are usually on an average 5–20 ft in length (exceptionally long species upto 30–75 feet have been on record). They are white & transparent. T. Solium is much smaller than saginata (6–10 ft) They have two basic parts, head and body consisting of proglottides, 1500 or more in T. Saginata, 1000 in T. solium. Tapeworms are hermophrodites.

Head or Scolex is different in the two species.

T. Solium has a typical, nonretractable rostellum one with 2 circles of 22–32 hooks. It has 4 circular suckers. It is spheroid in shape.

T. Saginata has no rostellum, but has 4 powerful suckers.

Proglottides or segments of T. solium are smaller than those of T. saginata and contain half the number of testes ($\leq$ 200). Eggs of both species are similar in morphology and will be discussed in detail under the diagnosis of taeniasis. Usually gravid proglottides are discharged in stool and these liberate ova. However occasionally eggs may also be found in stool.

Clinical Importance

(A) Common with T. Saginata & T. Solium

Life Cycle

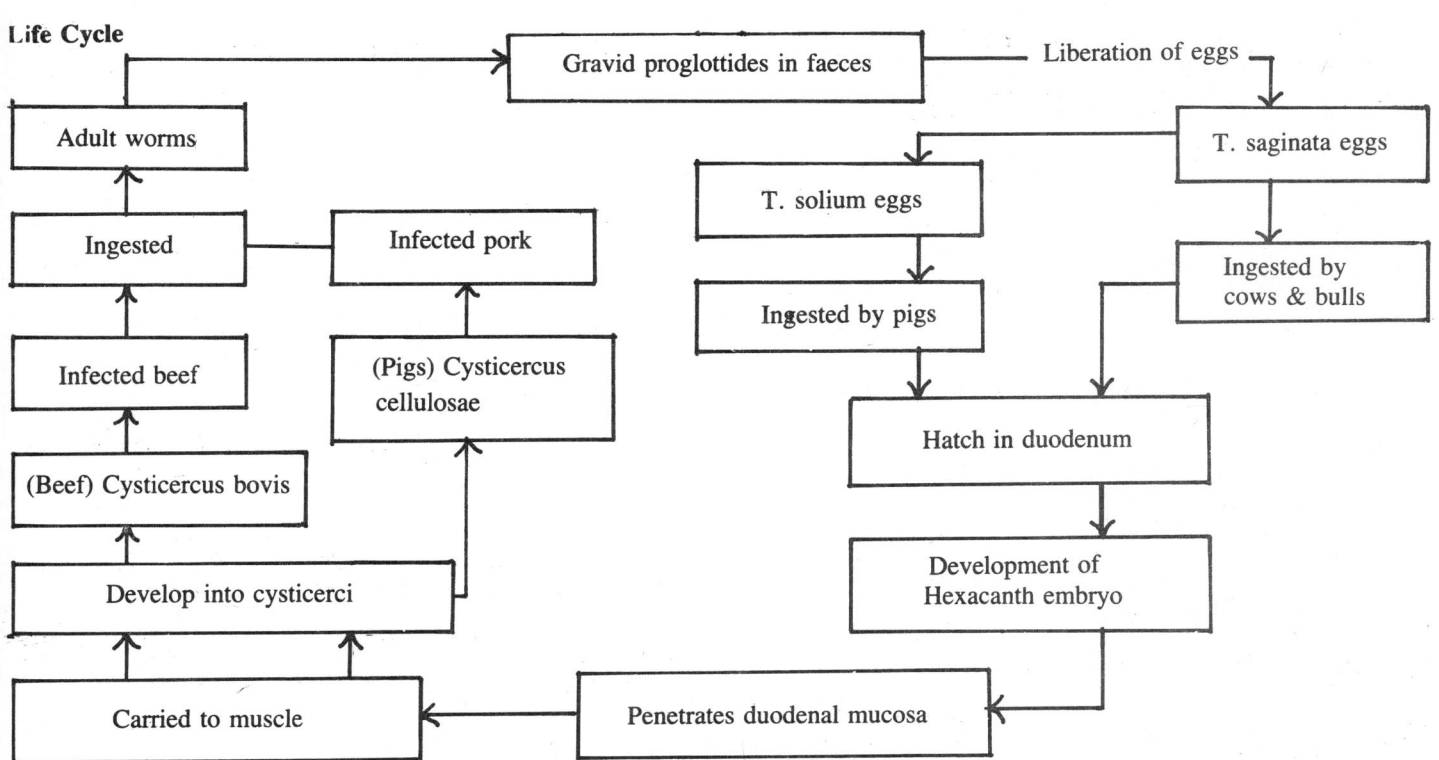

101

1. Verminous intoxication, caused by absorption of worm's excretory products, characterized by
   Dizziness
   Abdominal pain
   Headache
   Nausea & vomiting
   Diarrhoea/constipation
   Anorexia
2. Anaemia may occur
3. Infection may be asymptomatic

   Taenia solium is potentially much more dangerous since Cysticerci cellulosae can develop readily in human beings causing Cysticercosis.

   Infection occurs when embryonated eggs are eaten and hatch in the intestines. It may occur when
1. Eggs contaminate food articles
2. A gravid proglottide migrates to duodenum or stomach reverse peristalsis. This though is quite uncommon.

   In cysticercosis, virtually every organ/tissue may harbour cysticerci, though favoured sites are:
   (i) Subcutaneous connective tissue
   (ii) Eye
   (iii) Brain
   (iv) Muscles
   (v) Heart
   (vi) Lungs
   (vii) Liver

   A fibrous capsule of host origin surrounds the cystcercus in every organ except eye. Effects on host depend on site of localization of cystercerci & may include.
1. Visual impairment
2. Headache, Vomiting, Papilledema & Convulsion (due to Benign Intracranial hypertension B.I.H.)
3. Epilepsy of sudden onset (Most common manifestation).

   On dying a cysticercus produces a severe host inflammatory response which may prove fatal.

Diagnosis

1. OF SIMPLE TAENIASES: Diagnosis depends on stool examination

Gross/Naked eye Examination   Microscopic Examination of Ova

1. For Gravid proglottides
2. For scolices after giving antihelminthis drugs (Retrospective diagnosis)

1. Direct coverslip examination
2. Concentration methods
3. NIH Perianal Swab

Ova of taeniae

1. Spherical in shape
2. 31–43 μm in diameter
3. Bile stained
4. Does not float in saturated saline solution.
5. Consists of a thick embryspore which is brown in color & striated.
6. Contains an encosphere (14–20 μm) with 3 pairs of hooklets.
2. OF CYSTICERCOSIS: Diagnosis of cysticercosis, may really be quite difficult & in fact impossible. Various methods include.
   (i) Biopsy of subcutaneous nodule containing cysticerci
   (ii) Roentgenograms of skull & soft tissues may reveal calcified cysticerci
   (iii) Hemogram may reveal eosinophilia
   (iv) C.T. scan may reveal multiple small, opaque masses in the brain.
   (v) A positive indirect haemagglutination test using antigen from swine cysticerci.

Morphology of Cysticerci

   Cysticercus has a small unvaginated scolex & neck resembling an adult taenia. The external tissue consists of hair like processes, a peripheral collagenous fibrous layer, 2 muscle layers, peripheral cells, calcareous corpuscles.

2. ECHINOCOCCUS GRANULOSUS (HYDATID CYST DISEASE)

Geographical distribution

   Cosmopolitan. It is common in areas where there is a close relationship between man, sheep & dog. It is more common in temperate climates.

Habitat

   Man harbours only the larvae, adult worms reside in intestines of canine animals.

Life Cycle (E. Granulosus)

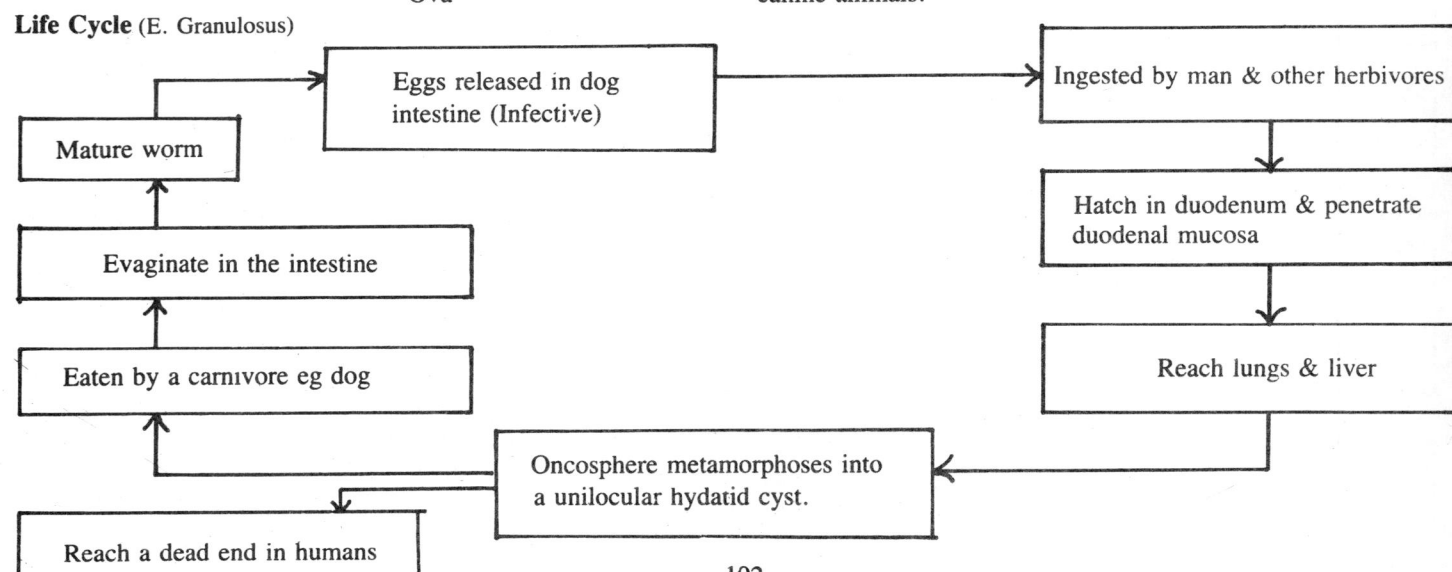

Morphology of Hydatid Cyst

Commonest sites for cysts are liver (50%) & lung (40%). Other uncommon sites include omentum, mesentery, peritoneum, pleura, skin, subcutaneous tissues, muscles, spleen, brain, kidney etc. Hydatid cysts may vary in size from being microscopic to very large containing upto 40 litres of fluid.

Contents of Cyst consist of hydatid sand & a clear, watery fluid of specific gravity 1007–1015 containing albumin, & a protein allied to casein, sodium chloride (0.5%), phosphates and sulphates of sodium & calcium, succinates, traces of sugar and a toxin allied to albumin.

Clinical features and importance

Hydatid cyst is usually asymptomatic because of its insidious growth. Once it is very large it becomes symptomatic depending on the site of involvement.

1. LIVER: It may appear as an insidiously increasing tumour of the liver. It can cause portal hypertension but jaundice is usually absent.
2. LUNG: Lung lesions are usually detected accidentally on routine X-Rays, although occasionally they may cause pressure on adjoining structures.
3. KIDNEY: Presentation resembles that of hypernephroma.
4. BRAIN: Presentation of a cerebral tumour.

If a hydatid cyst ruptures, it is a serious complication characterized by

i) Immediate pyrexia
ii) Urticaria
iii) Multiple cutaneous eruptions
iv) Anaphylactic shock
v) Peritonitis if cyst is on liver surface.

Diagnosis

1. Routine Roentgenograms — detect hydatid cysts quite often because of their typical radiological appearance. There is a smooth round outline. In lung a wavy line crosses the middle of the cyst, representing the holy sign.

2. Casoni's test — Inject 0.2 cc of sterile unpreserved fluid from a hydatid cyst intradermally into the patient. A positive reaction is the appearance of a urticarial wheel and flare in 20–20 mins.

Other immunological tests include

1. Complement fixation test
2. Precipitin test
3. Latex slide agglutination test.
3. Hemogram may show generalized eosinophilia (upto 20–25%)
4. Haemagglutination test — Formalinized sheep RBCs sensitized with tannic acid & antigen are used.

3. HYMENOLEPIS NANA

Geographical distribution

Cosmopolitan. It is the most common cestode in the world, especially in children.

Habitat

Human small intestine.

Morphology

Adult worm is 40 mm in length & 1 mm in width. Scolex bear 4 suckers & a retractable rostellum, armed with a single circle of 20–30 hooks. Proglottides are wider than long.

Clinical importance

It is rarely symptomatic. When present, symptoms represent those of simple taeniasis.

Diagnosis

Depends on identification of eggs in stool.
1. 30–47 μm in diameter
2. Floats in common salt soln (saturated)
3. Nonbile stained
4. Onosphere is covered with a thin, hyaline membrane
5. There is also an outer vitelline membrane.

Life Cycle (H. Nana)

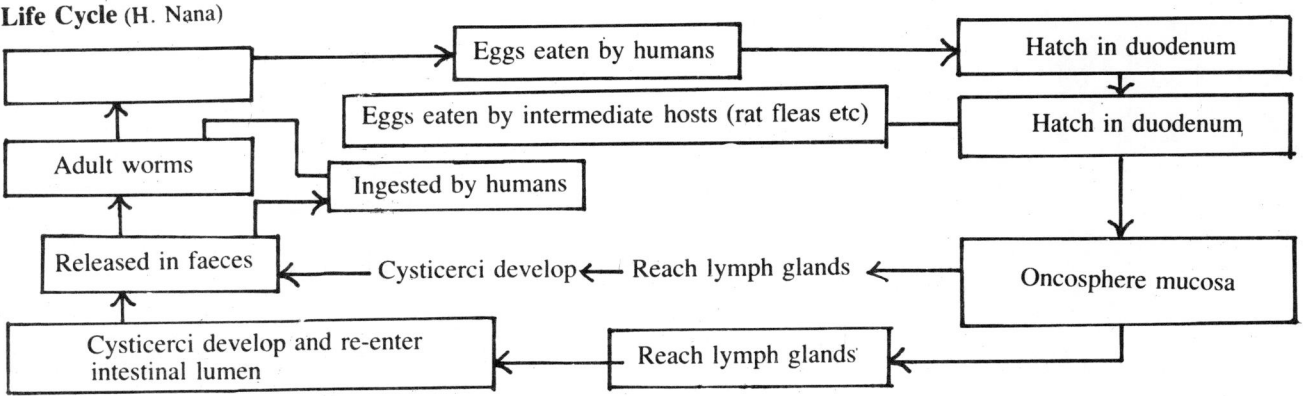

103

SECTION IV

IMMUNOLOGY

CHAPTER 16

BASIC FUNDAMENTAL TECHNIQUES

INTRODUCTION TO IMMUNOLOGY

Immunology is a young branch of medicine. The first effective immunization was performed by Edward Jenner (1749–1823), who introduced vaccination with cowpox in 1796 as a means of protection against small pox.

Immunity is of two types:

1. Cellualr Immunity

The concept was introduced by Metchnikoff (1887). Infective organisms are engulfed in the body by two types of circulating cells i.e. polymorphonuclear leucocytes and macrophages, the phenomenon known as phagocytosis.

2. Humoral Immunity

Introduced by Fodor in 1886, who observed a direct action of an immuneserum on microbes during the course of his studies on Anthrax bacilli. Before going further, certain terms used in immunology must be clarified as follows:—

1. **Antigen:** A substance that can induce a detectable immune response.
2. **Antibody:** A protein produced as a result of introduction of an antigen which has the ability to combine with that antigen.
3. **Anaphylaxis:** A reaction of immediate hypersensitivity which results from sensitization of tissue fixed mast cells by cytotropic antibodies following exposure to antigen.
4. **Allergy:** An altered state of immune reactivity, usually denoting hypersensitivity.
5. **Allergen:** Antigens that give rise to allergic reaction by IgE antibody.
6. **Anergy:** The inability to react to a battery of common skin test antigens.
7. **Antitoxin:** Protective antibodies that inactivate soluble toxic protein product of bacteria.
8. **Capping:** The movement of cell surface antigen toward one pole of a cell after antigens are cross-linked by specific antibody.
9. **Chemotaxis:** A process whereby phagocytic cells are attracted to the vicinity of invading pathogen.
10. **Complement:** A system of serum proteins that is primary humoral mediator of antigen-antibody reactions.
11. **Hapten:** A substance that is not immunogenic but can react with an antibody of appropriate specificity.
12. **Immunogen:** A substance that, when introduced into an animal provokes the immune response.
13. **Opsonin:** Substance capable of enhancing phagocytosis e.g. antibody & complement.
14. **Serology:** Determination of antibodies to infectious agents in serum, important in clinical medicine.
15. **Tolerance:** Condition in which responsive cell clones have been eliminated or inactivated by prior contact with antigen, with the result, that no immune response occurs on administration of antigen.
16. **Toxoid:** Antigenic but non toxic derivative of toxins.

IMMUNOLOGICAL APPARATUS

The immunological apparatus is a highly developed system belonging to reticulo-endothelial system which is diffusely scattered throughout the body. The two principal cells constituting this organ are macrophages and lymphocytes which are widely distributed through all the organs and tissues.

The principal cellular component in both types of reactions is the lymphocyte bursa dependent lymphocytes (B-cells) and thymus dependent lymphocytes (T-cells).

T. Lymphocytes

These are present in the peripheral lymphoid tissues as well as in blood. In blood, they constitute 70–80% of all lymphocytes.

Functions

1. Cellular Immune Reactions: Delayed hypersensitivity reactions.
— Resistance against infections by certain bacteria and viruses.
— Rejection of solid organ transplant.
— Resistance against tumors
2. Regulatory Functions: Modulation of immune response mediated by other T cells and B cells.

Function: B cells secrete immunoglobulins after they are transformed into plasma cells. Immunoglobulins, as will be discussed later, play the most important part in angigen-antibody reaction.

Macrophages

They are widely distributed in lymphoid tissues, blood and monocytes. They process and present the antigen to immuno competent cells. They also act as powerful effect on cells in cell mediated immune reactions. They also produce a number of soluble factors that influence the growth and functions of lymphocytes.

K Cells

They are characterized by the presence of Fc receptor but they lack Ig and surface markers of T cells and are non phagocytic. Functionally they are responsible for *Antibody Dependent cellular cytotoxicity (ADCC)*.

N.K. Cells: (Natural killer cells)

These are capable of lysing a variety of antigens, tumor cells and virus infected cells.

IMMUNOGLOBULINS

The immunoglobulins are the protein molecules that carry antibody activity. In serum electrophoresis, the majority of immunoglobulins migrate to γ globulin zone but significant amounts are also found in the β globulin zone. Immunoglobulins are glycoproteins composed of 82–96% polypeptide and 4–18% carbohydrate. The polypeptide component possesses almost all biological properties associated with antibody molecules.

The structure of immunoglobulin comprises of the following units:

1. **Basic Unit:** Each immunoglobulin contains at least one basic unit of monomer comprising of 4 polypeptide chains.

2. **H&L Chains:** Depending on the molecualr weight, the polypeptide chains are designated heavy (H) chains (one paid) and light (L) chains (one paid).

3. **V&C Regions:** Each polypeptide chain contains an aminoterminal portion called variable (V) region and carboxylterminal portion called *constant (C) region.*

4. **Domain:** The polypeptide chains do not exist 3–dimensionally as linear sequ-ence of amino acids but are folded by disulfide bonds into globular regions called *Domains.* The domains in H chain are called VH and CH 1, CH2, CH3, & CH4, and those L chains are designated VL & CL.

5. **Antigen binding site:** The part of antibody molecule which binds antigen is formed by only small numbers of amino acids in the V regions of H and L chains.

6. **Fab and Fc fraoments:** Digestion of an IgG molecule by papain enzyme produces 2 Fab fragments (Antigen binding) and one Fc fragment (Crystallizable).

7. **Hinge region:** The area of the H chains in the C region between first and second C region domains (CH1 and CH2) is the hinge region. It is more flexible and papain acts here to produce Fab and Fc fragments.

8. **Disulfide bonds:** Chemical disulphide (-S-S-) bonds between cysteine residues are essential for normal 3-dimensional structure of immunoglobulins.

Classes of Immunoglobulins

There are 5 classes of immunoglobulins IgG, IgA, IgM, IgD and IgE.

Biological Activities of different classes of Immunoglobulins

IgG: In normal human adults, IgG constitutes approximately 75% of the total serum immunoglobulins. There are 4 subclasses of IgG, IgG1, IgG2, IgG3 and IgG4. IgG is the only immunoglobulin that can cross the placenta, IgG is also capable of fixing serum complement.

IgA: IgA is the predominant immunoglobulin class in body secretions comprising 15% of the total immunoglobulins. Secretory IgA provides the primary defence mechanism against some local infections owing to its abundance in salvia, tears, bronchial secretions and mucous secretions of small intestine.

IgM: It is prominent in early immune responses to most antigens and predominates in certain antibody responses like natural blood group antibodies. IgM is the most efficient complement fixing immunoglobulin.

IgD: The main function of IgD has not been determined, though there are isolated cases reported of IgD activity against certain antigens like insulin, penicillin, milk proteins, diphtheria oxoid and thyroid antigens.

IgE: Its main function lies in allergic reactions.

MECHANISMS OF IMMUNOLOGIC TISSUE INJURY (HYPER SENSITIVITY REACTIONS)

The immune disorders are classified by the source of antigen as follows:—

IMMUNE DISORDERS CLASSIFIED BY SOURCE OF ANTIGEN

EXOGE-NOUS	:	Atopic disease (e.g. poison ivy contact dermatitis; reactions to plant pollens, sera and drugs)
HOMOLO-GOUS	:	Reactions to isoantigens (e.g. transfusion reaction, erythroblastosis -fetalis, transplant rejection).
AUTO-LOGOUS	:	Autoimmune diseases (e.g. systemic lupus erythematosus, rtheumatoid arthritis, Siogren's syndrome).

The second classification is based on the machanisms of immunologically mediated disorders as follows:—

It occurs as a systemic disorder or a Local reaction.

Systemic Reaction: It usually follows an intravenous injection of an antigen to which host has already become sensitized. This often leads to a state of shock, which is sometimes fatal,

Local Reaction: It depends on the portal of entry of the allergen and takes the form of localized cutaneous reaction, conjunctival discharge, nasal discharge or bronchial asthma or food allergy.

Type I, Anaphylaxis:

Mediators of Type I Reaction: Type I reactions are mediated by IgE antibodies produced by lymphocytes and plasma cells in response to an allergen. Once released, IgE antibodies attach to mast cells and basophils through cell surface receptors. Once attached, these cells release a variety of powerful vasoactive mediators after a series of reactions which are shown as follows:

Primary Mediators released	Secondary mediators
1. Histamine	1. Arachidonic acid metabolites
2. Eosinophil chemotactic factor of anaphylaxis (ECE-A)	2. Leukotrienes
3. Neutrophilic chemotactic factor	3. Platelet activating factors (PAF)
4. Neutral Proteases	

Reactions of Systemic Anaphylaxis: After administration of heterologous proteins e.g. antisera, penicillin, enzymes, within minutes there is itching, hives, skin erythema followed shortly by contraction of respiratory bronchioles leading to respiratory distress. There is vomiting, diorrhoea, laryngeal obstruction leading to shock and death.

Reactions to Local Anaphylaxis: These are exemplified by atopic reaction which is defined as a genetically controlled predisposition to the production of specific IgE antibodies upon inhalation or ingestion of minute amounts of antigen like pollen, dust, animal dander etc. Specific diseases like urticaria, allergic Rhinitis, angio-oedema and bronchial asthma.

Type II Hypersensitivity

This type is mediated by antibodies directed toward antigens present on the surface of cells or other tissue components. The antigenic determinants may be intrinsic to the cell membrane or extrinsic adsorbed on the cell surface. In either case the reaction takes place by the binding of antibody to normal or altered cell surface antigens.

There are two antibody dependent mechanisms as follows:

1. **Complement mediated cytotoxicity:** In this reaction, antibody (IgM or IgG) reacts with an antigen present on the surface of the cell, causing activation of complement system and resulting in direct membrane damage and lysis. At the same time, the antibody coated cells become susceptible to phagocytosis example of such reaction is seen in Good-pasteur's disease, Autoimmune haemelytic anaemia and erythroblastosis foetalis.

2. **Antibody dependent cell mediated cytotoxicity ADCC:** In this, the target cells coated with IgG antibody can be killed by a variety of non sensitized cells that have Fc receptors. This is carried out by K cells, eosinophils, neutrophils and monocytes which bind to the target cell by the receptor for Fc fragment of IgG and carry out lysis without phagocytosis.

This mechanism has been studied in vitro and whether it plays role in vivo is not known.

Type III Hypersensitivity (Immune complex mediated)

This type of hypersensitivity reaction is induced by antigen antibody complexes that produce tissue damage as a result of their capacity to activate a variety of serum mediators, principally complement system and biologically active fragments e.g. kinins. The toxic reaction is intiated when antigen combines with antibody, either within the circulation (circulating immune complexes) or at extra vascular sites (in situ immune complexes).

There are two types of antigens that cause such reaction.

Exogenous Antigen: eg. foreign protein, bacteria, viruses.

Edogenous Antigen: In which the individual can produce antibody against its own body component.

Type IV Hypersensitivity (Cell mediated)

This type of hypersensitivity is initiated by specifically sensitized T lymphocytes. It induces the classic delayed hypersensitivity reactions and cell mediated cytotoxic reactions.

(i) **Delayed Hyper-sensitivity:** The type of reaction is initiated by specifically sensitized T. Lymphocytes generated during the initial contact with antigen, some of the memory cells remain in the circulation for a long time. When the individual is re-exposed to the specific antigen, e.g. tuberculin, T. lymophocytes are stimulated to divide and release a variety of biologically active molecules K/a lymphokines. The lymphokines amplify the inflammatory response by recruiting inflammatory cells, activating them and keeping them it site. The most important result is stimulation and activation of macrophages within the lesion which further cause tissue damage and inflammatory reactions. Example of this type of reaction is Tuberculin Reaction.

(ii) **T-Cell mediated cytotoxicity:** The process of CTLs is complex and illunderstood. They however, once sensitized, kill the antigen bearing target cells. This group of T cells are characterized by the presence of OK T5/T8 antigens on their surface. The CTL after causing lysis of the target cell, survives the encounter and is then recycled to kill other target cells.

This CTL mediated lysis is highly specific and the cells are not affected.

It is now clear, that this specificity is due to the presence of cell surface HLA antigens by which CTLs recognize their target cells. It is suggested that the infection of the cell with the antigen e.g. virus, changes the cell surface HLA antigen, which is different from the normal self HLA antigen, so as to evoke the CTLs, capable of recognizing altered self and thereby kill the virus infected target cell. e.g. Transplant Rejection Reaction.

MEDIATORS OF IMMUNOLOGICAL REACTIONS

The complement system

The Complement system is the primary humoral mediator of antigen-antibody reactions. It consists of at least 20 chemically and immunologically distinct plasma proteins capable of interacting with each other. The various functions they carry out are increased vascular permeability, chemotaxis, opsonization prior to phagocytosis and lysis of target organisms.

Pathways: Activation occurs via two pathways:

(i) **Classic pathway:** Initiated by antigen-antibody complexes.

(ii) **Alternate Pathway:** Initiated by a variety of largely non-immunologic stimuli.

The Kinin system

This system results in the ultimate release of the vaso active nonapeptide *bradykinin,* a potent agent that increases vascular permeability; contraction of smooth muscle, dilatation of blood vessels and pain when injected into the skin.

The Lymphokines

When antigen is injected intradermally into an appropriate sensitized host, a delayed skin reaction may develop over the course of 24–48 hours, characterized by mononuclear cell infiltrate. The initial reaction of antigen with a few specifically sensitized lymphocyte results in the production of soluble mediators called lymphokines.

The functions of lymphokines are:

1. Recruit host inflammatory cells
2. Activate the inflammatory cells
3. Keep them at site of inflammation
4. Amplify the cell mediated hypersensitivity reaction (Type IV)

While these substances exert marked biological effects on the cells, they are produced in only minute quantities by activated lymphocytes.

A variety of lymphokines, detected usually by diverse functional assays has been described. It is not yet clear, how many chemically distinct molecules are involved, nor how many of the lymphokine activities detected in vitro are relevant in vivo.

The following table shows the various products of activated lymphocytes:

Some of the important lymphokines are described below:—

1. **Macrophage migration Inhibition factors:** This substance inhibits the normal active migration of macrophages.

It is of low molecular weight and lacks immunologic specificity. It is a glycoprotein which can be generated in vitro by interaction of immune T cells with antigen.

2. **Interferons:** They represent a family of molecules that can also exert immuno modulatory effects in addition to its antiviral activity.

It is of three types α, β and γ

The interferon produced by sensitized T cells is called *gammainterferon* which is chemically distinct from alpha and beta interferons induced by viruses.

Gamma interferon: can activate macrophages levels of metabolic activity accompanied by greater ability to kill tumour cells and ingested microbes.

3. Chemotactic factors: These are for neutrophils, eosinophils, basophils, monocytes and other lymphocytes.

4. Interleukin-2.: This substance also called T cells growth factor is produced by antigen of mitogen activated T cells. It, in turn, causes proliferation of the T cells involved in mediating cellular immunity.

5. Transfer Factor: This is an ill defined substance present only in humans, which has the ability to transfer delayed hypersensitivity and enables to prepare the non sensitized lymphocytes to respond to specific antigen without preparing the host to make antibody against the same antigen. The exact mechanism is not known, but it is postulated to be a *single-stranded polynucleotide* which either is informational or may provide some part of a receptor for antigen.

HISTOCOMPATIBILITY ANTIGENS (HLA)

Definition: The term HLA refers to *human leucocyte antigen displayed* on the various cell surfaces, that evoke the rejection of transplanted organs. This is brought about by the recognition of histocopatibility antigens displayed on the cell surfaces of the donor organ through the recipient's Immunesystem. It is called human leucocyte antigen because mhc encoded antigens were initially detected on white cells.

Structure & genetic Constitution: The structure and organization of HLA s and coresponding HLA genes is complex and still incompletely understood.

Several genes code for histocompatibility antigens, but those that code for the most important transplantation antigens are clustered on a small segment of *chromosome* 6. This cluster of genes constitutes the human *major histocompatibility complex (MHC) or HLA complex.*

The HLA complex is composed of four closely linked Loci called HLA *complex on chromosome 6.*

HLA-HLA loci show high degree of polymorphism i.e. the existence of multiple allelic forms in a population. Each of the several allelic determinants at these loci is identified by a number e.g. HLA—B5, etc.

Already, more than 40 antigens have been recognised at HLA—B locus. These antigens are designated by a *W* e.g. HLA—BW 21.

Antigens coded by HLA—A, B & C loci are called *Class I Antigens* and those coded by HLA—D/DR loci are called *Class II* Antigens. These are ME,—MT and SB antigens.

Distribution: Class I Antigens are present on virtually all the nucleated cells. They evoke the formation of humoral antibody in genetically non-identical recipients.

Class II Antigens: are present on mainly B lymphocytes, monocytes/ macrophages, dendritic/Langerhan's cells and some endothelial cells. Class II Antigens are products of Ir (Immune response) genes, which determine individual pattern of responses to foreign antigens.

Inheritance of HLA Haplotype: A set of closely linked genes on one chromosome constitutes a haplotype and these tend to be inherited enbloc including one gene each from HLA—A, B, C, D and DR loci. Parents share one haplotype with all children and differ in the other. However if both parents had shared one haplotype, there would be a 1 in 2 chance of parents and offspring being identical. This degree of haplotype sharing is of fundamental importance in predicting graft survival.

Significance of HLA complex:

1. Organ Transplantation: In organ transplantation, HLA antigens of the graft evoke both humoral and cell mediated response, which leads to graft destruction, if there is a disparity between donor and recipient. Hence, HLA typing is very important in the selection of donor–recipient combinations.

2. Regulation of Immune Responses: Class II Antigens having a Ir gene control, regulate the immune response of an individual.

3. **Cell to Cell Interaction in Immune Response:** The ultimate expression of immune response both humoral and cellular results from interaction of various immunologically active cells. These interactions are critically dependent on the recognition of class II HLA antigens.

4. **Role in Host Defence:** The T cell mediated lysis of the virus and tumor cells by cytotoxic T cells; is brought about in the presence of class I antigen as follows:

DIAGRAM 66

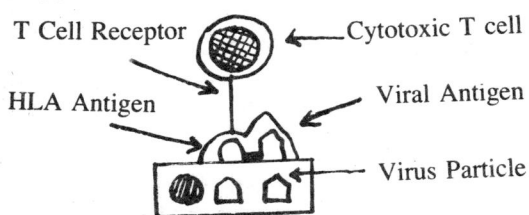

As we can see, it is the HLA antigen present on the surface of virus infected cell which is recognized by the cytoxic-T cell via, its surface receptor for the same, that the Olysis is brought about cytotoxic T cell cannot recognize viral antigens independent of HLA Antigen (*HLA Restriction*)

5. **HLA and Disease Association:** A variety of diseases have been found in association with certain HLA types.

Selected Examples of H.L.A. and disease association
Table 29

Disease	HLA	Estimated Relative Risk
Ankylosing spondylitis	B 27	90
Reiter's disease	B27	48
Acute anterior uveitis	B27	16.9
Rheumatoid arthritis	DW4/DR4	4.2
Hashimoto's disease	DR3	2.6
Addison's disease	B—8, DW3	4.0
Hemochromatosis	BW A3	6.3
21-Hydroxylase Deficiency	A3, BW 47	4, 15
Dermatitis herperiformis	B8, DW3	8.7, 13.5

The best known is the association of *Ankylosing spondylitis* and *HLA—B 27.*

In view of physiologic role of HLA complex in regulation of immune response, the following two mechanisms are postulated in their association with immunologically mediated diseases.

(i) involvement of Immuno Response genes which regulate the levels of auto-antibody responses. Hence association with auto immune diseases.

(ii) Direct participition of HLA macromolecule in disease in which pathogens may share cross—reacting antigens with HLA or molecule may provide receptors for viruses and this may facilitate virus cell interaction leading to disease process.

IMMUNOLOGIC LABORATOTY TESTS

Clinical Laboratory Methods for Detection of Antigens and Antibodies:

In the past two decades, immunologic laboratory methods have gradually become increasingly more refined and simplified. In the present chapter, test for detection of antigens and antibodies are discussed.

The topic covered in this chapter include the following:
1. Immunodiffusion
2. Electrophoresis
3. Immunoelectrophoresis
4. Radio immunoassay
5. Immuno chemical and physicochemical methods.
6. Immuno fluorescence
7. Agglutination
8. Complement fixation

The important, and commonly used techniques will be described:—

IMMUNODIFFUSION

Principle: The antigen and antibody are detected by their reaction to form a *precipitate line*. It is the most common technique. It may be *Single* or *double*. In Single Immunodiffusion, the antigen or antibody remains fixed and the other one is allowed to move in agar filled tube and form precipitate complex with it, *Double immunodiffusion:* Both reactants are free to move towards each other and precipitate.

Movement in either form may be radial or linear.

Clinical Application: Most important application is in estimation of *Serum immunoglobulins* or serum proteins.

Technique: *Quantitative determination of the immunoglobulins IgG; IgA & IgM; by Tri-partigen-Plates:—*

Composition of Tri-Partigen Plates: Tripartigen immunodiffusion plates contain a prepared agar gel in which H—chain specific antiserum to the respective immunoglobulins is incorporated. (The antiserum is produced by immunization of sheep and goats)

Preservative — Sodium azide 1 mg/ml.
Sodium P–ethyl mercury
mercapto benzene sulfonate $\leq$ 0.1mg. per ml.

Method:

1. Open the plate & leave the opened plate to stand for about 5 mins. at room temp. to allow any condensation water that may have accumulated in the walls to evaporate.
2. IgA & IgM are determined with undiluted serum. Only when IgG is to be determined, sera to be tested and control serum used must be diluted 1: 10 with normal saline.

Procedure

1. Well 1 is filled with 5 μl of control serum. Well 2–12 are each filled with 5 μl of sera under tests.
2. Close the plate tightly & leave it to stand at room temp.
3. Diffusion time of 50 hrs. (IgG & IgA) & 80 hrs. (IgM).
4. At the end of the given diffusion time, the diameter D of the precipitin rings should be measured accurately to 0.1mm. using a suitable calibrated instrument.
5. The immunoglobulin concentrations related to the measured diameters are read directly from the tables of reference values.

(The results are reliable only when the value found for the control sera applied to well 1 lies within the confidence range taken from the table of values enclosed with each pack of control sera.

Confidence range with Hoechst packing = 15% of immunoglobulin concentration with each pack.

When determining IgG, value found must be multiplied by the dilution factor 10.

6. If the protein concentration of the sera samples diverge considerably from normal value, this means that resultant ppt. rings will fall outside the assay range of the plate. In this case examination is repeated using high dilution. (Tripartigen IgM is not suited for IgM determination in seminal fluid).

Immunoelectrophoresis: (IEP)

Principle: Immuno electrophoresis combines electrophoretic separation diffusion in the electric field and immune precipitation of proteins simultaneously. Hence both identification and approximate quantities can thereby be accomplished for individual proteins present in serum, urine or other biologic fluid.

Immunelectrophoresis as described by Graber and Williams (1953) added the immunological discrimination of double diffusion to zone electrophoretic separation of protein solutions. The original method was rather cumbersom and demanded large volumes of antiserum. Scheidegger (1955) modified the method by scaling the whole technique down to the 76x26 mm microscope slide. This allowed the initial electrophoretic separation to be conducted in 45 min. instead of 6 hour and the diffusion phase to be completed in 24 hrs. instead of 10 days. The restricted space available on 76x26 mm glass slide did, however, make for difficulties in comparison between separation pattern and was restrictive when non-specific antisera were used to identify individual precipitin arcs.

Materials

1. **Electrophoresis apparatus:** any low voltage power pack is suitable provided it can produce a maximum of 50 MA or 50 V current or voltage stabilised (Shandon Southern VOKAM).

2. **Universal electrophoresis tank** (Shandon Southern). Electrophoresis wicks: filter paper or lint laid over the Electrophoresis bridge supports of the electrophoresis tank.

3. **Gel Punch and suction device** and suitable template. Glass plates 80x80 mm. The plates should be precoated with 2-5% agar and dried. This skinning process make the gel adhere to the plate so that it does not become detached during subsequent washing procedures.

4. **Wooden blocks** 10x2x2 cm metal rule double bladed knife for through cutting. A double bladed knife can be made by blotting two surgical scalpel blades on either side of a 1 mm metal spacer bar. Water bath. horizontal table micropipette.

5. **Agar:** Various commercial agar preparations are suitable including Difco Special Agar—Noble and behringwerke purified Agar Noble in barbiturate buffer is dispensed in 6 ml. aliquots. Difco special Agar Noble, 3.6g Barbitone buffer PH 8.6, 150ml. and distilled water 150ml.

6. **Barbitone buffer** (Venoral) PH 8.6, (dilute stock solution 1 in 2). (Stock Solution): Sodium barbitone 154g. Barbitone 27.6g distilled water to 10 litre. Add sodium azide, 10G. as an antimicrobial preservative). Stain solution: ponceau S 2g. Trichloracetic acid 30g. distilled water to 1 litre. Dissolve and leave overnight before use. Staining time: 10 min. Destain solution: 5% acetic acid.

7. **Anti serum in appropriate quantity**

Method

1. Preparation of the gel: 6 ml of predispensed agar is melted in the water bath and pour into the "Preskinned" glass plate on a horizontal table. The gel is left to set and then allowed to harden at 4°C in a moist chamber.

2. Origin wells: Place the gel over the template and cut origin wells 1–2 mm diameter according to template. The wells should be evacuated by suction.

3. Samples loading: the origin wells are filled to the brim with the test samples. One well should be reserved for a control sample stained with Bromophenol blue to provide a marker of electrophoretic migration.

4. Electrophoresis: the gel is inverted and placed in the electrophoresis tank so that the agar is in direct contact with the wicks or the support bridges. A constant current of 1.5 MA/Cm gel (12ma per 80 mm plate) is applied and or until the Bromophenol blue mark has migrated to within 1 cm. of anode wick.

5. On completion of the electrophoretic separation the gel is removed from the tank and placed over the templates. The wooden blocks are placed on either side of the gel and the metal rule supported over the gel. With the rule as a guide cut the antiserum troughs with the double bladed knife. Gently lift out the & remove the agar from the troughs.

6. Fill the troughs with antiserum (Aprox 100 μl).

7. Place the gel in a moist chamber to diffuse for 18-24 hrs. at ambient temperature. The gel should be maintained horizontal during this diffusion phase. On completion of diffusion the precipitin lines can be examined by incident light illumination against a dark background.

8. To prepare permanent preparations, unreacted protein must be washed from the gel. This is achieved by washing in saline for 24 hrs. and in distilled water for 1hr. The gel is covered either with filter paper and dried in a warm air oven or with three layers of Whatman 3mm paper and press dried. The plat can be now stained, excess stain being removed by washing in 5% acetic acid.

Possible Sources of Error

1. Electrophoretic separation must be adequate. Too long or too short separation will lead to difficulties in interpretation.

2. Too short an antiserum trough or irregularities in cutting it, will distort the precipitin pattern.

3. Bacterial contamination or proteolytic degradation of the serum sample will distort the pattern and alter the electrophoretic mobility of many proteins.

4. Diffusion will occur more rapidly at a high temperature. With a high ambient temperature precipitin pattern should be examined sooner than the usual 18-20 hours.

5. When testing for small molecular weight proteins, such as Bene-Jones protein, the precipitin pattern should be examined at 30 min. intervals to avoid loss of the preciptin lines due to rapid diffusion of the antigen towards the antiserum trough.

Identification of Precipitin Lines

The analysis of a precipitin pattern requires a certain degree of practice and familiarity. Albumin, transferrin & the major immunoglobulin lines are readily identified, but other lines often need other techniques to aid their identification.

Specific antisera–The use of two antisera in troughs on either side of an electrophoretic separation allows the direct comparison of the precipitin lines produced by a polyspecific antiserum and the corresponding line produced with a monospecific antiserum. The advantage of the 80x80 mm plate over the 76x26 mm slide can be seen where direct comparison can be made between different test samples developed against monospecific and polyspecific antisera.

Specific stains–Certain plasma proteins can be stained with specific stains. Liporoteins can be stained with oil red or Sudan black. Haptoglobin and haemopexin can be stained with benzidine which identifies the haemoglobin or haem-components. Ceruloplasmin can be stained with Litatic P–phenylenediamine

Purified proteins–In certain instances where purified proteins are available these can be used to identify precipitin arcs in an immunoelectrophoretic pattern. Method utlising purified proteins have been described by Clausen and Hermans (1960) and Osserman (1960).

Counter Current Immuno electrophoresis: (CIEOP)

Principle: The basic principles of the method involve electrophoresis in a gel medium of antigen and antibody in opposite directions simultaneously from separate wells. With resultant precipitation line at a point intermediate between their origins.

Clinical Applications: In detection of the following
— HBs Ag (Australia Antigen)
— Cord IgM in Intrauterine infection
— α (Alpha) fetoprotein
— Fungal Precipitins

Prozone Phenomenon: It refers suboptimal precipitation which occur in the region of antibody excess. Thus dilution of antisera need to be reacted with fixed amounts of antigen in order to obtain maximum precipitation line. This is a common to phenomenon seen in paraproteinemias.

Hepatitis B Surface Antigen (HBs Ag) Detection

There are 3 tests done in routine for detection of HBs Ag in serum:—
1. Immuno–diffusion (I.D.)
2. Counter Current immuno–electrophoresis (C.I.E.O.P.)
3. Reversed passive Haemagglutination (R.P.H.A.)
4. Latex Agglutination tests
5. ELISA
6. Immuno Assays

C.I.E.O.P.

Principle: Under appropriate electrophoretic conditions HBs Ag (Hepatits B–Surface antigen) moves like an Alpha 2, globulin towards the anode, the HBs AB (Hepatitis B–surface antibody) a gamma globulin, moves towards cathode. A line of precipitation is formed perpendicular to the direction of flow of current where these fractions meet.

Procedure: The C.I.E.O.P. technique consists of following 3 steps.
1. Preparation of slides.
2. Charging of samples.
3. Operation of equipment.

Preparation of Slides

i) Place clean glass slide on horizontal surface.
ii) Pour 2.5 ml of hot 1% agarose on slide and allow it to solidify.
iii) Place the slide in moist petri dish & keep it in refrigerator (2-8°C) for further solidification.

Charging of Samples

i) Punch two holes for each test & positive control with punch (Diameter 4 mm) at a distance of 8mm on the agarose glass slide.

ii) Remove agarose medium by suction in order to produce holes.

iii) Fill the wells on LT side with respective patient's serum & HBs Ag positive serum (Positive control) using seperate capillary for each test.

iv) Fill the Rt side wells with HBs Ab positive serum.

Operation of Equipment

i) Fill the chamber of electrophoresis tank with Barbitone buffer PH 8.6 (equal amount in both the chambers).

ii) Place the slide in the Electrophoresis tank in such a way that wells containing HBs Ag serum point towards cathode and HBs Ab wells towards anode.

iii) Connect the slide with buffer in each chamber using moist filter paper wicks.

iv) Apply 7 MA current per slide at 120 volts & continue the run for 40-60 minutes.

Other Methods for Detection of HBs Ag

(a) **Immuno Diffusion:** i) Preparation of slide & charging of sample is done in the same way as in C.I.E.O.P.

ii) After charging the sample, keep the slides in moist petri dish for 48 hrs.

Interpretation: i) A faint white line of precipitation (in a direction perpendicular to that of flow of current) between test well and HB Ab well indicates the presence of Hbs Ag in the samples (Positives result).

ii) A line of precipitation between positive Hbs Ag & positive HBs Ab serum indicates a satisfactory positive control.

1% Agarose: Dissolve 1 gm Agarose in 100 ml of barbitone buffer by heating.

Barbitone Buffer: pH 8.6; 0.0 5M.

Composition

Barbituric Acid	— 1.830 gms.
Sodium-Diethylbarbiturate	— 10.3 gms.
Distilled Water	1000 ml.
Sodium Azide (preservative)	100 gms.

(b) R.P.H.A. (Raphadex B):—

This is a 3rd generation test for detection of HBs Ag.

Principle: It is based on the principle that R.B.C.s coated with anti HBs will agglutinate in the presence of Hepatitis B surface antigen. The reactive specimen show agglutination which is exhibited by a diffused cell pattern upon settling. A non reactive specimen does not cause agglutination and settles into a compact cell button.

Procedure

i) Put 25 μ litre specimen diluent in each well for test serum as well as for positive & negative control well.

ii) Add 7 μl of test serum with separate capillary.

iii) To positive control well add 7 μl positive control serum.

iv) To negative control well add 7 μl negative control serum.

v) MIX

vi) Add 25μl cells to each well (Antibody to Hbs Ag) Chimpanzee coated human red Blood cells (Lyophilized).

vii) Mix Again

viii) Stand at room temperature for 2 hours.

ix) Read.

Interpretation: The cell settling pattern of a strongly reactive specimen will appear as a large diffused pattern of cells with an irregular periphery.

The cell settling pattern of a weakly reactive specimen will appear as smaller, more dense pattern of cells with a slightly irregular periphery, and larger than negative control.

Moderate reactive specimen show cell settling pattern intermediatory to the above two.

Non–reactive cell settling pattern is a distinct, compact button of cell with a smooth, regular periphery (No agglutination).

AGGLUTINATION TECHNIQUES

Agglutination and precipitation reactions are the basis of most commonly used, techniques in laboratories.

The agglutination of insoluble native antigens or antigen coated particles can be simply assessed with or without the aid of a microscope. *Requirements* in agglutination tests are three:—

(1) Stable cell or particle suspension.

(2) Antigen close to the surface.

(3) The knowledge that incomplete or non-agglutinating antibodies are not detectable without modifications.

Types of Agglutination Reactions:—

(1) **Direct Agglutination Test:** In this, red blood cells, bacteria, fungi etc. can be agglutinated by serum antibody. The clumping can be seen directly or under microscope after incubating for some time.

(2) **Indirect (Passive) Agglutination Test:** In this, the soluble antigen is passively absorbed or chemically coupled to red blood cells or other inert particles and thereby form stable reagents for antibody detection.

Agglutination tests may be performed in tubes or microtitre plates.

Clinical Applications

In detection of Rheumatoid factor, Anti streptolysin—O (ASL-O); C—reactive protein (CRP), coomb's Test. Detection of HBs Ag, Factor VIII Antigen in haemophilia and related clotted diorders, HCG detection in urine.

Latex Agglutination inhibition Test: In this test, instead of red blood cells, latex particles are used as the agent for coating the antigen. The most important clinical application of this test is the *Pregnancy Test* or the detection of Human chorionic gonadotrophin (HCG) in the urine of pregnant female. The test employs antiserum (anti-HCG produced in female rabbits) and antigen which consists of latex particles coated with HCG.

ELECTROPHORESIS

Electrophoresis is the separation of proteins in an electric field on the basis of the surface charge. It was perfected in 1937 by Tiselius. Generally paper, agarose or cellulose acetate strips are employed as supporting media which do not interfere in the flow of molecules in the electric field.

Electrophoresis of Serum Proteins

Principle

Various charged fractions of serum proteins are separated by subjecting serum to an electric field.

Paper Electrophoresis

Reagents

(1) Venoral buffer (ionic strength 0.05, PH 8.6 Diethyl barbituric acid 1.84g. Sod. Die-thyl barbiturate 10.3g. in water. Add water to 1 litre.

(2) Staining solution: 0.01% bromphenol blue, 5 gm. of $Zn SO_4$ $7H_2O$ added and dissolved in 5% acetic acid. Made to 100ml. with 5% Acetic Acid.

(3) Wash solution: 5% acetic acid.

(4) Fixative solution: 5% acetic acid containing 0.3% Sod. acetate.

Execution: Buffer is poured into two tanks of electrophoresis apparatus (vertical type, horizontal type–vertical type discussed here). Whatman 1mm. Filter paper strips (4cm. x 32cm.) are moistened with buffer, removing the excess buffer with a blotting paper. 20µl of serum are applied exactly on the line drawn previously on the middle of the paper. The paper is mounted on the apparatus.

The apparatus is closed tightly and the electrophoretic run is started.

Voltage applied: 150 volts.

Current Strength 1 to 1.5 milliamps. for a 4 cm. strip. Time of run : 6 hours.

At the end of the run, the strips are removed and dried at 110°C for 20 mts. They are then washed for 6 mts., each time in two changes of wash solution. Subsequently the strips are washed with the fixative solution for 6 mts. and dried at room temperature or at 100°C for about 15 mts.

Scanning/Elution:

The stained bands on the strips can be scanned directly in a densitometer.

Cellulose Acetate Membrane Electrophoresis

Requisites: (1) Cellulose acetate membrane:
(2) Filter paper strips
3) Venoral buffer (pH 6.6, 0.07M)
Barbituric acid 0.38g.
Add distilled water to 500 ml.
Add Thiomersal 0.01% for preservative purposes.

(4) Staining solution: 0.8% Poneau 3R in 6% Trichloroacetic acid.

(5) Decolourization solution: 1% Acetic acid.

(6) Alkaline solution for elution: 0.01 N–NaOH solution.

Execution

(1) Pretreatment of cellulose acetate membrane (6 cm × 3.4 cm) with buffer.

(2) Preparation of Electrophoretic bath; Set the apparatus & connect with electricity. Pour buffer solution in the tanks and mount the membrane on the supporter bridge of the apparatus and wet by buffer solution.

(3) Sampling: Apply 0.0006—0.0012ml. per lcm. of membrane.

(4) Pass a constant current at 0.4–0.8 mA per lcm, of membrane for 45–60 mts.

(5) Staining: After time-up, separate the membrane from bath and put in the staining solution for 3 mts.

(6) Decolourise the background of the membrane with 1% acetic acid using several changes of acetic acid.

(7) Scanning by densitometry or elution with 0.01 N NaOH, as described previously.

Clinical Laboratory Methods for Detection of Cellular Immune Function

The immune system in humans can be divided into 2 major parts, one involving *humoral immunity* (antibody and complement) and the other *immuno–competent cells i.e cellular immunity* The present chapter reviews the tests that have medical application in the detection of cellular immune function. This is studied through the following tests:—

1. Delayed hypersensitivity skin tests.
2. Lymphocyte Transformation Test.
3. Assays for T and B lymphocytes.
4. Neutrophil Function.

(1) Delayed Hypersensitivity Skin Tests:

Principle: The tests is based on recall of T lymphocyte immunologic memory and thus overall T lymphocyte function is assessed. The postulated sequence of events leading to the appearance of the delayed hypersensitivity type skin test is that circulating T lymphocytes come into contact with antigen (mainly held by skin macrophages) and pre–sensitized cells present are stimulated to lymphokine production and blast cell transformation. The lymphokines encourage the trapping of circulating mononuclear cells at the site of antigen and the activation of non–sensitized by stander cells in to the reaction. A cascade effect is produced with increasing localization of mononuclear cells which is clinically manifest as induration. Local persistence of antigen favours the production of a more vigorous response and Vica versa. Thus, subcutaneous (instead of intradermal) injection of antigen result in its rapid removal before a local response is apparent. The presence of oedema of the skin will result in false negative results due to increased lymphatic clearance of antigen.

Method

The volar aspect of the forearm is the most convenient site for testing.

1. Prepare the arm by shaving and cleaning with isopropyl alcohol, finally drying thoroughly with a sterile swab.

2. Mark out the area to be tested with the code numbers of the antigens to be tested with a skin pencil or suitable non-washable marker (e.g. Ball-point pen).

3. Inject the appropriate antigen solution using a disposable syringe. The skin is stretched taut with the free hand and then, with the needle of the syringe at a very shallow angel with the bevel uppermost, the needle is introduced, intradermally. Care should be taken not to inject subcutaneously causing bleeding, or not to penetrate enough resulting in an exit puncture and leakage of antigen solution over the skin. Once the needle is in place the solution is gently injected & the skin should blanch and a small bleb is rainsed. Some of the antigen solution are painful on injection and the subject should be warned in advance to obviate inadvertent movements of the arm. When the needle is withdrawn, ideally there should be no bleeding at the site of injection indicating that dermal vessels have not been punctured. There may occasionally be very slight blood leakage with good technique but persistent oozing suggests that the injection has been subcutaneous and not intradermal; a false negative result may thus be obtained.

4. The test sites are examined 48 hours later. If problems are

expected in distinguishing Arthus reactions, the tests can be read at 6 and 24 hours.

5. Both erythema and induration are measured in mm. The response is not always symmetrical and irregular induration can be measured in two directions at right angles & the result averaged. A positive response is conventionally assessed as one giving 7.5 mm induration. Response can be graded with 3-4 mm = ±, 5-8mm = +, 9-11mm = + +, 12mm or more = + + + +.

Comments

There are no normal values as such available for skin test responses and there is very little information as to the percentage of normal population responding to the various antigens. It is for this reason that a battery of antigens is used with the expectation that, at least one positive result indicates normal cell mediated immunity.

It is conventional to mesure a positive response as one with 5 mm or more of induration, although again information is lacking as to the normal range of induration in those giving a positive response.

Elisa Test

The ELISA TEST (Enzyme linked immunosorbant assay) is one of the most widely employed variants of enzyme immunoassay. Enzyme immunoassays have emerged as quantitative techniques for detection of antigens, haptens and antibodies. They all employ various enzymes linked to either antigen or antibody as a label which can easily be detected by measurement of enzyme activity.

Principle: The ELISA assay can be used to measure either antigen or antibody. To measure antigen, the antibody is bound to solid phase, incubated with test serum and then a second enzyme labelled antibody is added, Substrate is then added and enzyme activity is related to antigen concentration.

Clinical Applications: In detection of HBs Ag, HCG levels in urine or blood, CEA levels, Steroid hormones, immunoglobulins, antibodies to bacteria, viruses, DNA and allergens.

Procedure

Material and Methods

1. **Test sample:** Serum sample stored at — 75°C till the time test is performed.

2. **Enzyme Conjugate:** Antibody to the specific antigen is conjugated to enzyme. The commonly used enzyme being horse–radish peroxidase. Other are alkaline phosphatase, Lysozyme and glucose-6 phosphate dehydrogenase. The enzyme is coupled to antigen or antibody by various cross–linking agents e.g. glutaral-dehyde and dimaleimide.

3. **Substrate —** Ortho phenylene diamine. (OPD) or 5—amino salicylic acid.

4. **Antibody Microtest Plate:** Precoating of antibody carried out in flat bottomed, 96 well microtest plates with specific dilution.

5. **Diluent:** Phosphate buffer saline (PBS) pH 7.2, 0.1 M or carbonate buffer pH 9.5 or Normal saline with 0.1% sodium azide.

Method

1. The antibody is diluted to 1:500 in PHS at pH 7.2 and 75 μm is added to the bottom of each well.
2. Incubate the plates at 4°C in a moist chamber overnight for 18-20 hrs.
3. Wash the plate three time with PBS supplemented with 0.05% Tween 20 (BS-T) for 5 minutes each.
4. Add 200 μl of 1% bovine serum albumin in each well and incubate overnight at 4°C in a moist chamber.

5. Add 25 μl of the test samples positive and negative control in to the test plates coated with antibody.
6. Incubate the plate for 2 hours at room temperature.
7. Wash three times with PBS—T and add 50 μl of peroxidase conjugated antibody to each well.
8. Incubate the plates at room temperature for 2 hours and wash five times with PBS—T.
9. Add 100 ml of freshly prepared substrate i.e. orthophenyl diamine in citrate buffer pH 5.0 and hydrogen peroxide.
10. After 30 minutes incubation at room temperature in a dark box, add 75 μl of 2 M Sulfuric acid to stop the reaction.
11. Add 75 μl of PBS to make final volume of reaction mixture as 250 μl.
12. A positive test is indicated by the production of yellow colour as a result of the product of enzyme reaction. This is read by the naked eye against a white background or by measuring the optical density at 492 nm in a spectro photometer using a microcuvette or a micro elisa reader.

Calculations

$$\frac{O.D. \text{ Test} - O.D. \text{ Blank II}}{O.D. \text{ Blank I} - O.D. \text{ Blank II}} = \frac{O.D. \text{ of sample}}{> O.D. \text{ mean}}$$

Interpretation of Results

A sample is labelled positive if the yellow colour is stronger than that of the negative control and if the optical density, measured as the ratio of test to negative control is more than 2:1

(O.D. of Blank I is the average optical density of 5—7 negative controls and O.D. of Blank II is the optical density of 100 μl substrate, 75 μl of 2M sulphuric acid and 75 μl of PBS)

A test sample with a ratio between 1.5 and 2.1 is repeated and if the ratio is still less than 2.1 the test should be considered negative.

Advantage of ELISA technique

1. Simple and easy to perform
2. Sensitivity at low cost,
3. Stability of reagents
4. Lack of radiation hazards
5. Potential for automation
6. Relatively inexpensive equipment.

EIA Assays Currently Available

1. Hepatitis	:	HBs Ag, anti-HBs Ag, Anti — HBc Ag, IgM anti — HBc Ag HBe/anti HBe, anti—HA V anti-Delta
2. Cancer	:	CEA, AFP, Beta HCG, Estrogen Receptor, TdT, PAP
3. STD	:	N. Gonorrhoeae Chlamydia Trachomatics
4. Infections	:	Rubella, Rotavirus cytomegalovirus, IgE, Toxo — G
5. Metabolic	:	Ferritin, Prealbumin
6. Thyroid	;	TSH
7. AIDS	:	HTLV — III

Useful Stock Solutions

1. Ficoll Hypaque

11. 40gm. of Ficoll is dissolved in 160ml. of distilled water. Add 40ml. of Conray 280
or
22ml. of Conray 420

2. Phosphate Buffers:

0.2 M—   Soln. A — Na_2HPO_4 — 14.32 gm/200ml.
           Soln. B — KH_2PO_4 — 5.44 gm/200 ml.
0.15 M — Soln A — Na_2HPO4, $12H2O$ — 53.70 gm/L
      30   Soln B — KH_2PO4 — 20.41 gm/1.

TABLE: 30

S.N.	SOLUTION (A) ml.	SOLUTION (B) ml.	pH
1.	0.25	9.75	5.29
2.	0.50	9.50	5.59
3.	1.0	9.0	5.91
4.	2.0	8.0	6.24
5.	3.0	7.0	6.47
6.	4.0	6.0	6.64
7.	5.0	5.0	6.81
8.	6.0	4.0	6.98
9.	7.0	3.0	7.17
10.	8.0	2.0	7.38
11.	9.0	1.0	7.73
12.	9.5	0.5	8.04

3. Phosphate buffered saline — (PBS) pH 7.2

18 ml. of 0.2M Soln. A
7 ml. of 0.2M Soln. B
4.38 gm Nacl.
   Add. distilled water to make upto 500ml.
   Store in refrigerator. Make a fresh every third day.

4. Hank's Solution:

1. 775ml. distilled water in a flask.
2. Dissolve by shaking after each addition — A
   80 gm. NaCl
   4 gm. KCl
   2 gm. Na_2HPO_4 $12H_2O$
   1 gm. KH_2PO_4
   (Slight heating may be used to dissolve the last two)
3. To 100 ml. distilled water, add 2 gm. $CaCl_2$ without heating.
Add to A — Gives B.
4. To 100 ml distilled water, add 2 gm. $MgSO_4$ without heating.
Add to B—Gives C.
5. Add 20gm Glucose to C — Gives D (Dissolve without heat)
6. To 25 ml. distilled water add 200 mg phenol red. Dissolve by
stirring & pulverising. Add to D & make volume to 1000ml. Filter
using a millipore filter. Store in refrigerator. Make a fresh after 2
— 3 weaks, unless sterile.
   For use dilute 1: 10 in distilled water & adjust pH with $NaHCO_3$
(2.8 gm/100ml).

5. Alsever's solution:—

For storing sheep red cells
24.6 gm glucose
9.6 gm Trisodium citrate (dihydrate)
5.04 gm NaCl.
Dissolve in 1200 ml. distilled water
Adjust pH to 6.1 with 10% citric acid.
Use 50 ml. of Alsever's solution for 50 ml. of whole blood.

116

SECTION V

BACTERIOLOGY

CHAPTER 17

INTRODUCTION TO MICROBIOLOGY

Compared to the wide spectrum of diseases to which mankind is exposed, we have knowledge about the etiopathogenesis of very few, of which one group is diseases caused by microbes.

The study of microbes is very important because diseases caused by microbes are potentially curable and preventable.

Microbiology has very close link with curative medicine in regard to the precise diagnosis and the rational treatment of disease which are:

A) Microbial — Caused by
1. Bacteria
2. Spirochaetes
3. Rickettsiae
4. Fungi
5. Viruses
6. Mycoplasma (PPLO Pleuropneumonia like organisms)
7. Chlamydiae
B) Parasitic — Caused by
1. Protozoa
2. Helminths

Before discussing further, certain terms in common use need be clarified.

1. **Saprophytes:** Organisms that grow on decaying matter.
2. **Parasites:** A microbe or larger specie that lives in or on and obtains its nourishment from a living host. Parasites may be:
i) Commensals — Constitute normal flors of body.
ii) Pathogens — microbes invading the tissues producing disease.
3. **Opportunistic Pathogens:** Commensals which, as and when body defences are impaired, may invade and cause disease.
4. **Toxins:** Poisonous substances, produced by microbes that cause manifestations of diseases.
5. **Infection:** The process of microbial invasion of the body is called infection.
6. **Infectious/Contagious Disease:** Infective diseases that are readily communicable from person to person.
7. **Sources of Infection:** Habitats in which the pathogens ordinarily grow and from which they are disseminated to susceptible hosts.
8. **Vehicles Of Infection:** Inanimate objects responsible for transfer of pathogens also called fomites e.g. Towels and Linen.
9. **Vectors:** Living organisms which transmit disease. Microbes are able to grow in the vectors.
10. **Zoonoses:** Infections prevalent primarily in animals, which accidentally are transmitted from animal to man but not back.
11. **Exogenous infection:** Infections from external sources.
12. **Endogenous infection:** Infection due to opportunistic invasion of tissues by a commensal.
Nosocomial infection: Hospital infection.
Infectivity: Ability of pathogenic microbes to initiate infection.
Virulence: A measure of the infectivity.

Invasiveness: Capacity of microbes to invade and multiply in healthy tissues.

SOURCES OF INFECTION

Exogenous
1. Patients
2. Carriers
   (a) Healthy carriers
   (b) Convalescent carriers
   (c) Contact carriers
   (d) Paradoxical carriers
3. Infected animals
4. Soil

Endogenous
1. Bowel e.g. E. Coli
2. Nasopharynx eg. Pneumococci

3. Skin e.g. staph albus
4. Nostrils e.g. staph aureus

MODES OF SPREAD

1. **Respiratory infection**
   i) Direct contact with infected secretion e.g. kissing/hugging.
   ii) Indirect contact involving fomites
   iii) Dustborne
   iv) Droplet spray

2. **Skin, Wound & burn infection**
   i) Contact — Direct, Indirect.
   ii) Dust borne
   iii) Contamination with droplets

3. **Venereal infection**
   i) Sexual intercourse
   ii) Communal use of bathing facilities and towels

4. **GIT infections**
   Transmission is by faeco-oral routes, may be:
   i) Water borne
   ii) Hand infection
   iii) Food borne
   iv) Vectors e.g. Housefly (Musca domestica)

5. **Arthropod borne blood infection**
   i) Mosquitoes (malaria, yellow fever)
   ii) Flea (Plague).
   iii) Louse (Epidemic typhus, European relapsing fever)
   iv) Tsetsefly (Trypanosomiasis).

6. **Laboratory infections**
   i) Artificial cultures.
   ii) Diagnostic/necropsy materials (Brucellae, Rickettsiae & Francisella tularensis are especially liable to cause laboratory infections).
   iii) Used syringes.
   iv) Blood and blood products.

CHAPTER 18

THE MICROSCOPE

MAGNIFICATION BY A MICROSCOPE

Magnification at 105 mm. Initial Magnification of the objective multiplied by the magnification of the eyepiece.

Objective (Focal length)	Magnification of the objective Eye-piece		Total Magnification
2/3 or 16mm	10	10x	100
1/6 or 4mm	45	10x	450
1/12 or 1.8mm	100	10x	1000

USE OF MICROSCOPE

Put the slide on the stage and focus under low power and then under high power or oil immersion as the case may be.

Focussing: At first use the coarse adjustment and then the fine (micrometer) adjustment. When examining a slide under low or high power, lower the condenser and work with concave mirror. In case of an unstained Specimen, close the diaphragm for better definition of the object. Diaphragm and condenser should be manipulated each time for critical illumination of the object to be examined.

USE OF OIL IMMERSION LENS

A suitable field is found under low power. A drop of oil placed, objective lowered until it is in contact with the oil and almost touches the slides. This is observed with the eye on the level with the stage. Then looking through the microscope the objective is raised by course adjustment until the object is in focus, final focussing is done by fine adjustment, immersion oil should always be removed after work is over with a little xylol. On no account use alcohol.

Causes of failures to focus under the oil-immersion
1. Quick movement of the coarse adjustment.
2. Viewing the wrong side of the slide.
3. Too thick a coverslip.

After working, immersion oil is removed with a little Xylol Never use alcohol.

DARK GROUND ILLUMINATION

The light which illuminates the object must not enter the objective directly. The only light admitted must be that which has been reflected by the object itself. A special condenser is used which allows a wide cone of light and then stops that portion which normally enters the front of the objective. The oblique rays which normally miss objective when scattered by the object, enter the objective to illuminate image of the specimen against an entirely dark background. It is used to examine organisms in living state without staining. It increases visibility without increase in resolving power.

CARE OF MICROSCOPE

(1) Keep it free from dust (2) Handle the microscope by the handle supporting the base with hand in an erect position (3) Avoid jerks (4) Draw tube may be used by a spiral motion (5) Systems should never be separated (6) Lens should be cleaned by Xylol (7) Oil Immersion lens must be cleaned after using

PROBLEM WHILE USING MICROSCOPE

1. Light too strong — Lower condenser
   too faint — 1. Use condenser of higher aperture
   2. Adjust Mirror.
2. Under Oil immersion the field appears dark with moving shadows of bubble of air in oil. Oil has left the space between the slide and lens.
3. Definition is poor: Objectives have been insufficiently cleaned. If speacks appear in field and float about they are usually in your eyes. If stationery but revolving with the eye piece, clean the eye piece. If they do not move they are due to dust on back of objectives.

SPECIAL TYPES OF MICROSCOPE

1. Phase contrast microscope

It is method of illumination which enables observation of entirely transparent objects without staining.

Principle: Ordinary specimens are visible because they have an amplitude or intensity contrast. Many specimens do not change the amplitude of light but change the phase of light waves. These phase changes are converted into amplitude changes which are visible to the eye. Special phase contrast apparatus in place of condenser and phase contrast objectives are required.

2. Electron Microscope

In principle it works by using light of shorter wave length to increase resolving power. A powerful electron beam is passed in vacuum through magnetic fields which replaces the usual optical system of the microscope and image of the material under examination is photographed. The lenses are circular electro magnets whose focus varies as the strength of applied magnetic field. A magnification of 10,000 to 50,000 can be obtained in practice and objects as small as 1–2 micron photographed.

3. Fluorescent Microscope

Some substances emit light when stimulated. The source of light is UV lamp or a carbon arc. The filter used in the system permits only short wave blue rays to fall on the object, if the object is autofluorescent, it emits colour. Alternatively the object can be stained by fluorescent dyes; Rhodamine, Auramine or Flurocin isothiocynate; making them visible under fluorescent microscope.

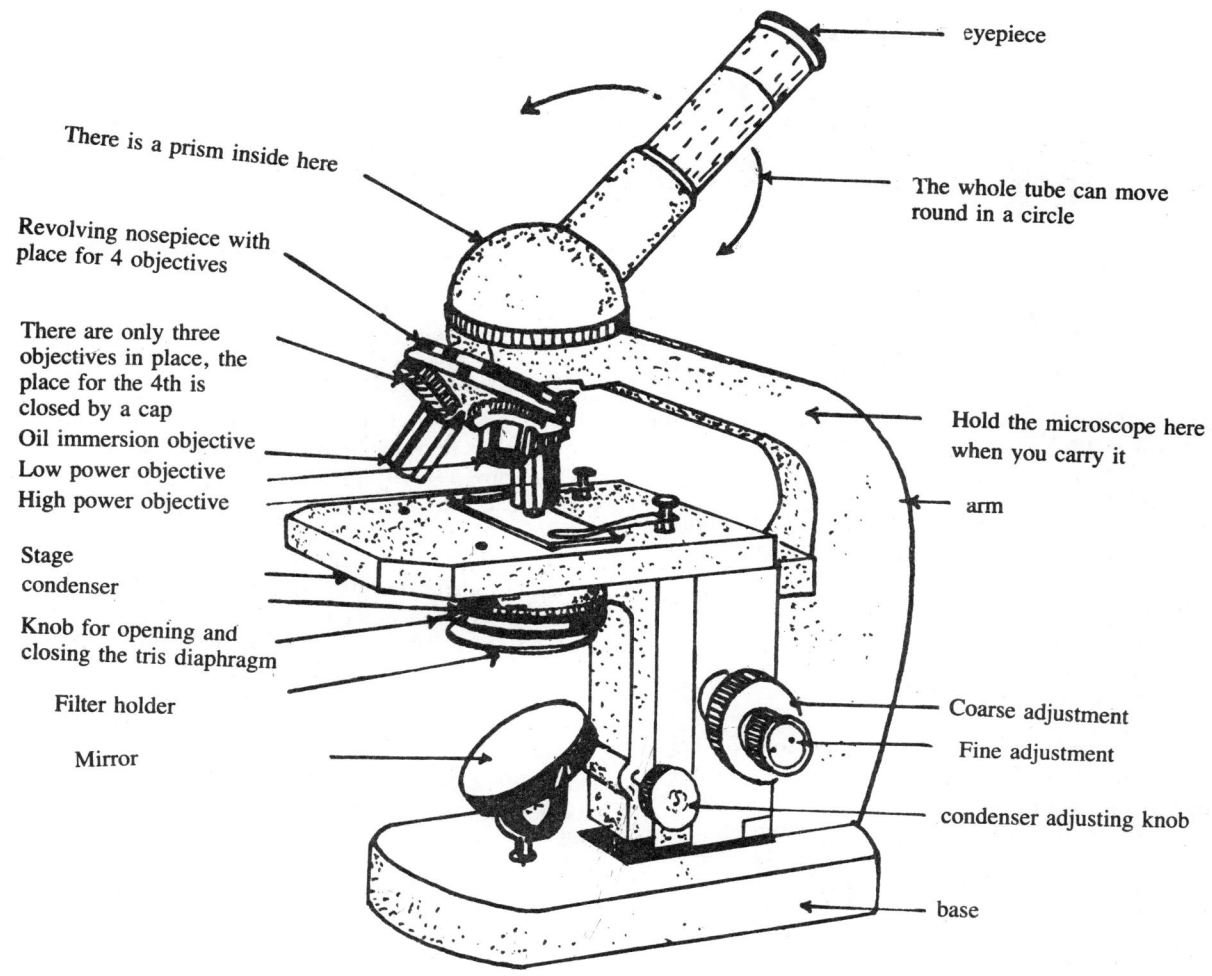

There is a prism inside here

Revolving nosepiece with place for 4 objectives

There are only three objectives in place, the place for the 4th is closed by a cap
Oil immersion objective
Low power objective
High power objective

Stage
condenser

Knob for opening and closing the tris diaphragm

Filter holder

Mirror

eyepiece

The whole tube can move round in a circle

Hold the microscope here when you carry it

arm

Coarse adjustment
Fine adjustment

condenser adjusting knob

base

DIAGRAM 1 The Microscope

The metnod is widely used for many immunological investigations.

MICROMETRY

Measurement of objects is important in microscopic work. Measurement methods are comparative methods so that degree of magnification is immaterial and need not be known.

Measurement by Means of Mechanical stage is used for objects not less than 100–200 microns.

SAFETY PRECAUTIONS IN THE LABORATORY

Over 4000 laboratory associated infections have been reported and many more still go unreported. Laboratory acquired infections may be different from natural infections in pathogenesis and clinical presentation.

Biosafety in a microbiological laboratory is very essential and basically depends on three components:

a) Basic standard of laboratory design, operation and equipment.
b) Selection and use of essential biosafety equipment.
c) Safe laboratory procedures.
Some practical and easily safe laboratory rules are:

i) Avoid mouth pipetting.
ii) Avoid smoking and eating in the laboratory.
iii) Decontaminate working are at least once a day.
iv) Wash hands with soap and water after handling infectious material.
v) Always wear laboratory coats in the laboratory only.
vii) Decontaminate all waste materials before disposal.
viii) Perform all technical procedures in a way to minimise aerosol formation.
ix) Provide adequate safety training to the laboratory staff.
x) Actively immunize the workers against specific diseses handled.

121

CHAPTER 19

EXAMINATION OF SPECIMENS FOR MICROBIOLOGICAL INVESTIGATION

Examination of specimens for this purpose are divided into three headings:
A.   Examination of Materials from Sites Normally Sterile
B.   Examination of Materials from Sites Possessing Normal Flora
C.   Examination of Pus from Abscesses and Swabs from Wounds

A.   EXAMINATION OF MATERIALS FROM SITES NORMALLY STERILE

1.   Blood Culture

i) Incubate the blood culture bottle containing blood sample at 37°C in an incubator till growth appears for a maximum of 7 days.
ii) After 24 hours incubation, a loop ful of material is cultured on blood agar and Mac-Conkeys' agar plate.
iii) Incubate the plates at 37°C overnight.
iv) Examine next day for growth. If growth is positive, proceed accordingly.
v) If no growth is obtained incubate culture plate for a further 24 hours.
vi) If still no growth inoculation of sample may be repeated after 7, 14 and 21 days of incubation of original sample.
vii) If still no growth, sample should be reported as sterile.

2.   Examination of Cerebral Fluid (C.S.F.)

i) **Macroscopic examination:** Examine and record appearance and volume of the fluid.
ii) **Microscopic examination:** If the clot is present transfer small pieces of clot on slide, tease it and let it dry. Then perform staining. If no clot is observed centrifuge a part of specimen under sterile conditions and make three smears from deposit, one each for gram staining, Leishman staining and Ziehl-Neelsen staining.
iii) **Cell Count:** Performed on an uncentrifuged specimen in Neubauer's chamber.
Culture: Culture should be done immediately on its arrival in the laboratory. Deposit is seeded on blood agar and chocolate agar, incubated in presence of 5–10% CO_2 achieved by keeping a lighted candle and closing the lid. The uncentrifuged fluid should be incubated overnight. When the primary culture is sterile, it may be possible to recover pathogen by repeating culture from incubated fluid.

3.   Examination of Serous Fluids

Various fluids include pleural, pericardial, ascitic, synovial and hydrocoele fluids.
i) Describe volume, color and appearance. Look for sulphur granules.
ii) Centrifuge, deposit is used for staining.

iii) Culture on Mac Conkey Plate, two blood agar plates and a tube of Robertsons meat medium. Incubate one blood agar plate anaerobically.
iv) Examine culture plates and proceed accordingly.

4.   Examination of Urine

For diagnosis of urinary tract infection the presence of pus cells in the urine is important but more than half the patients of U.T.I. may not show a state of pyuria. A count of over 10^5 bacteria per ml is significant and indicates urinary tract infection. A count of less than 10^5 ml. is considered to be due to contamination.

Culture of urine sample should be done within one hour of collection, otherwise refrigerate at 4°C.

Use bacteriological loop with 4mm internal diameter. Inoculate one loopful, each on blood agar and MacConkey plates. Incubate at 37°C overnight. Examine for bacterial growth. Count number of colonies and give the count as:

No. of colonies × 100 = No. of Bacteria/ml. If the growth is confluent, it is always significant. If no growth occurs in 24 hours and if still no growth is observed report as sterile after 48 hours. If repeated cultures are sterile, isolate for Mycobacterium tuberculosis.

B.   EXAMINATION OF MATERIALS FROM SITES POSSESSING NORMAL FLORA

The processing of specimen from sites which are normally not sterile differs in the following ways:
a) Direct microscopic examination of the material is not very conclusive except Mycobacterium tuberculosis in sputum or corynebacterium in throat swab.
b) Isolation of the pathogens which are less in number becomes difficult so invariably enrichment media have to be used.
c) The skill to distinguish normal flora from the pathogens on the basis of colony characterisitics needs to be developed.

1.   Gastrointestinal Tract

a) **Macroscopic examination:** Make gross examination of stool, noting color, consistency and presence of blood or excess mucus.
b) **Microscopic examination:** Make a light emulsion of stool in saline. Look for blood, pus, ova and cysts. Gram staining is of little value.
c) **Culture procedure:** Inoculate a sample of faeces onto several types of solid media and into fluid enrichment medium. On the third day, suspicious colonies can be inoculated alternatively into this system and confirmed by serology.

First Day
a) Plate on bile — lactose media (Mac Conkey and Blood Agar)

122

b) inoculate small piece into selenite F broth or GN broth.

Second Day

c) After overnight incubation at 37°C, examine blood agar plate for staphylococci & candida. Transfer non-lactose fermenting colonies from bile-lactose media to a set of five tubes, one tube each of SIM medium, Koser's citrate, urea agar and Russle's double sugar agar and small tube with charcoal gelatin disc in 1 ml of peptone water.

d) Subculture selenite F broth or GN broth to bile lactose medium.

Third Day

e) Note the pattern of reaction in five tubes. If reactions are suggestive of salmonella or shigella, perform slide agglutination test.

f) Inoculate non-lactose fermenters from step (d) into sets of five tubes.

Fourth Day

g) Read reactions from procedure (e). Complete identification may be made at this stage.

h) Read the five tubes from step (f) and if indicated, inoculate as in (e) and continue as in (g). If there is possibility of staphylococci or clostridial food poisoning, stool should be treated accordingly.

2. **Female Genital Tract**

Studied under 3 headings

a) **Acute Cervicitis and Vaginitis:** If clinically gonorrhoea is suspected a swab is obtained and inoculated into Thayer-Martin medium.

b) **Chronic Vaginitis:** A saline soaked swab should be taken. Make a hanging drop preparation. Look for Trichomonas vaginalis. Examine gram stained film. If positive for T. vaginalis, culture in special media for this. For bacterial and fungal causes, plate the Swabs onto blood agar, Mac Conkey and Transgow media. Examine after 24 hours of incubation at 37 degree C.

c) **Puerperal Sepsis and Septic Abortion:** A high vaginal swab is taken, smear is made, examined for streptococci, gram-positive rods and pus cells. Plating is made onto 2 blood agar plates (One for Anaerobic culture), a Mac-Conkey plate and Robertsons meat medium. Incubate blood agar and Mac-Conkey agar plates at 37°C. Look for growth the next day. Normal flora is excluded.

3. **Sputum**

The objective of culturing the sputum is to diagnose bacterial infection of lung. Open case of pulmonary tuberculosis can be diagnosed by direct microscopy.

Select purulent or bloody flecks and transfer a loopful to a clean slide, press another slides over it. Press the slide together and then pull them apart. Flame both slides after drying. Stain by gram's stain and look for bacteria. Inoculate a blood agar and MacConkey agar plate with a small loopful of sputum specimen. Put blood agar plate in a candle jar. If incubated plates show no acceptable pathogens, subculture meat medium both aerobically and anaerobically. If no growth, re-examine meat medium by gram stain and re-culture if necessary.

Processing of Sputum for AFB: A biological safety cabinet (U.V. sterilized) is used. Small portion of the material is transfer-red to a clean slide. Prepare the smear with a bacteriological loop or by pressing glass slide on it. Label the slides, air dry and flame immediately.

Stain by Ziehl Neelsen's stain.

Examine under oil immersion.

Culture: Mix equal volumes of sputum and 3–4% sodium hydroxide containing 0.004% phenol red in a centrifuge tube. Centrifuge at 3000 rpm for 20–30 minutes. Discard supernatant. Add 2N HCl dropwise from a pipette to achieve yellow end point. Add 4% NaOH to get faint pink end point. Inoculate two slants of L-J medium. Observe culture every week. If there is growth around 3–4 weeks, stain by Z–N stain. Discard the tube after ten weeks if there is no growth.

4. **Throat Swab/Nasal Swab**

Inoculate blood agar and Mac Conkey agar by rolling the swab over small portion of agar surface and by streaking a sterile wire loop to develop isolate colonies. Incubate at 37°C aerobically overnight. Examine plates next morning for the presence of pathogens.

5. **Nasopharyngeal Swab**

It is especially useful in study of meningo coccal carriers where throat swab is not satisfactory.

Seed blood agar and chocolate agar preferably on bedside. Incubate these plates in air plus 10% CO_2 at 37°C. If growth is obtained, proceed for further identification.

6. **Skin**

General procedure of skin culture involves inoculating skin onto a portion of blood agar, Mac-Conkey and colistin — nalidixic acid agar plate. Make incisions into surfaces of plates for demonstration of haemolysis. Incubate at 37°C for 24 to 48 hours. If positive growth, perform subculture for identification.

7. **Conjunctiva Culture**

These are best taken with a sterile bacteriologic loop and plated directly on chocolate and blood agar plates incubated in 10% CO_2. Viral inclusions are shown by Giemsa stain in inclusion conjunctivitis.

8. **Male Urethral Discharge**

Urethral Discharge from patients with urethritis is used for making smears directly on slide. After heat fixation, stain by Gram's method. Presence of gram negative diplococci is strongly suggestive of gonorrhoea. Culture on chocolate agar and incubate in 10% CO_2.

C. EXAMINATION OF PUS FROM ABSCESS AND WOUNDS

Procedure: A gross examination is made for volume, colour and consistency. A gram film preparation is made. Examine for pus cells and bacteria. A Z-N preparation should also be made. A drop of pus should be mixed with 10% potassium hydroxide for fungi. Plate out on blood agar and Mac-Conkey plate and inoculate meat medium. Incubate one blood agar plate anaerobically.

The plates are examined after 24–48 hours of incubation at 37°C. If positive growth, then identification is carried out by subcultures and gram's staining.

If plates are found to be sterile, further aerobic and anaerobic subcultures are made from meat medium.

CHAPTER 20

STERILIZATION AND DISINFECTION

DEFINITIONS

1. Sterilization : Sterilization is the freeing of an article from all living organisms including bacteria and their spores.
2. Disinfection : Disinfection is a process having a narrow spectrum of activity, effective principally on non acid fast vegetative organisms and with an uncertain action on bacterial endospores.

STERILIZATION AND DISINFECTION

PHYSICAL METHODS	CHEMICAL METHODS
1 **Heat:** (a) Dry heat	**1 Bactericidal**
1. Flaming	
2. Hot air oven	
3. Red heat	**2 Bacteriostatic**
(b) Wet heat	
2 **Radiation:** (a) Inonizing	
(b) Nonionizing	
3 **Filteration**	

Note: Sterilization in the strict sense is effected only by physical means. Chemical means are effective only in certain cases in which physical means cannot be employed.

1. STERILIZATION BY HEAT

Heat is the most certain method of sterilization. Sterilization by heat can be effected in 2 ways:
- A. Dry Heat
- B. Wet Heat

A. Sterilization by Dry Heat

It is suitable for glassware, syringes, metal instruments, paper-wrapped goods which are not spoiled by high temperature and water impermeable oils, waxes and powders. It can be done in 5 ways:

i) **Red Heat:** This is done by holding articles, in the flame of burner until hot.

ii) **Flaming:** Here sterilization is effected by passing the article through the bunsen flame without allowing it to become red hot.

iii) **Burning of Sprit:** It is not an effective method.

iv) **Hot Air Oven:** This allows controlled application of dry heat.

It is the best method for sterilizing dry glassware such as test-tubes, petri-dishes, flask, pipettes and instruments, such as forceps, scalpels, throat swabs and assembled all glass syringes; dry materials sealed in containers and powders, fats, oils and greases that are impermeable to moisture.

Glass-ware should be perfectly dry. Before sterilization plug test-tubes and flasks with cotton wool stoppers. Other glassware may be wrapped in kraft paper or sterilized metal cans. Time the holding period of 1 hr. at 160 degree C when the thermometer first shows that oven air is at 160°C

v) **Infra-Red Radiation:** Infra-radiation generates high temperatures and can be employed in central sterile supply departments only.

B. Sterilization by Moist Heat

Moist heat can be employed in 3 ways.
- i) At temperatures below 100°C.
- ii) At temperatures of 100°C.
- iii) At temperatures above 100°C.

i) **At Temperatures Below 100°C:** These are not reliable. Best known is pasteurization of milk. Vaccines prepared from cultures may be sterilized in a special bath (Vaccine bath) at a comparatively low temperature, 1 hour at 60°C being usually sufficient.

ii) **Moist Heat at a Temperature of 100°C:** It can be done in 2 ways:

a) **Boiling at 100°C:** Boiling at 100°C for a minimum of 10 mins. is sufficient to kill all non-sporing and many, but not all sporing organisms.

b) **Steaming at 100°C:** Pure steam in equilibrium with water boiling at normal atmosphere pressure has normally, a temperature of 100°C. Steaming at 100°C. is employed commonly for culture. There are 2 ways:

1. **By a Single Exposure at 100°C for 90 Mins:** The spores of some thermophilic and rare mesophilic bacteria survive this treatment.

2. **Tyndallization:** Intermittent exposure at 100 degree C for 20–45 mts. on 3 successive days. First exposure kills the vegetative forms. Between heating the spores become vegetative forms which are killed during subsequent heating.

iii) **Moist Heat above 100°C or Sterilization in Autoclave:** Water boils when its vapour pressure equals the pressure of atmosphere. Thus when pressure is increased water boils at a higher temperature thereby raising the temp. of steam above 100°C. It is especially suitable for culture media. aqueous solns, the steam preventing evaporation during heating. In the autoclave all parts of the load must be permeated by steam. Once heated up, there is a minimum holding time, given as follows:

Pressure lb/in^2	Temperature In C	Holding Time In minutes
0	100	—
10	115	45
15	121	18
30	134	3

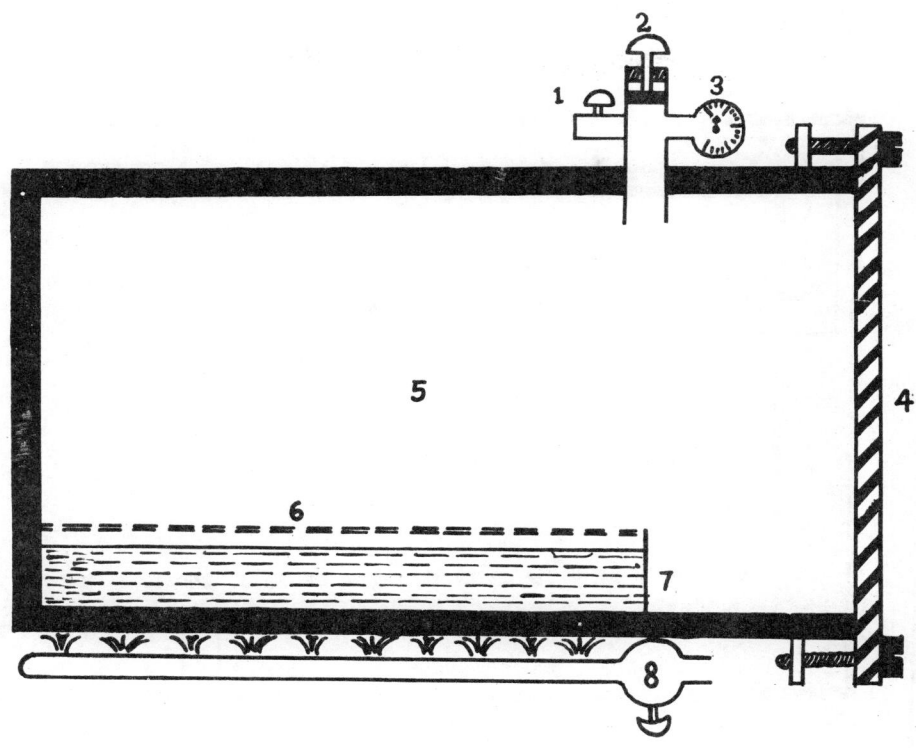

DIAGRAM 2 Simple Non Jacketed Autoclave.

1. Chamber discharge tap.
2. Adjustable safety valve.
3. Pressure gauge.
4. Chamber door.
5. Chamber.
6. Perforated tray.
7. Water.
8. Gas Burner

a) **Simple Non Jacketed Laboratory Autoclave:**
It is of two types:
1. Horizontal type.
2. Vertical type.
Both are pressure cooker types and have a similar basic structure.

Deficiencies of Simple Autoclave: The mothod of air discharge is inefficient. It also lacks means for drying the load after sterilization.

b) **Steam Jacketed Autoclave With Automatic Air and Condense Discharge:** Most are horizontal cylinders or rectangles (20″ × 50″) of rustless metal e.g. monel metal. Rectangular chambers are more conveniently loaded. At the front is a swing door, fastened by a capstan head which operates radial bolts and automatically remains locked while the chamber pressure is raised.

C. HIGH PREVACUUM STERILIZERS

They are the most advanced surgical sterilizers. They are equipped with electrically driven pumps capable of exhausting the chamber almost to a perfect vacuum, thus removing about 98% of the air. The absence of air enables the steam to penetrate very rapidly and heat up all parts of the load.

1) Autoclave Control and Sterilization Indicators

1. **Automatic process control:** It carries out the whole sterilization cycle.

2. **Recording thermometer:** It makes a graphic timed record of temperature changes

3. **Thermocouble:** It discovers the heating up time required for a given kind of load.

4. **Chemical indicators:** Browne's sterilizer control tubes used contain a red solution which turns green when heated at 115 degree C for 25 minutes (Type-I) o 15 min (Type-II) or at 160 degree for 60 minutes (Type-III).

5. **Adhesive tape:** Brown Bowie Dick autociare tape test for steam penetration is used extensively.

6. **Spore indicators:** A preparation of dried bacterial spores in placed within the load in the autoclave and after autoclaving is tested for viability e.g. Bacillus stearothermophilus spores are killed at 121°C in about 12 mins. The indicators are placed in the centre of the largest and most densely packed items of the load and some in the coolest part.

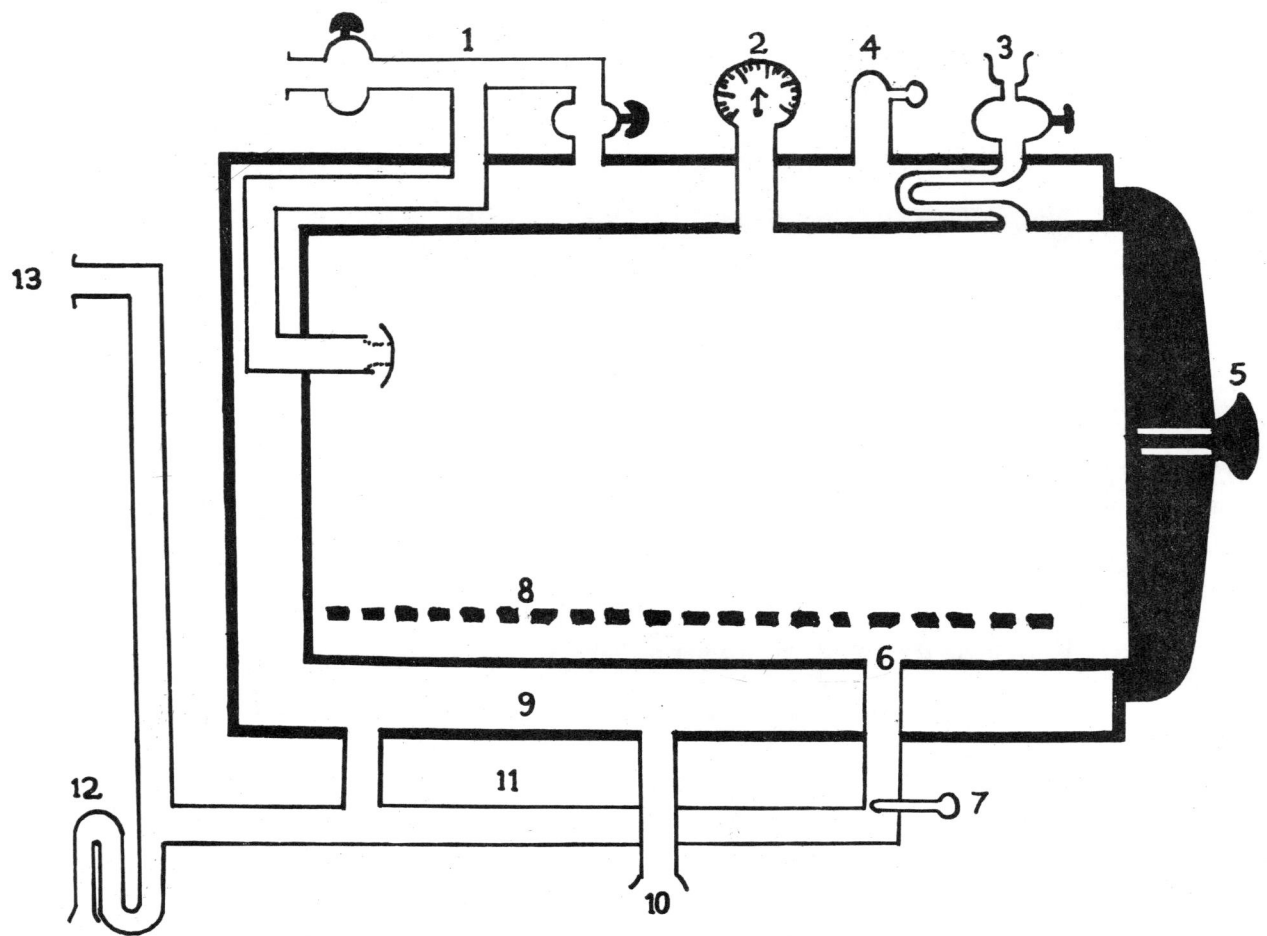

DIAGRAM 3 Steam Jacketed Autoclave
1. Venturi Tube.
2. Pressure gauge.
3. Air filter intake.
4. Safety Valve.
5. Chamber door.
6. Discharge channel.
7. Thermometer.
8. Perforated tray.
9. Jacket.
10. Steam supply.
11. Jacket steam trap.
12. Drain.
13. Discharge to atmosphere.

2) Sterilization by Radiation

Ultraviolet Radiation: Effectiveness of U.V. light increases with decrease in wave-length.

UV radiation is equally effective against Gram positive and Gram negative bacteria, spores are 10 times and viruses are 200 times more resistant.

But UV radiation has a low to nil penetrating power.

Ionizing Radiation: They are not used because they cause mutations and are not safe for workers.

3) Sterilization by Filtration

Filtration is the only means of sterilizing heat labile fluids e.g.:
i) Serum
ii) Antibiotic solution.
iii) Some culture media.

The British Pharmaceutical codex test for bacteria proof filters requires that efficient filters should be able to return serratia marcesciens. This indicates a diameter of 0.75 m or less.

However sterilizing filters render a liquid bacteria free but not virus-free.

Types of Filters

i) **Earthenware Candles:** They are of 3 types.
a) Berkefeld filters.
b) Mandler filter
c) Chamberland filters
These filters may be used for the removal of organisms from fluid cultures to obtain the bacterial toxin.

ii) **Asbestos or Seitz Filter:** These consist of a disc of an asbestos composition through which fluid is passed. The discs are available in three grades namely:
a) K or Clarifying
b) N or Normal
c) EK or special.

iii) **Sintered Glass Filters:** They are made of finely ground glass fused sufficiently to make the small particles adhere.

iv) **Cellulose Membrane Filters:** Three types are available:
a) Gradocol membranes
b) Modern membrane filters.
c) Oxoid membrane filters made of cellulose acetate. They are much less adsorptive and rate of filtration is much greater. Also

bacteria retained on the surface of a membrane filter can be grown by placing in a culture media.

Technique of Filtration: As fluids do not readily pass through filters by gravity, it is necessary to use positive or negative pressure. Suction is the most convenient method of filtration, the fluid being drained into a sterile filtering flask, which is a conical flask of thick glass with a side-arm.

A negative pressure of about 100–200 mm of mercury is applied

4) Chemical Methods

1. **Acids:**

   i) **Inorganic Acids:**
      a) Boric Acid: 2–3% aq. soln.,
         Dusting powder and Borax -glycerine.
         Bacteriocidal & antifungal.
      b) Chromic Acid: Powerful germicide.

   ii) **Organic Acids:**
      a) Benzoic acid   Anti fungal and Bacteriocidal plus
      b) Salicylic acid   Keratolytic action
      c) Mandelic Acid
      d) Nalidixic acid

2. Alkalies NaOH and KOH

Potent germicides used to disinfect excreta samples, sputum samples, effective against all forms of life.

3. Alcohols

i) Ethanol: Maximum activity at 70% concentration. Ineffective against spore forms.

ii) Isopropyl alcohol: More potent than ethanol.

4. Aldehydes

i) Formaldehyde: This irritant water soluble gas is highly lethal to all kinds of microbes and spores.
   a) Disinfection with formalin: Commercial formalin is a 40% solution of HCHO in H_2O, containing 10% Methanol.
   b) Disnfection by HCHO gas: Atmosphere must have a RELATIVE HUMIDITY OF 60%, a temperature of 18 degree C. Conc. should be 2mg/litre of air. It is used to disinfect Blankets, mattresses, rooms, operation theatres and smaller articles like hair brushes.

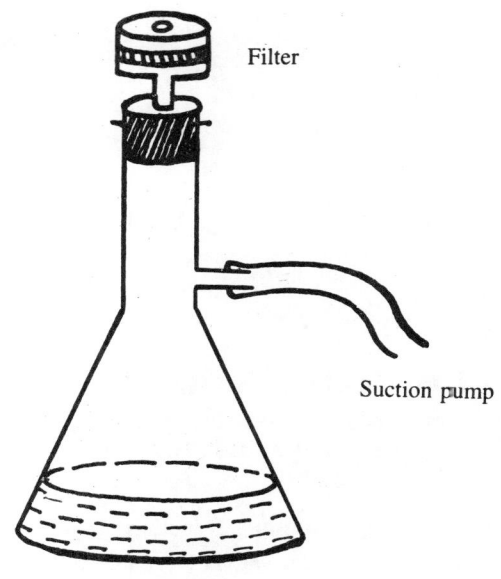

DIAGRAM 4

ii) Glutaraldehyde: Less irritant than HCHO.

iii) Methenamine

5. Phenols and Derivatives

   i) Phenol: Oldest antiseptic, introduced by Joseph Lister. It is outdated.

   ii) Cresol: Ortho-para-methyl derivative of phenol. Used as 0.1% soln.

   iii) Lysol: Cresol on saponification gives lysol. Used as 3% soln.

   iv) Chlorzylenol (Dettol): 1–1.5% Skin antiseptic prior to surgery. 6% Sterilization of surgical instruments

   v) Picric Acid: Trichlorophenol.

   vi) Hexylresorcinol: Weak antiseptic.

   vii) Thymol.

   viii) Bithinol.

   ix) Hexachlorophane: It is a Chlorinated phenol.

   x) Chlorehexidine: Contains Cetrimide as well.

   xi) Hycolin: 2% hycolin is suitable as a disinfectant in hospitals.

CHAPTER 21

IDENTIFICATION OF BACTERIA AND PREPARATION OF CULTURE MEDIA

IDENTIFICATION OF BACTERIA

There are numerous methods on the basis of which bacteria can be differentiated and identified. They together form a complete system of identification.

i) Morphology and Staining Reactions

A Gram stained smear shows the (i) Gram reaction; (ii) Size; (iii) Shape and (iv) grouping

A hanging drop preparation may be used to demonstrate motility.

ii) Cultural Characters

Including growth requirements and appearance of cultures to the naked eye. Attention is paid to; (a) Size of colonies; (b) outline of colonies; (c) elevation; (d) translucency; (e) Colour and (f) Hemolysis on Blood Agar.

iii) Biochemical Reactions

a) **Fermentation reactions:** It depends on whether or not a bacterial growth in a liquid medium will ferment particular sugar. There may be production of acid or of acid plus gas.

b) Tests dependent on particular end products: Indole, H_2S and nitrities, in certain bacteria.

c) **Certain enzymatic activities:** Such as oxidase, catalase, urease, gelatinase, collagenase, lecithinase or lipase.

d) **Specialised techniques:** Thin layer chromatography (TLC) and gas liquid chromatography.

iv) Antigenic Characters

Species can be identified by specific antibody reactions observed in serological tests.

v) Fluorescence Microscopy and Fluorescent Antibody Procedures

When certain dyes are exposed to UV light, they absorb energy and emit visible light. Such a dye is said to fluoresce. When tissue cells or organisms are stained with such a dye and examined with UV light they are seen as fluorescent.

Antibody molecules can be labelled by conjugation with such a dye. When fluorescent antibody is allowed to react with homologous antigen on a cell surface, this direct immunofluorescence procedure affords a highly sensitive method for identification.

vi) Typing of Bacteria

The typing of strains may depend upon special biochemical or serological tests or highly specialized bacteriophage and bacteriocin typing.

vii) Animal Pathogenicity and Toxigenicity

In case of certain organisms the inoculation test provides a reliable method of identification. In case of involved toxins, by use of specific neutralising antisera identification is highly specific.

viii) Antibiotic Specificity

The organism is tested for its ability to grow on artificial nutrient media containing different concentrations of antibiotics, thereby determining the minimum inhibitory concentration.

GENERAL TYPES OF MEDIA

1. Defined Synthetic Media

They are prepared exclusively from pure chemical substances and their exact composition is known. It is of two types:

a) **Simple synthetic media:** They contain a carbon and energy source, an inorganic source of N.P.S. and various inorganic salts in a buffered aqueous solution.

b) **Complex synthetic media:** Incorporate in addition to basic necessities, certain amino acids, purines, pyrimidines and other growth factors.

2. Routine Laboratory Media

a) **Basal media:** eg. nutrient broth and peptone water are simple routine media and are called basal media;

b) **Enriched media:** Prepared to maintain the nutritional requirements of more exacting.

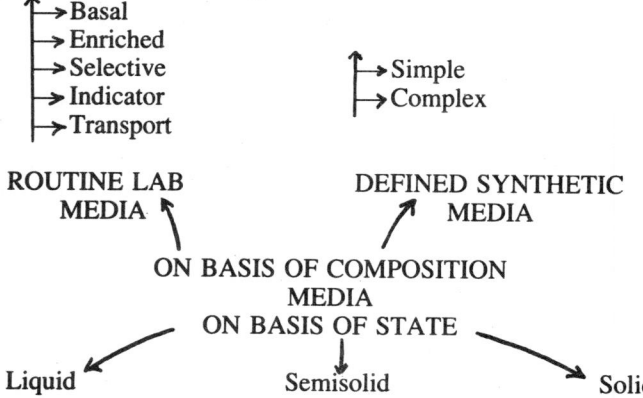

Liquid media are disadvantageous because growth exhibit no speficity and organisms cannot be separated.

Substances used to solidify media

i) Gelatin

ii) Pieces of potato impregnated with nutrient solutions.

iii) Coagulated serum
iv) Inspissated egg
v) Agar

c) **Selective media:** Contains substances that inhibit all but a few bacteria. An enrichment medium is liquid selective medium.

d) **Indicator media:** Incorporate substances that change visibly as a result of metabolic activities of particular organisms.

e) **Transport media:** Used to sustain sensitive organisms for a short period.

CONTAINERS FOR MEDIA AND CULTURES

Flasks stoppered with cotton wool, test tubes stoppered with cotton wool or with slip-on metal caps, and Screw capped bottles of different capacity and shape can be used as containers of media and cultures. Glassware must be thoroughly cleaned before use for culture media and new glassware requires special treatment to remove free alkali. Sterilization of glassware is brought about by dry heat in a hot air oven.

The use of plastic petri-dishes e.g. sterilin, Dyos is a substantial saving of labour since they are supplied sterile by the manufacturer and are disposable after one use.

Common ingredients of culture media

i) **Water:** Tape water is suitable if low in mineral content. But otherwise glass distilled water may be used.

ii) **Agar:** It is prepared from a variety of sea-weeds. The product is available as dried strands or powder. At concentrations normally used most bacteriological agars melt at about 95°C & solidify only when cooled to about 42°C. Main agars used are:
Japanese agar in conc. of 2% and
Newzealand agar in conc. of 1.2%.

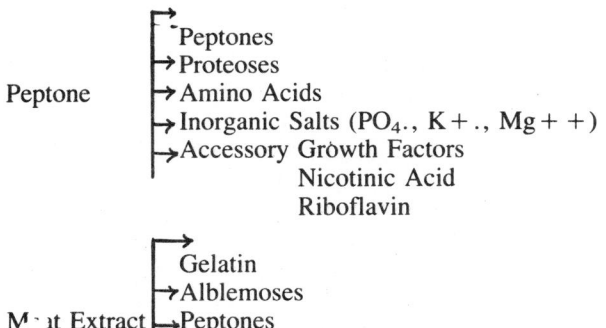

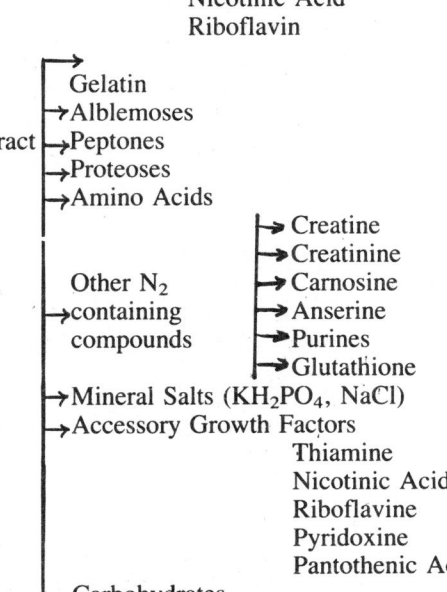

iii) **Peptone:** It consists of water soluble products obtained from lean meat or other protein material, such as heart msl, by digestion with proteolytic enzymes.

iv) **Casein Hydrolysate:** It consists largely of amino-acids obtained by hydrolysis of milk protein casein.

v) **Meat Extract:** Finely divided lean beef is held in boiling water for a short time. After removal of extra fat, it is concentrated by evaporation to a dark viscid paste containing 70–80% solids.

vi) **Yeast Extract:** Commercial yeast extract is prepared from washed cells of brewers or bakers yeast.

vii) **Blood:** Blood for use must be collected with aseptic precautions, from man, horse, rabbits or sheep.

viii) **Fildes Peptic Digest of Blood:** It is better because peptic digestion of blood liberates nutrients from red cells.
Saline 0.85% + HCl + Defibrinated sheep blood + Pepsin

Heat at 55°C for 2 hrs
+ 20% acq. NaOH
+ HCl drop by drop
+ Chloroform → Shake Vigorously

ix) **Serum:** Serum obtained is sterilized by filtration through a seitz-filter.

COMMON MEDIA IN USE IN LABORATORIES

1. **Nutrient Broth:** It is of 3 types
i) Meat infusion broth consisting of a watery extract of lean meat to which peptone is added.
ii) Meat extract broth prepared as a mixture of commercial peptone and meat extract.
iii) Digest broth consisting of a watery extract of lean meat that has been digested with a proteolytic enzyme so that additional peptone is not required.

2. **Nutrient Agar:** Nutrient agar is nutrient broth solidified by the addition of agar.

3. **Semi Solid Agar:** Agar is added to media concentrations too low to solidify them.

4. **Peptone Water:** It is used as basal medium for carbohydrate fermentation tests and formation of indole.

10 gm Peptone + 5 gm NaCl, 1 litre Warm Water, pH 7.4–7.5 → Filter → Autoclave for 15 minutes

5. **Blood Agar:** It is especially suitable for gonnococcus and other delicate pathogens. It is also an indicator medium showing hemolysis. The medium is prepared by adding sterile blood to sterile nutrient agar that has been melted and cooled to 50°C. Blood is used at a conc. of 10%.

6. **Chocolate Agar:** It is suitable for H. influenzae. During heating red cells are ruptured & nutrients are liberated. It is prepared by heating 10% of sterile blood in sterile nutrient agar at 75°C.

7. **Serum Agar:** It is prepared by adding 10% of sterile serum to sterile nutrient agar that has been melted and cooled to 50°C. It is generally used as slopes.

STAINING PROCEDURES

As bacteria consist of clear protoplasmic matter, it is difficult with ordinary microscope to see them in the unstained condition.

Staining, is therefore, of primary importance for the recognition of bacteria.

METHODS OF MAKING FILM OR SMEAR PREPARATION

Film preparations are made either on cover slips or on $3 \times 1''$ glass slides, usually the latter. It is essential that the coverslips or slides should be perfectly clean or free from grease, otherwise, films will be uneven.

For ordinary use, wipe the slide with a clean dry cotton cloth and then, holding its end with forceps roast it free from grease by passing it 6–12 times through a Bunsen's flame.

Alternatively moisten the finger with water, rub on the surface of a fine sand soap and then smear the surface of the slide. After removing the soapy film with a clean cloth, the surface is clean and free from grease.

The slides should not be cleaned and used again since it is difficult to ensure that all organisms are removed.

Coverslips should be 3/4 or 7/8 inches square and 0.1 mm thick. They are cleaned by the dichromate sulphuric acid solution. They are then well washed first in tap water and then in distilled water and stored in stoppered jar in 50% alcohol.

PREPARATION OF FILMS

In the case of fluid material, loopful is taken up, spread thinly on the slide. The slide is then dried by keeping it high on a Bunsen flame. The film is then dried by heating through the glass slide.

Solid Material: Cultures on agar. A loopful clean water is placed on the slide. The loop is then sterilized and a minute quantity of material is transferred to the drop, thoroughly emulsified and mixture is spread evenly on the slide. The film is then fixed and dried as above.

A. Simple Stains

These show not only the presence of organisms but also the nature of cellular content in exudates. Commonly used one are as follows:

i) **Methylene blue:**
Saturated solution of loffler's
Methylene blue in alcohol.
Procedure
1. Stain for 3 min. with methylene blue stain.
2. Wash with water.
3. Examine directly or after mounting in glycerine.

ii) **Dilute Carbol Fuchsin**
Ziehl-Neelsen's stain diluted with water, 10–15 times its valume.
Procedure
1. Stain for 10–15 sees.
2. Wash well with water.
3. Airdry and examine directly.

B. Gram's Staining Method

A.	Methyl Violet	— 0.5 gm
	Distilled Water	— 100 ml
B.	Iodine	— 1.0 gm
	Potassium Iodide	— 2.0 gm
	Distilled Water	— 100 ml

Grind potassium iodide and iodine in a mortar and dissolve in not more than 20 ml of distilled water. Make up to 100 ml with distilled water. Store in coloured glass bottles.

C.	Basic fuchsin	— 0.1%
	Or safranine	— 0.5%

Basic Fuchsin: Dissolve 0.1 gm basic fuchsin in 10 ml alcohol, allow to stand over night and make volume to 100 ml with distilled water.

Safranin: Grind 0.5 gm Safranine in 10 ml alchol and make up the volume to 100 ml with distilled water.

Procedure

i) Cover the slide with methyl violet solution and allow to act for about 10 seconds.
ii) Pour off stain and wash with Gram's iodine solution thoroughly.
iii) Cover the whole slide with Gram's iodine solution and leave it for about 2 minutes.
iv) Decolorize with acetone (100 percent). Decolorization is very rapid and complete in 2–3 seconds. After this period of contact, wash thoroughly with water under a running tap, which should be running before the acetone is applied to the slide.
v) Wash with water.
vi) Apply counterstain for 20–30 seconds.
vii) Wash with water and dry between blotting paper.
viii) Examine under oil immersion without mounting.

Results: Gram positive bacteria are stained violet while Gram negative are Reddish pink.

C. Ziehl-Neelsen Method: Used for staining acid fast bacilli

Preparation of solutions

1. Ziehl — Neelsen's (Strong) carbol fuchsin

Basic fuchsin	—	10 gm
Absolute Ethanol	—	100 ml
5% Solution of Phenol (in water)	—	1000 ml

Dissolve the dye in alcohol and add to the phenol solution.
2. Sulphuric Acid — 20% solution
Place 800 ml water in a large flask. Add 200 ml Conc. Sulphuric Acid — about 50 ml at a time, gently puring down the side 10% and 5% are also used in special situations mentioned elsewhere in the text.
3. Alcohol — 95%
4. Counterstain Loffler's methylne blue or Malachite green

Procedure

1. Cover slide with carbol fuchsin and heat until steam rises. Allow to stain for 5 min., heat being applied at intervals to keep stain hot. The stain must not be allowed to evaporate dry.
2. Wash with water.
3. Cover with 20% sulphuric acid. Red colour of the preparation is changed to yellowish brown. After about a minute in acid, wash with water and pour more acid — Repeat till, the film is very faintly pink.
4. Treat with 95% alcohol for 2 minutes.
5. Wash well with water.
6. Counter stain with loffler's methylene blue or dilute malchite green for 15–20 seconds.
7. Wash, blot, dry and mount as mentioned.

Results: Acid fast bacilli stain bright red and the background tissue, cells and other organisms are stained blue or green.

Modification of Ziehl — Neelsen Method

1. Leprosy bacilli are also acid fast, but usually to a less degree so that 5% sulphuric acid is used for decolorization.
2. Actinomcyes and Nocardia can be treated with 1 percent H_2SO_4 to demonstrate the acid fastness.
3. Cultures of some Nocardia are acid fast with 0.5 percent H_2SO_4.
4. **Brucella differential stain:** Dilute (1 in 10) Carbol fuchsin, allow to stain without heat for 15 min. Decolorize with 0.5% acetic acid solution for 15 seconds, wash and counterstain with loffler's methylere — blue for 1 min.

D. **Albert — Staining:** For corynebacterium diphtheriae.

A. Albert's I

Tolu dine Blue	1.5 gm
Malachite Green	2.0 gm
Glacial Acetic Acid	10 ml
Alcohol (25% ethanol)	90 ml
Distilled water	1000 ml

Dissolve the dyes in alcohol and add to the water and acetic acid. Allow to stand for one day and then filter.

B. Albert's iodine (Albert's II)

Iodine	6 gm
Potassium iodine	9 gm
Distilled water	900 ml

Procedure

1. Cover the slide with Albert's stain 1. and allow to act for 3–5 min.
2. Wash in water and blot dry.
4. Cover the slide with albert's iodine and allow to act for 1 min.
5. Wash and blot dry.

Result: By this method volutin granules with in bacilli stain bluish black, the protoplasm green and other organisms mostly light green.

E. Staining of Spores

Spore bearing organisms, when stained with grams; are deeply coloured, where as the spore is unstained and appears as a clear area in the organism. For the staining of spore. *Acid Fast Stain* is used in the following manner:

1. Stain with Ziehl — Neelsen's carbol fuchsin for 3–5 min, heating until steam rises.
2. Wash with water.
3. Treat with 0.5% percent sulphuric acid for 1–5 minutes. Wash with water. Counterstain with 1% methylene blue for 3 min. Wash in water, blot and dry.

Result: Spores are stained bright red and protoplasm blue.

F. Staining of Capsules

Capsules: The capsules of bacteria present in body fluids and pus are often clearly stained when treated by common stains like methylene blue. Artificial cultures, do not stain for capsule by the common stains. For this purpose, special methods are employed known as relief staining. The methods adopted for staining of capsules are:

1. Wet film India ink method
2. Dry film India ink method
3. Relief staining with Eosin.

Wet Film India Ink Method

Is the method of choice.

Procedure

1. Clean a slide, put a loopful of India ink on it.
2. Place a small portion of bacterial culture on India ink and emulsify.
3. Place a clean coverslip and press through the sheet of blotting paper so that the ink film becomes very thin and pale in colour.
4. Examine under oil immersion.

Results: Bacteria is seen as a highly refractile outline against dark background of ink particle. The capsular zone is visualized as a clear space between the refractile portion and the dark background of India ink.

Demonstration of Flagella by Modified Leifson's Method

The stain, basic fuchsin with tannic acid is deposited on the bacteria and flagella from an evaporating alcoholic solution. The degree of staining is controlled by an exact determination of duration of exposure.

Procedure

1. Clean the glass slide with absolute alcohol and then with conc. H_2SO_4 saturated with potassium dichromate by immersing for several days. Rinse with water, dry in air and flame.
2. Fix broth culture by 1–2% formalin (W/V).
3. Sediment the bacilli by centrifuging at 2000–3000 rpm.
4. Decant supernatant and suspend bacteria in distilled water.
5. Centrifuge again and gently resuspend in distilled water to obtain a final slightly cloudy suspension.
6. With a flamed platimum look, place a loopful of suspension on prepared slide and gently spread over as $2cm^2$ area.
7. Allow to air dry at room temperature.
8. Place slide horizontally on a staining rack and put exactly 1 ml of stain on slide to cover whole of the surface.

Stain is prepared as follows:

Tannic Acid	—	10 gm
Sodium Chloride	—	5 gm
Basic Fuchsin	—	4 gm

Prepare the solution by adding 1.9 gm of powder mixture to 33 ml of 95% ethyl alcohol and add distilled water to make volume to 100 ml. Adjust pH to 5.0.

9. Leave at room temperature for exactly required time.
10. Rinse off excess stain through slowly running tap water.
11. Counter stain with methylene blue for 30 min.
12. Wash with water, drain, dry and examine under oil immersion.

Romanowsky Stains

Romanowsky stains impart a reddish-purple colour to chromatin of malaria and other parasites due to a substance which forms when methyline blue is ripened either by age or by heating. Various Romanowsky stains are leishman's; Wright's, Jenner's and Giemsa stains.

Leishman's Stain

(For protozoa in blood films)

Reagents:

Leishman dye	—	3.8 g
Methyl Alcohol	—	250 ml
Glycerol	—	250 ml

Preparation of Stock Solution

1. Grind 3.8 g of leishman stain and add glycerol in a mortar slowly.
2. Add half of methyl alcohol and continue grinding.
3. Transfer to a glass stoppered bottle.
4. Pour remainder methyl alcohol into mortar and grind the residue. Transfer this to the bottle.

Preparation of Buffer Solution

Potassium dihydrogen phosphate — 0.7 gm } Adjust pH to 7.2
Disodium hydrogen phosphate — 1.0 gm
Distilled water — 1000 ml

Preparation of Working Solution

1. Filter the stock solution.
2. Add 3 drops of stain for 1 ml of buffer solution.

Procedure

1. Fix thin films with methyl alcohol.
2. Pour off alcohol.
3. Pour 3 ml of diluted stain for 30 min.
4. Differentiate by holding under a stream of water for approx. 15 seconds.
5. Allow slides to drain and dry before examination.

Results: Malarial parasite will to be seen as per stage and species.

Giemsa Stain

(For Protozoa and spirochaetes)

This consists of a number of compounds made by mixing different proportions of methylene blue and eosin. These have designated as Azure I, Azure II and Azure II Eosin: The following method by Lillie is recommended for preparation:

Contents

Azure A eosinate	—	0.5 gm
Azure B Eosinate	—	2.5 gm
Methylene Blue Eosinate	—	2.0 gm
Methylene Blue Chloride	—	1.0 gm
Glycerol	—	375.0 ml
Methyl Alcohol	—	375.0 ml

Procedure

Rapid Method

1. Fix films in methyl alcohol for 3 min.
2. Stain in a mixture of 1 part stain and 10 parts of phosphate buffer pH 7.0 for 1 hour.
3. Wash with buffer solution, allowing the preparation to differentiate for about 30 secs.
4. Blot and allow to dry in air.

Slow Method

Valuable for demonstrating spirochaetes:—
1. Fix films in methyl alcohol for 3 min.
2. Make a mixture of 20 ml of buffer (pH–7.0) and 1 ml of stain in petridish.
3. Place a thin glass rod in petridish.
4. Place slides in petri dish with one end on the glass rod.
5. Stain for 16–24 hours

6. Wash in buffer solution.
7. Allow to air dry, mount and examine under oil.

Field's Stain (For Staining Thick Blood Films For Malarial Parasite)

Reagents

Solution A (Methylene Blue)
Methylene blue — 1.3 gm
Na_2HPO_4 anhydrous — 5 gm
— Dissolve in 50 ml Distilled Water,
— Bring to boil and evaporate to dryness;
— Add KH_2PO_4 6.25 gm
— Add 500 ml of boiled, warmed, distilled water.
— Keep for 24 hours.
— Filter

Solution B (Eosin)

Eosin	—	1.3 gm
Na_2HPO_4 (An-hydrous)	—	5.0 gm
KH_2PO_4 (Anhydrous)	—	6.25 gm
Distilled Water		
Filter before use	—	500 ml

Procedure

1. Dip the slide in solution A for 1–2 sec.
2. Rinse in distilled/tap water until the stain ceases to flow from the film.
4. Dip the slide in solution B for 1–2 sec.
4. Rinse in clean water for 2–3 sec.
5. Place vertically on rack to drain and dry.

J.S.B. Stain (For Malarial Parasite) Devised by Jasbir Singh and Bhattacharji

Reagents

Solution-I

Methylene Blue	—	0.5 gm
Sulphuric Acid 1%	—	3 ml
Potassium Hydroxide 1%	—	10 ml
Distilled water	—	500 ml

Solution-II

Eosin	—	1 gm
Tap Water	—	500 ml

Procedure (For thick film)

1. Put the slide in solution I for 10 seconds.
2. Wash for 2 seconds in a jar containing acidulated water (pH 6–6.6).
3. Stain with solution II for 1 second.
4. Wash in jar (2) for 5 seconds.
5. Immerse in solution I again for 10 secs.
6. Wash as above for 10 sec. or till the smear gives a pink background.
7. Dry and examine.

Staining of Spirochaetes: Fontana's Method

Reagents

a) **Fixative**

Acetic Acid   1 ml

Formalin	—	2 ml
Distilled Water	—	100 ml

b) **Mordant**

Phenol	—	1 gm
Tannic Acid	—	100 ml
Distilled Water	—	100 ml

c) **Ammoniated Silver Nitrate**

10% Ammonia dissolved to 0.5% sol. of AgNO$_3$ in distilled water till the precipitate formed just dissolves, ADD AgNO$_3$ drop by drop, till precipitate reappears, and does not dissolve.

Procedure

1. Treat the film three times for 30 sec. each with fixative.
2. Wash off the fixative with alcohol and allow to act for 3 min. Drain excess alcohol.
3. Pour on mordant, heating till steam rises and allow to act for 30 sec.
4. Wash well in distilled water and dry the slide.
5. Treat with ammoniated silver nitrate, heating till steam rises for 30 sec., when film becomes brown in colour.
6. Wash well in distilled water, dry and mount in Canada balsam.

Results: Spirochaetes are stained brownish black
Background is brownish yellow.

Levaditi's Method (For staining Spirochaetes in Tissues)

Procedure: (Pyridine modification).
1. Fix the tissue in 10% formalin.
2. Wash the tissue for 1 hour in water.
3. Place in 96–98% Alcohol for 24 hours.
4. Place in 1% solution of silver nitrate (to which 1/10th volume of pure pyridine is added) for 2 hours at room temperature and thereafter at 50°C for 4–6 hours.
5. Rapidly wash in 10% pyridine solution.
6. Transfer to reducing fluid, which consists of 4% Formalin — 100 parts.

Add just before	Acetone	— 10 parts
use Pyridine		— 15 parts

Keep the tissue in fluid for two days at room temp. in dark.
7. Wash well with water, dehydrate in increasing strength of alcohol and embed in paraffin.
8. Cut the section, mount in usual way with Canada balsam.

Staining of Fungi in Wet Mounts with Lacto-Phenol Blue

Reagents:

Phenol crystals	—	20 gm
Lactic Acid	—	20 ml
Distilled Water	—	20 ml
Cotton Blue/Methyl blue	—	0.075 gm

Phenol crystals dissolved by gentle warming.

Procedure

1. Place a drop of 95% alcohol on slide.
2. Gently tease out a fragment of culture in alcohol and allow alcohol to evaporate.
3. Add a drop of strain.
4. Apply a cover slip and gently press.
5. Remove excess stain around the edges of cover slip.
6. Examine after a few minutes.

Result: Fungal hyphae stain blue black.

Staining of Virus Inclusion and Elementary Bodies

Inclusion Bodies

Basophilic Inclusion Bodies — Giemsa's stain
Acidophilic Inclusion Bodies — Manus methyl blue Eosin stain.

Elementary Bodies

— Giemsa's stain (Useful for vaccinia and psittachosis)
— Brucella Differential stain (Useful for chlamydia)
— Gutsteins Method (Useful for variola — vaccinia group).

CHAPTER 22

PRINCIPLES OF MICROBIOLOGICAL DIAGNOSIS

Best way of diagnosing any infectious disease is to directly demonstrate the causative organism either in direct microscopy or in culture. But this is not always possible due to a variety of reasons.

DIAGNOSIS OF A DISEASE

DIRECT EVIDENCE
1. Demonstration by naked eye e.g. various intestinal worms.
2. By microscopic evidence e.g. stained smear showing gonococci in urethral pus and A.F.B. in sputum.
3. Culture best way of diagnosis specially for bacteria and fungi.

INDIRECT EVIDENCE
1. Demonstration of specific antigen e.g. by latex agglutination, ELISA etc.
2. Specific e.g. Serological tests.
3. Non-specific e.g. E.S.R., T.L.C., D.L.C.

In routine practice both types of evidences should be attempted, and the two should act as complementary to each other for making a final diagnosis.

Morphological Classification of Bacteria

A. True Bacteria

I. COCCI

i) Gram positive
1. Streptococci (Arranged in chains)
2. Staphylococci (Grape like Clusters)
3. Micrococci (Irregular clusters)
4. Sarcina (Cubical packets of 8)
5. Pneumococci diplococci

B. Higher Bacteria
(Filamentous)

1. Actinomycetes.
2. Nocardia
3. Streptomyces

ii) Gram Negative
1. Neisseria — Intracellular diplococci
2. Veillonella — Irregular clusters.

II. BACILLI

i. Gram positive
a) Sporing
   1. Bacillus
   2. Clostridia
b) Nonsporing
   1. Corynebacterium
   2. Erysipelothrix
   3. Lactobacillus
   4. Listeria

ii) Gram negative
a) Polar flagella
   Pseudomonaccae
b) Peritrichous flagella
   1. Enterobacterioceae
   2. Achromobacteriacae
   3. Brucellaceae
   4. Bacterioidaceae

iii) Acid Fast
   1. Mycobacterium

III. VIBRIOS AND SPIRILLA

1. Vibrios
2. Spirillum

IV. SPIROCHAETES

1. Borrelia
2. Tereponema
3. Lepotospira.

Isolation Of Bacteria

In this chapter, the identification points of most commonly isolated bacterial pathogens in routine hospital practice shall be discussed.

Table 31
Identification Of Gram +ve COCCI Colonies In Blood Agar

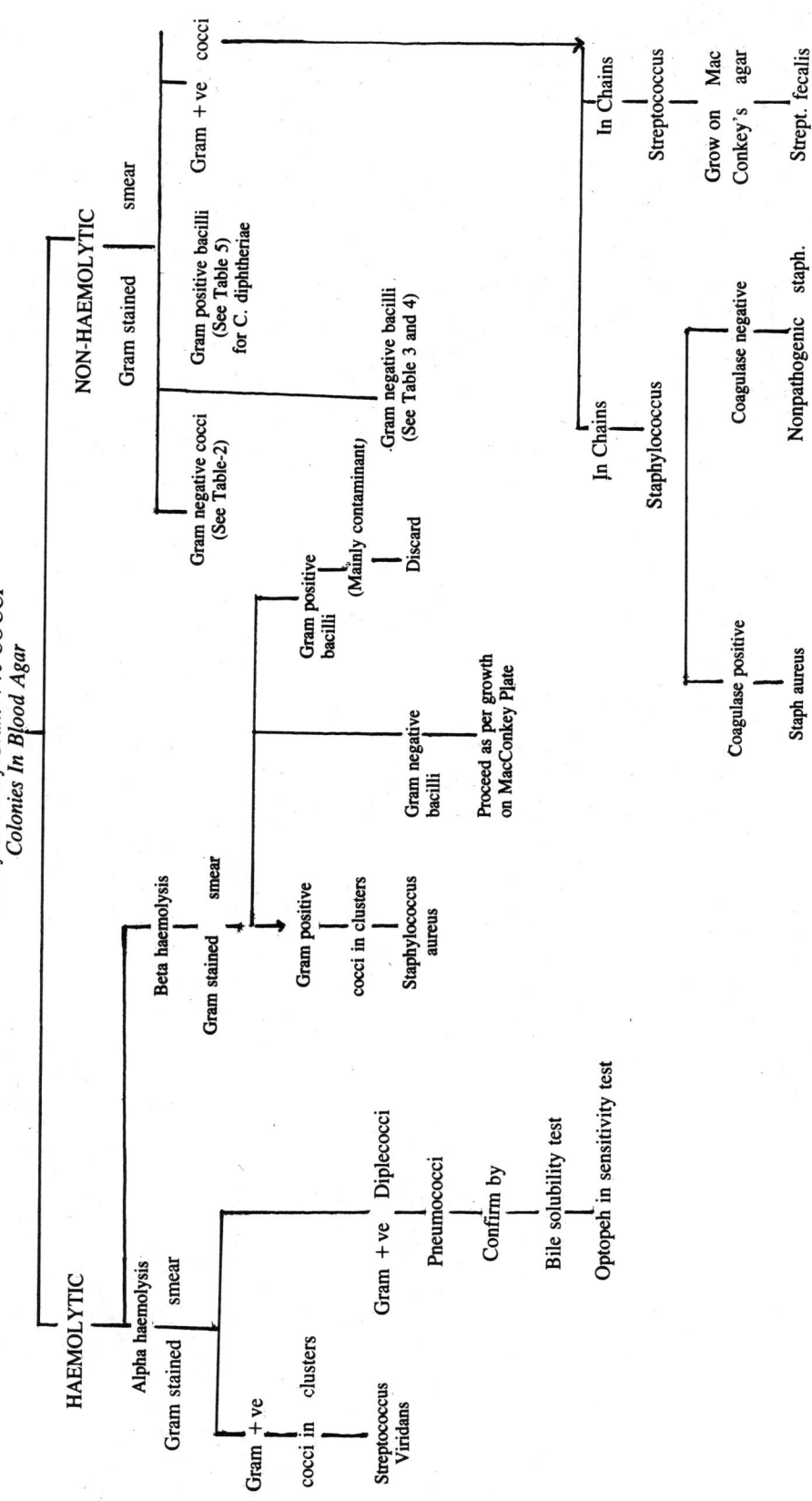

Footnote
1. Alpha haemolysis means partial haemolysis and on plate is visible in the form of greenish discolouration.
2. Beta haemolysis means complete haemolysis and on plate is visible in the form of a clear halo around the colony.

135

Table 32 *Identification of Gram Negative COCCI — Oxdiase Positive*

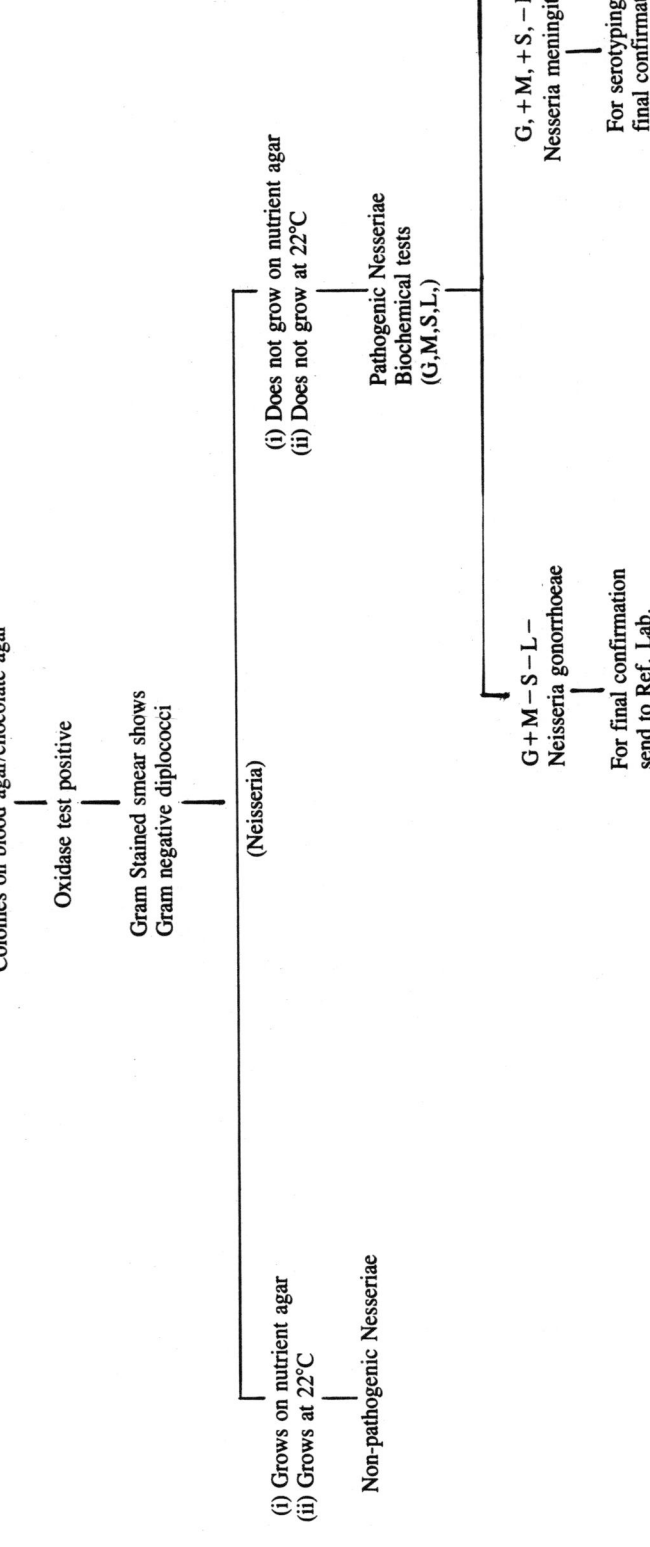

Colonies on blood agar/chocolate agar

Oxidase test positive

Gram Stained smear shows
Gram negative diplococci

(Neisseria)

(i) Grows on nutrient agar
(ii) Grows at 22°C

Non-pathogenic Nesseriae

(i) Does not grow on nutrient agar
(ii) Does not grow at 22°C

Pathogenic Nesseriae
Biochemical tests
(G,M,S,L,)

G+M−S−L−
Neisseria gonorrhoeae

For final confirmation
send to Ref. Lab.

G,+M,+S,−L−
Nesseria meningitidis

For serotyping and
final confirmation
send to Ref. Lab.

(G — Glucose, M — Maltose, S — Sucrose, L — Lactose)

Table 33. *Identification of Gram Negative Bacilli*
Growth on Mac Conkey's agar/DCA
Gram stained smear
Gram negative bacilli

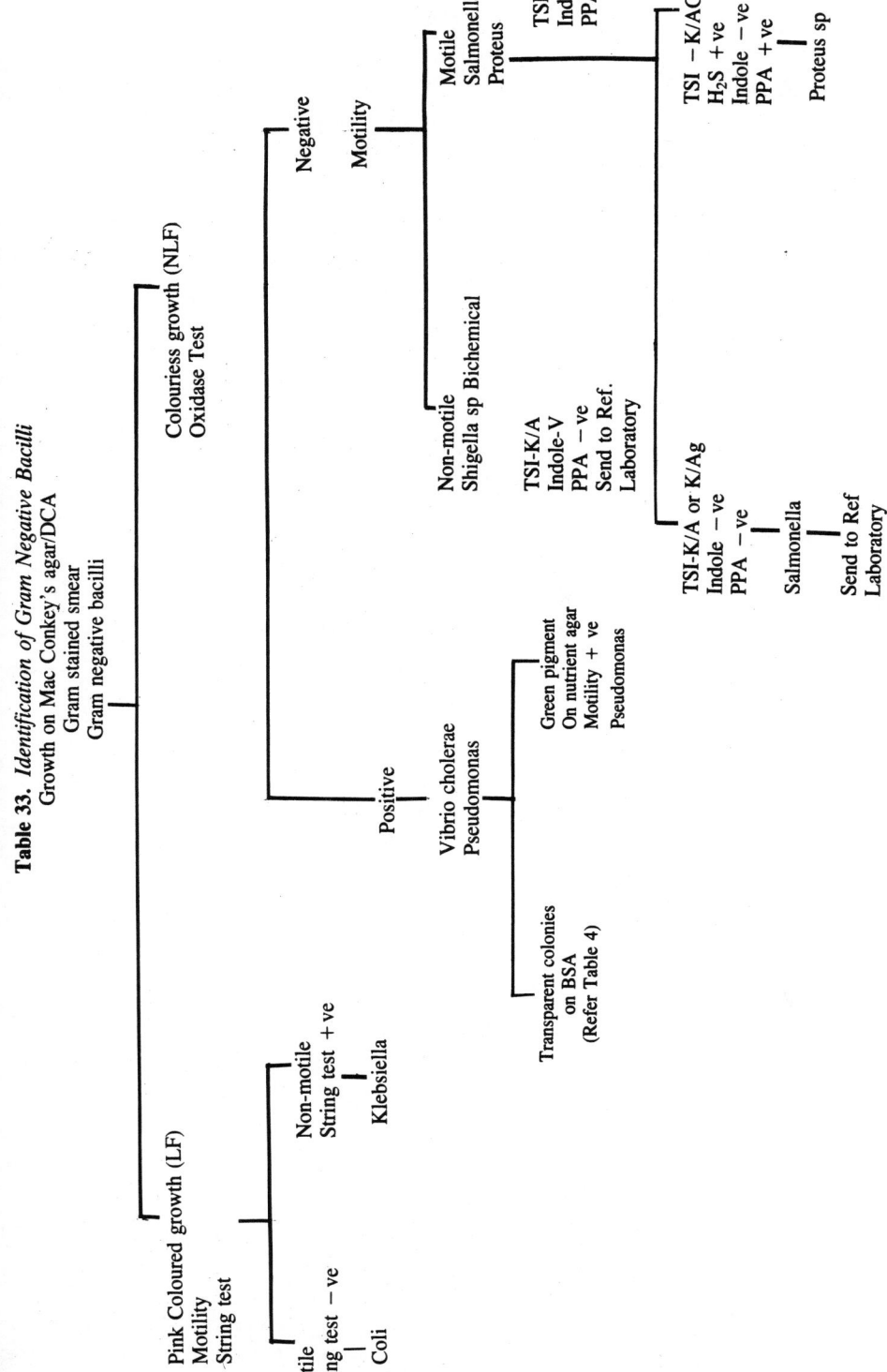

Table 34 *Identification of Gram Negative Bacilli — Oxidase Positive* Growth on B.S.A.

Translucent/Transparent

Motility

Typical darting Motility

Vibrio cholerae

Send to Reference Lab For agglutination with specific antiserum

Opaque

Motility positive

Green pigment on Nutrient Agar

Pseudomonas sp.

Table 35 *Laboratory Diagnosis Of Diphtheria*

The only important becterium of Gram positive bacilli group is Corynebacterium which shall be discussed here. Since the rapidity of diagnosis in this case is of paramount importance, we shall discuss the diagnosis from the smear level:

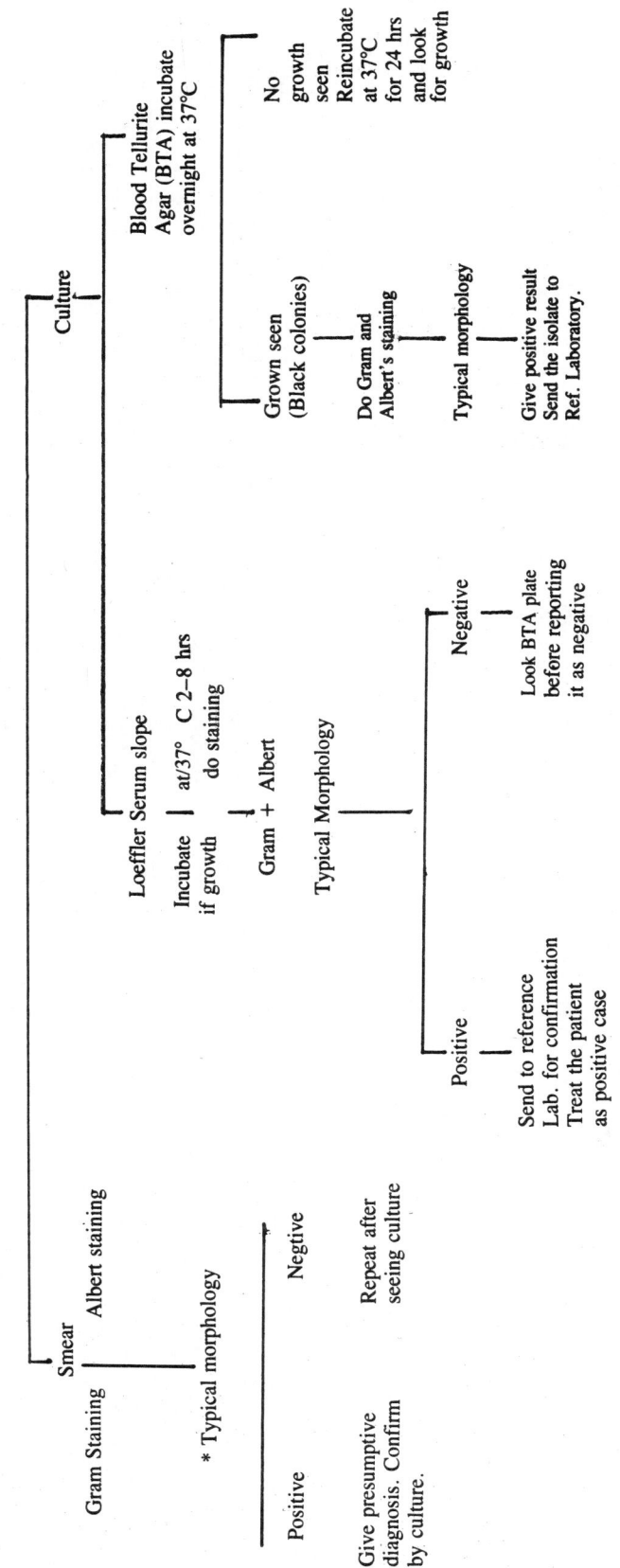

Throat Swabs (two in No.)

Smear

Gram Staining | Albert staining

* Typical morphology

Positive → Give presumptive diagnosis. Confirm by culture.

Negtive → Repeat after seeing culture

Culture

Loeffler Serum slope → Incubate if growth at/37° C 2–8 hrs do staining → Gram + Albert → Typical Morphology

Positive → Send to reference Lab. for confirmation. Treat the patient as positive case

Negative → Look BTA plate before reporting it as negative

Blood Tellurite Agar (BTA) incubate overnight at 37°C

Grown seen (Black colonies) → Do Gram and Albert's staining → Typical morphology → Give positive result. Send the isolate to Ref. Laboratory.

No growth seen → Reincubate at 37°C for 24 hrs and look for growth

* Thin slender bacilli, pleomorphic, with one and clubbed, weakly Gram positive and with metachromatic granules. Diphtheroids are thick, short mostly of uniform size and usually without metachromatic granules.

Note: If the Gram positive bacilli isolated on blood agar not confirmed as C. diphtheriae, then do not attach much importance, discard them.

Antibiotic Sensitivity Tests

Antimicrobial agents include basically 2 groups of drugs
1. Disinfectants
2. Chemotherapeutic agents.

Assessment of the range of sensitivity of pathogenic bacteria isolated from patients to different antimicrobial agents, performed in-vitro is of importance to the physician for prescribing the chemotherapeutic agents. However it has to be kept in mind that in-vitro result may not be 100% applicable in-vivo (in the human body).

Principles: A wide range of tests is available, each of which is appropriate for a different purpose. Tests most commonly used are.

1. Minimal Inhibitory concentration

It measures the lowest concentration of antimicrobial agent that will inhibit the growth of a known strain of bacterium.

In this test we use different concentrations of a drug to prevent the growth of an indicator bacterium in solid or liquid media.

These test are of importance mainly in pharmacology especially for determining dosage of drugs.

2. Rideal Walker test

This tests the potency of disinfectants to kill bacteria in reference to a standard (phenol in this case).

Phenol Cofficient: It expresses the bactericidal power of a particular disinfectant as compared with pure phenol.

Rideal walker test measures the phenol coefficient of disinfectant under standard conditions.

3. Chick Martin & Garrod tests:

They also determine the phenol coefficient of the disinfectant in presence of a standard amount of organic matter.

4. Tests for disinfecting actions on surfaces.

5. Capacity use-dilution test: Measures effect of repeated challenge by bacteria.

6. **Stability test:** Measures stability & long time effectiveness of a diluted disinfectant.

7. **The in-use test:** Determines the presence/absence of bacteria in-use disinfectants.

What we will discuss in detail here are the antibiotic sensitivity tests as carried out in routine in a microbiology laboratory. These are the DISK-DIFFUSION TESTS OF SENSITIVITY TO ANTIBIOTICS, which are simple, reliable and specially applicable in routine clinical bacteriology.

Disk Diffusion Tests

Principle

Disk diffusion method consists of impregnating small disks of a standard filter paper with given amounts of chosen range of antibiotics. These are placed on plates of culture medium previously spread uniformly with an inoculum of bacterial isolate. After incubation, degree of sensitivity is determined by measuring visible areas of inhibtion of growth produced by diffusion of antibiotic into the surrounding medium.

Preparation of Disks

It is most conveniably available to use commercial dry disks. These are 6 mm in diameter and consist of absorbent paper, impregnated with antibiotic. They are marked with letters showing name of antibiotic.

Preparation of Wet Disks

Punch disks 6.25 mm. in diameter from no 1 whatmar filter paper, dispense in batches of 100 in screw capped bottles and sterilize by dry heat at 140°C for 2 hrs. Prepare solutions of antibiotics so that 1 ml. solution contains 100 times the amount of antibiotic required for 1 disk. Add 1 ml solution to each bottle and store in wet conditions. They retain their potency for several months at 40°C (in contrast, dry disks expire very quickly).

Disks: containing different antibiotics can be recognised by:
1. Typed/printed letters
2. Colour applied to plain paper.
3. Paper on which black spots/lines have been stencilled.

Colouring is done with cotton dyes which are fast and do no interfere with action of antimicrobial agents.

Choice of drugs for disk test:

When large numbers of sensitivity tests have to be done on isolates from clinical specimens, it is convenient to restrict the routine tests to the number of first line antibiotics that can be conveniently tested on a single culture plate. Preferably 6 and at most 8 disks are used on one plate. Different appropriate first line sets of 6 or 8 drugs may be selected for use with different types of clinical specimen e.g. exudates/sputum/urine/Blood Selection is also guided by the nature of isolates obtained. The set should depend on frequency of usage by clinicians.

1. For Cultures Other Than Urine

Sets of antibiotics include Ampicillin; cotrimoxazole (Septran) Erythromycin; Benzylpenicillin; Tetracycline; Cephalexin & Streptomycin.

2. Cultures From Urine

High content disks are used. Set includes Ampicillin; Cotrimoxazole (Septran); Nalidixic acid; Nitrofurantion; Gentamicin; Kanamycin; Cephalexin & Tetracycline.

Staphy-lococci	Othercocci & Gram + ve bacteria	Most Gram − ve	For Hemophilus	For Pseudomonas	For Clostridia & Gram − ve anaerobes
1. Erythromycin	Ampicillin	Ampicillin	Ampicillin	Carbenicillin	Ampicillin
2. Fucidin	Cephalexin	Cephalexin	Cephalexin	Gentamicin	Clindamycin
3. Benzylpenicilin	Cotrimoxazole	Cotrimoxazole	Coloramphenicol	Kanaycin	
4. Ampicillin	Erythromycin	Streptomycin	Cotrimoxazole	Polymyxin B	Fucidin
5. Lincomycin	Benzylpencilin	Gentamincin	Tetracycline		Benzylpenicillin
6. Tetracycline	Kanamycin			Tetracycline	
7. Cotrimoxazole		Chloramphenicol			Metronidazole
8. Gentamicin		Chloramphenicol			

Drug concentrations used for common antibiotics

Drug	Normal Conc (pg)	High Content (pg) For Urine.
1. Ampicillin	2	30
2. Benzylpenicillin	1	30
3. Carbenicillin	100	100
4. Cephalexin	5	30
5. Erythromycin	10	—
6. Gentamicin	10	30
7. Kanamycin	10	30
8. Nalidxic acid (Gramoneg)	—	30
9. Nitrofurantoin	—	200
10. Septran (Cotrimoxazole)	1.25 Trimet 23.5 hoprim Sulfamethoxazole	1.25 23.5
11. Streptomycin	10	30
12. Tetracycline	10	30

Culture medium used

A nutrient agar medium should be used which is as far as possible free from substances inhibitory to action of antibioties. Suitable sensitivity test agars are available from commercial suppliers. pH should be 7.2 — 7.5. Blood should be added when testing strept. Pyogenes or pneumococci. Chocolated blood should be used with Hemophilus. A vol. of 20 ml. medium is poured in 8.5 cm. petridishes with flat bottoms to obtain a 3–4 mm. deep layer.

Test procedure

(1) Dry culture plate in incubator, until surface is free from moisture. Inoculate test bacteria by any of the following procedures

For test on primary cultures

Sample is placed over culture plate and spread uniformly with a dry sterile swab.

For tests on pure Subcultures

Inoculation by flooding

Place 2ml of inoculate Tip in different directions to spread it. Remove excess fluid with pipette. Dry the plate inverted in an incubator for 30 mins.

Inoculation by Spreading

Place loopful of culture & spread with loop or swabstick.

(2) After plate is dried after inoculation, apply the chosen disks with proper disk spacing, with sterile fine pointed forceps.
(3) Incubate for 18–24 hrs at 37°C.
(4) Measure the diameters of zones of inhibition of growth including 6 mm. diameter of disk by callipers or viewing against a ruler.
(5) Simultaneously a control of known sensitivity is run.
a) Oxford strain of staph aureus (Type 6571)
b) Eschirichia coli (NCTC 10418)
c) Pseudomonas aeruginosa (NCTC 10662)

Reading interpretation

1) Report the test stain as sensitive if diameter of its zone of inhibition by a drug is greater than, equal to or ≤4mm less than that on control culture.
2) Report as follows:
>12 mm. — sensitive
>10 mm — <12 mm — Moderately sensitive
<10 mm — Resistant

CHAPTER 23

BACTERIOLOGICAL DIAGNOSIS FOR SYPHILIS AND CLOSTRIDIA

I. DIAGNOSIS OF SYPHILLIS:

DARK FIELD EXAMINATION TECHNIQUE:

A. Surface of suspected ulcerated lesion should be cleaned with saline & gauze, then gently abraded further with dry gauze, without bleeding. The lession is then squeezed to espress a serous transudate & a drop of transudate is picked up on the surface of a glass slide
Mix a drop of saline with it.
Cover it with coverslip & examine immediately for Tr. pallidum with a dark field or contrast microscope
A single examination does not exclude syphilis. Prior use of topical antiseptic may interface with the examination.

B. In case of secondary syphilis, organism may be demonstrated by saline aspiration of lymph nodes.

ii) SEROLOGY:

Serology is very important becasue after primary syphilis it is almost impossible to demonstrate treponemes. At this point it is necessary to perform serological tests to diaganose the condition.

Lipoidophil
Nonsepecific antibody test (STS)
Serological Tests
1. Flocculation (VDRL)
2. CFT (Wasserman Kalmer)
3. Agglutination
Specific Treponemal Antibody tests
1. FTA-ABS
2. Tr. Pallidum I (TPI)
3. Hemagglutination

LIPOIDOPHIL ANTIBODY TESTS (STS)

1. **VDRL:** Carried out on 76 × 50 mm slides with ceramic rings or 3 × ½" tubes

Transfer 0.5 ml of inactivated serum to tube and add 0.5 ml of diluted antigen (cardiolipin).
Shake for 5 min in a Kahn shaker.
Centrifuge at 2000 rmp.

Place 0.016 ml serum & 0.01 ml. diluted antigen on to the slide with ceramic ring.
Rotation is carried out by a mechanical slide rotator.

Visible aggregation
is taken to be positive.
VDRL titers reach 1.32 during sec. syphilis.

2. COMPLEMENT FIXATION TEST: Reagents are added as follows

Tube 1 (Control)~serum 0.2 ml.
Salin @ 2 ml
Compiement (Serum control) 1 ml.
TUBE 2 (test)~Serum 0.2 ml
Saline 1 ml
complement (test) 1 ml
Antigen 1 ml
~Place the tubes in water bath for 1 hr at 37°C
After this to each tube add 1 vol. of sensitized RBCs & place in water bath for another 30 mins.

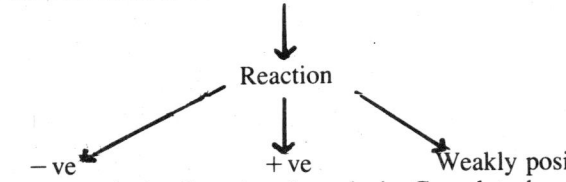

Reaction

−ve
complete hemolysis in both tubes.

+ve
Complete hemolysis in control tube with no hemolysis in test tube.

Weakly positive
Complete hemolysis in control tube with partial hemolysis in test tube.

This test can be quantitative if doubling dilutions of serum in saline from 1 in 5 to 1 in 160 are used.

TERPONEMAL ANTIBODY TESTS

1. **FTA — ABS TEST** (Absorbed Flourescent Treponemal Antibody test):

The patients serum is first absorbed with a non-pathogenic treponemal antigen to remove group specific antibiotics which may be produced against saprophytic treponemes.

The patients absorbed serum is then placed on a slide containing Tr. pallidum (dried). Any specific Ab. in the serum is fixed to Treponsemes. It is then detected by addition of flourescin labelled AHG.

2. TREPONEMA HEMAGGLUTINATION ANTIBODY TEST

Formolized tanned sheep R.B.Cs. are conjugated with the antigens of a lysate of Nicol's strain of Tr. pallidum. Results of the reaction between antibody & coated cells give clear cut & reproducible results.

Specificity is similar to TPI test & sensitivity comparable to FTA tests.

3. TPI TEST:

Points serum is incubated with living virulent treponemes (NICHOL'S STRAIN) in the presence of complement. When specific antibody is present the spirochaetes are killed & immobilized.

Current routine practice of sera examination:

1) VDRL slide test
ii) Treponema hemagglutination Antibody test.
iii) Absorbed Flourescent Treponemal Antibody test.

False +ve serological tests for syphilis:

ACUTE (Disappear with in 6 months) Occur in	CHRONIC (Persist for 6 months) occur in
1. Mycoplasma pheumonia	1. Drug addicts
2. Malaria	2. Autoimmune diseases e.g. SLE
3. Acute viral infections	3. Ageing
4. Acute bacterial infections	
5. following small pox vaccination.	

TABLE 36   CLOSTRIDIA

	Morphology in culture	Colonies on Blood Agar	Cooked meat medium	Milk Medium	Liquefaction of coagulated serum	Fermentation of CLSMSa	Pathogenicity to guinea pigs and mice
Tetani	Slender bacilli with round terminal spores, usually gram negative	Transparent, haemolytic Swarming, with feat-hery projection	Slight digestion blackening & pungent odour	Unaltered	–	– – – – –	Tetanus produced +
Welchii	Large, thick stubby bacilli, Spores usually absent	Large, circular regular outline haemolytic	Gas, No digestion meat Reddened	Acid, Gas Rapid Clotting	–	+ + + + –	+
Septicum	Pleomorphic short with central or sub terminal spores	Transparent, projection haemolytic swarming	Gas, No digestion meat Reddended	Acid, Gas, Slow clotting	–	+ + – + +	+
Oedematiens	Large, Gram positive rods, Central or subterminal spores	Trens-lucent convex, haemolytic, spreading	Gas, No digestion meat Reddened	Slow Clotting	–	+ – – + –	+
Botulinum	Large, pleomorphic bacilli oval spores subterminal	Large, Irregular, feathery projections Opaque, pseudo-haemolytic	Gas, Types vary in Proteolytic Activity	Casein precipitated No digestion	±	+ – – + –	+

GLSMSa = G = Glucose, L = Lactose, S = Sucrose, M = Maltose, Sa = Salioin.

LAB DIAGNOSIS OF GAS GANGRENE

Causative Organisms:

Cl. Welchii (60%)

Cl. Oedematiens (20–40%)

CL. Septicum (10–20%

Material Processed: Wound exudate or tissue

Procedure: Specimen of exudate or tissue

```
                    │
        ┌───────────┴───────────┐
        ▼                       ▼
     Culture                Microscopy
        │                       │
  ┌─────┴─────┐          ┌──────┴──────┐
  ▼           ▼          ▼             ▼
Aerobic   Anaerobic   Gram        Immunofluo
          +10% CO₂    smear       nescence
              │       Gram        Preparation
              ▼       Positive    in selected
                      Bacilli     cases
```

Aerobic   Anaerobic + 10% CO₂   Gram smear Gram Positive Bacilli   Immunofluo nescence Preparation in selected cases

Blood Agar Firm Blood Agar, Neomycin Blood Agar Egg yolk Agar Neomycin egg yolk agar with Antitoxin

Cooked Meat Broths

Unheated (1 sample)

Heated after Inoculation at 70°C for 20 min. (2 samles)

All incubated anaerobically with 10% CO₂

Subsequent Microscopy & Subculture on lactose egg yolk Milk Agar medium

Lactose fermenting colonies with Nagler effect

LAB. DIAGNOSIS OF Cl Welchii Food Poisoning.

Faeces or suspected food

(1) Culture by selective heating procedure

(2) Microcosiopic examination for spore forms

(3) Serological Tests for typical food poisoning by slide Aggiutination Test (Hobbs' types)

CHAPTER 24

VARIOUS COMMON BIOCHEMICAL TESTS AND REACTIONS

TESTS FOR METABOLISM OF CARBOHYDRATES & RELATED COMPOUNDS

These tests are as follows:
1. Tests to distinguish between aerobic and anaerobic breakdown of a carbohydrate.
2. Fermentation Reactions (To show the range of carbohydrates and related compounds that can be attacked).
3. Tests for specific breakdown products.
4. Tests for ability to use a specific substrate.
5. Tests for metabolism of proteins and amino acids.
6. Tests for production of Enzymes.
7. Miscellaneous tests

1. TESTS TO DISTINGUISH BETWEEN AEROBIC & ANAEROBIC BREAKDOWN OF A CARBOHYDRATE

For this Hugh & Leifson medium is used. It is a semisolid tube medium containing
1. Peptone 2 gm
2. NaCl 5 gm
3. K_2HPO_4 300 mg
4. Agar gel 3 gm
5. 1% aqueous
Bromothynol blue 3 ml.

Make to 1 litre with distilled water (Adjust pH to 7.1 before adding indicator). Autoclave at 121°C for 30 mins. Carbohydrate to be added is sterilized separately and added to give a final concentration of 1%. The medium is then tubed to a depth of 4cm using a Durham's tube.

Method: Duplicate tubes of medium are inoculated by stabbing. One tube is promptly covered with a layer of sterile melted petroleum jelly to a depth of 5–8 mm. Incubate for upto 30 days.

Fermenting organism produce a colour change throughout the medium while oxidising (aerobic organisms) produce colour change only on the surface of uncovered tube.

2. FERMENTATION REACTIONS

Majority of these tests are simply for the production of acid & gas or acid alone when a pure culture grows in the presence of test compound.

Carbohydrate or related compounds under test.

1. Monosaccharides Pentoses (Arabinose, xylose)
   Hexoses — Glucose
   — Fructose
   — Mannose
   — Galactose
2. Disaccharides — Sucrose
   — Maltose
   — Lactose
   — Trehalose
3. Polysacoharides — Starch
   — Inulin
   — Dextrin
   — Glycogen
4. Polynydric alcohols — Glycerol
   — Mannitol
   — Dulcitol
   — Sorbitol
   — Inositol
5. Organic acids — Citrate
   — Tartarte.
   — Gluconate
   — Malanate

Media Used for test

1. PEPTONE WATER (Most commonly used) (950) ml − 50ml 10% test soln + Indicator)
Indicators are:
 i) Andrade's indicator 10ml or
 ii) Bromocresol purple 25ml.
2. BROTH MEDIA: (Bromothymol blue as indicator).
3. SERUM BASES (Phenol Red as indicator).
 i) Serum Peptone water.
 ii) Hiss's Serum water.
(25% serum in distilled water).

Indicators used with end points

1. Andrade's indicator — (yellow to Reddish pink). 1 N NaOH + 0.5%. Acid fuschin till light yellow colour develops.
2. 0.005% Bromocresol purpla (Violet to yellow).
3. 0.01% Phenol red Pink purple to yellow).
4. 0.0025% Bromothymol blue (Blue to yellow).

A small inverted tube (DURHAM TUBE). Completely filled with liquid & containing no air bubbles is usually included in each culture tube to detect gas.

Method: Inoculate each culture tube with a speck of pure solid culture or a loopful of liquid culture. Incubate for 24 hrs or (48hrs) for slow growers. Late fermentation may take upto 40 days.

Colour codes for Common fermentation Reactions:

Glucose — Green
Lactose — Red
Maltose — Blue/white
Sucrose — Blue.
Mannitol — Mauve
Sorbitol — Black/Blue
Dulcitol — Pink

3. TESTS FOR SPECIFIC BREAKDOWN PRODUCTS

i) Methyl Red Test (MR reaction)

It is employed to detect the production of sufficient acid during fermentation of glucose and maintenence of conditions such that pH of old cultures is maintained at 4.5

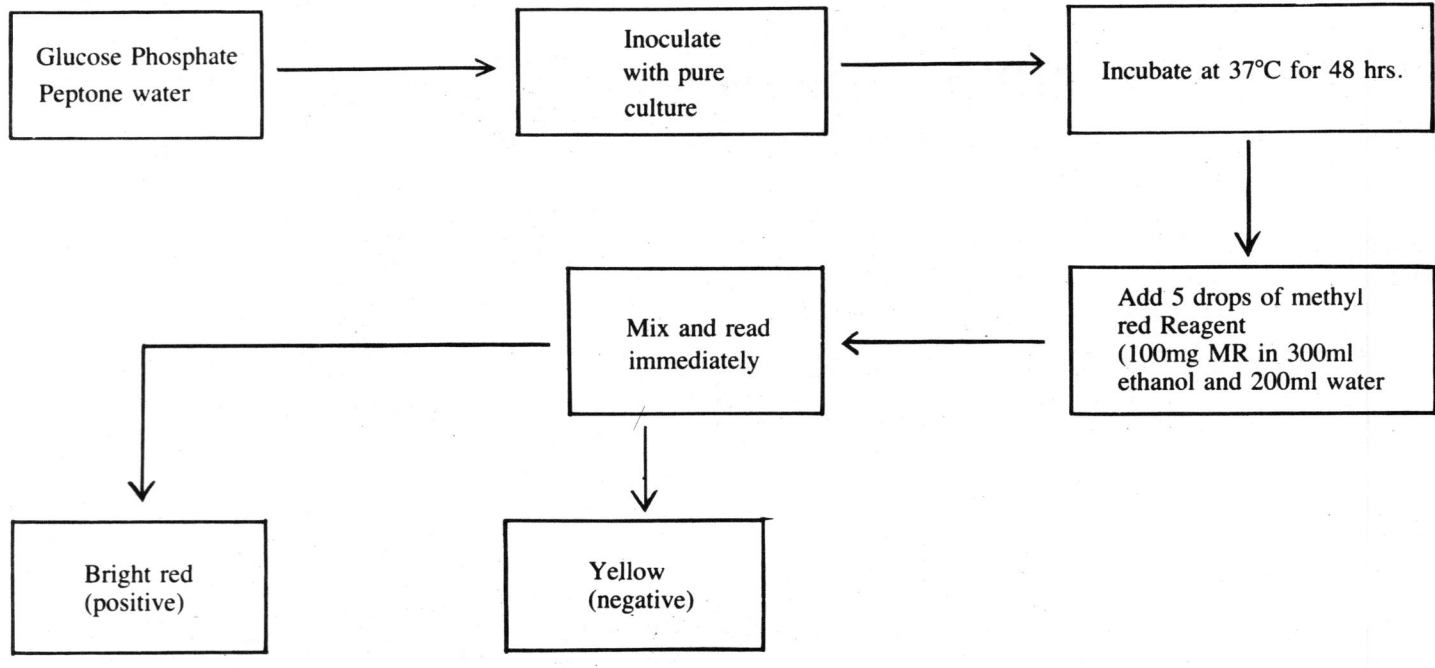

ii) Voges Proskauer (VP) test

PRINCIPLE

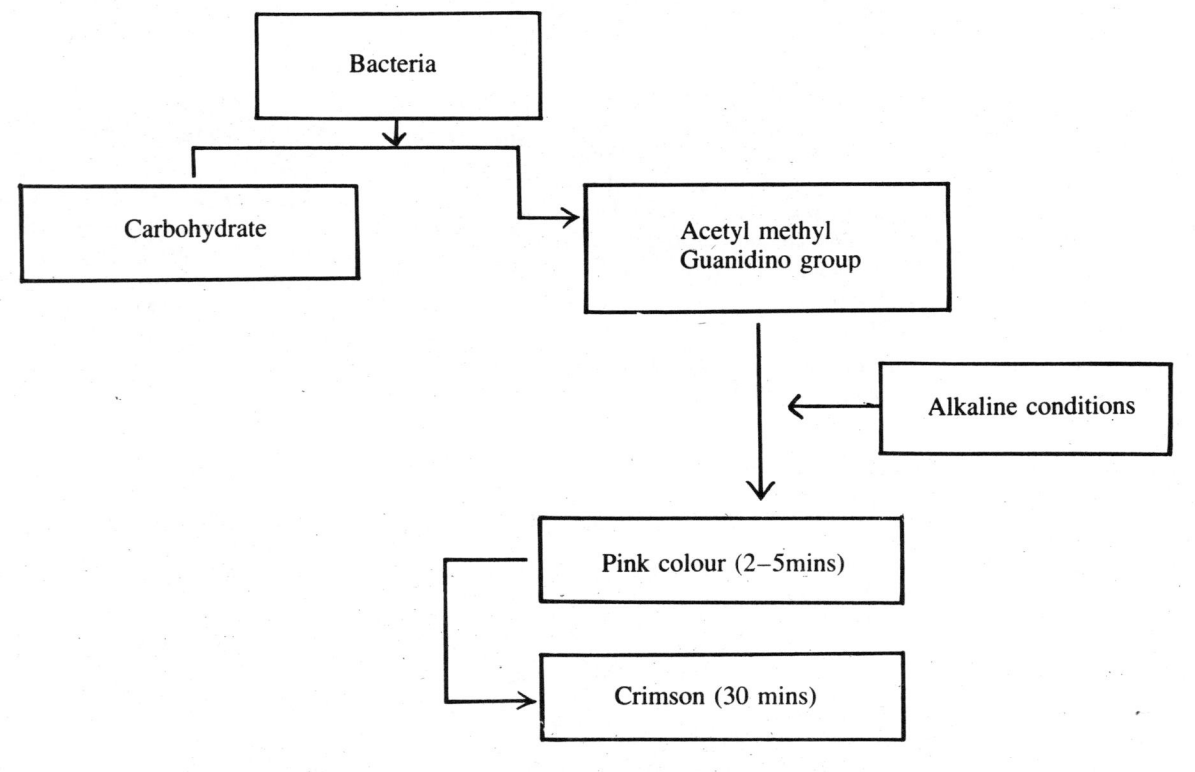

METHOD

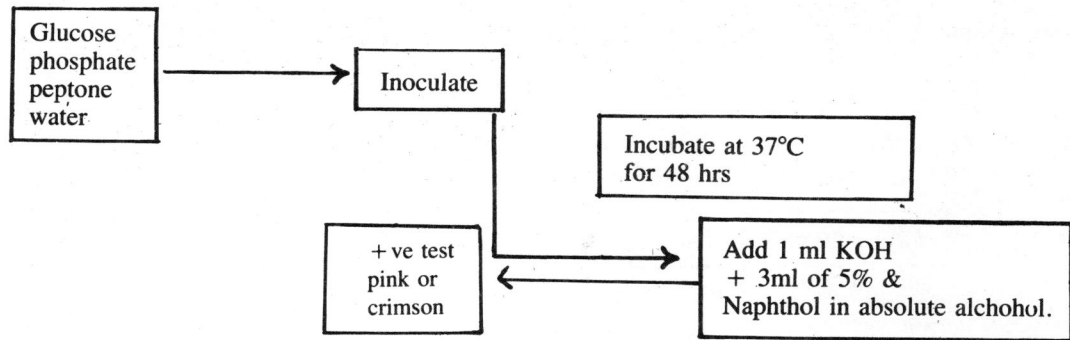

* An organism of enterobacterial group is usually either MR prositive & VP negative or vice-versa.

iii) GLUCONATE TEST

This tests the ability of an organism to oxidize gluconates to 2-Keto-gluconate. (Gluconate is non-reducing while 2-K-gluconate is reducing.

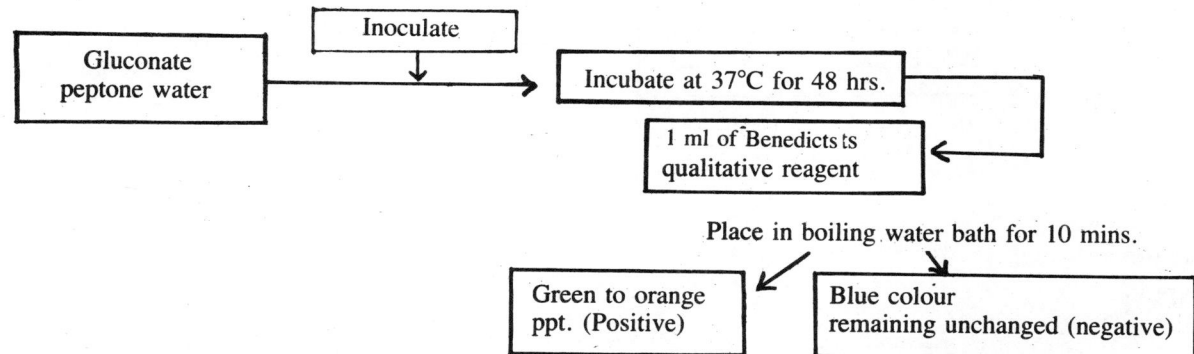

4. TESTS TO SHOW ABILITY TO USE A SPECIFIC SUBSTRATE

i) Citrate Utilization test

This tests the ability of an organism to use citrate as the sole source of carbohydrate and energy.

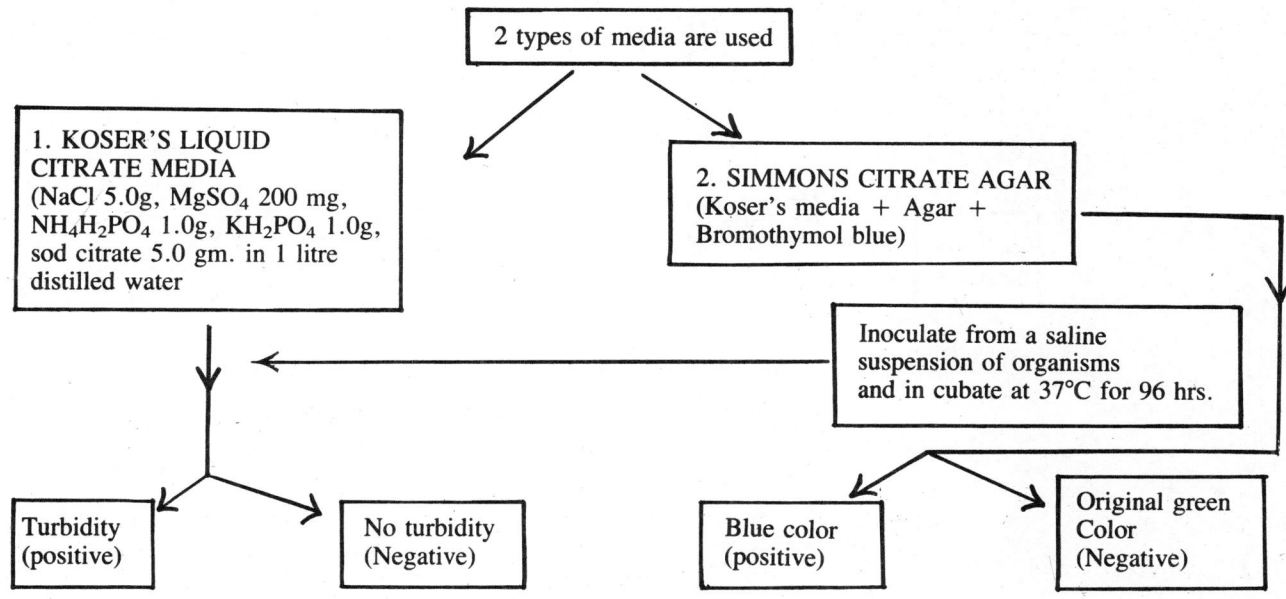

5. TESTS FOR METABOLISM OF PROTEINS & AMINO ACIDS

(i) Gelatin Liquefaction

2 methods of demonstrating
1) Using Nutrient broth + gelatin
2) Using gelatin agar

1-Gelatin broth (Nutrient broth + Gelatin + Egg albumin)
          (1 litre)   (120gm)   (2 egg whites)

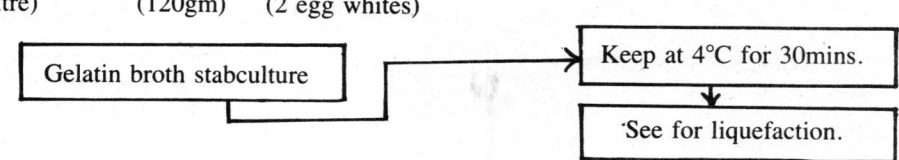

2-Gelatin agar (Nutrient agar 11, KH_2PO_4 500mg, K_2HPO_4 1.5g, gelatin 4.0gm, Glucose 50mg).

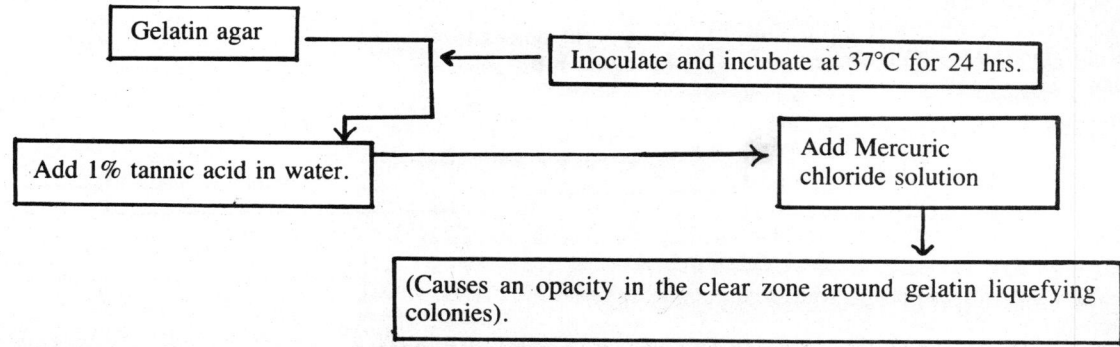

(ii) Indole test

PRINCIPLE:

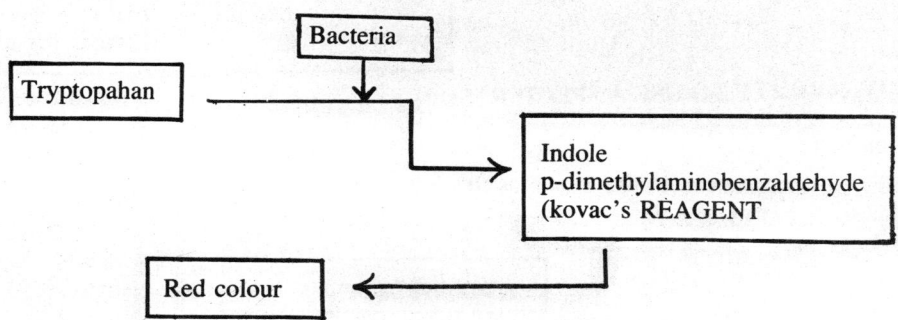

METHOD

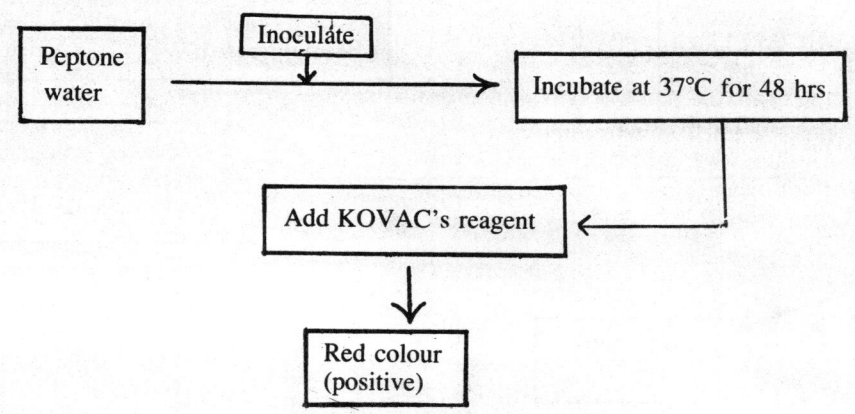

(iii) Urease test

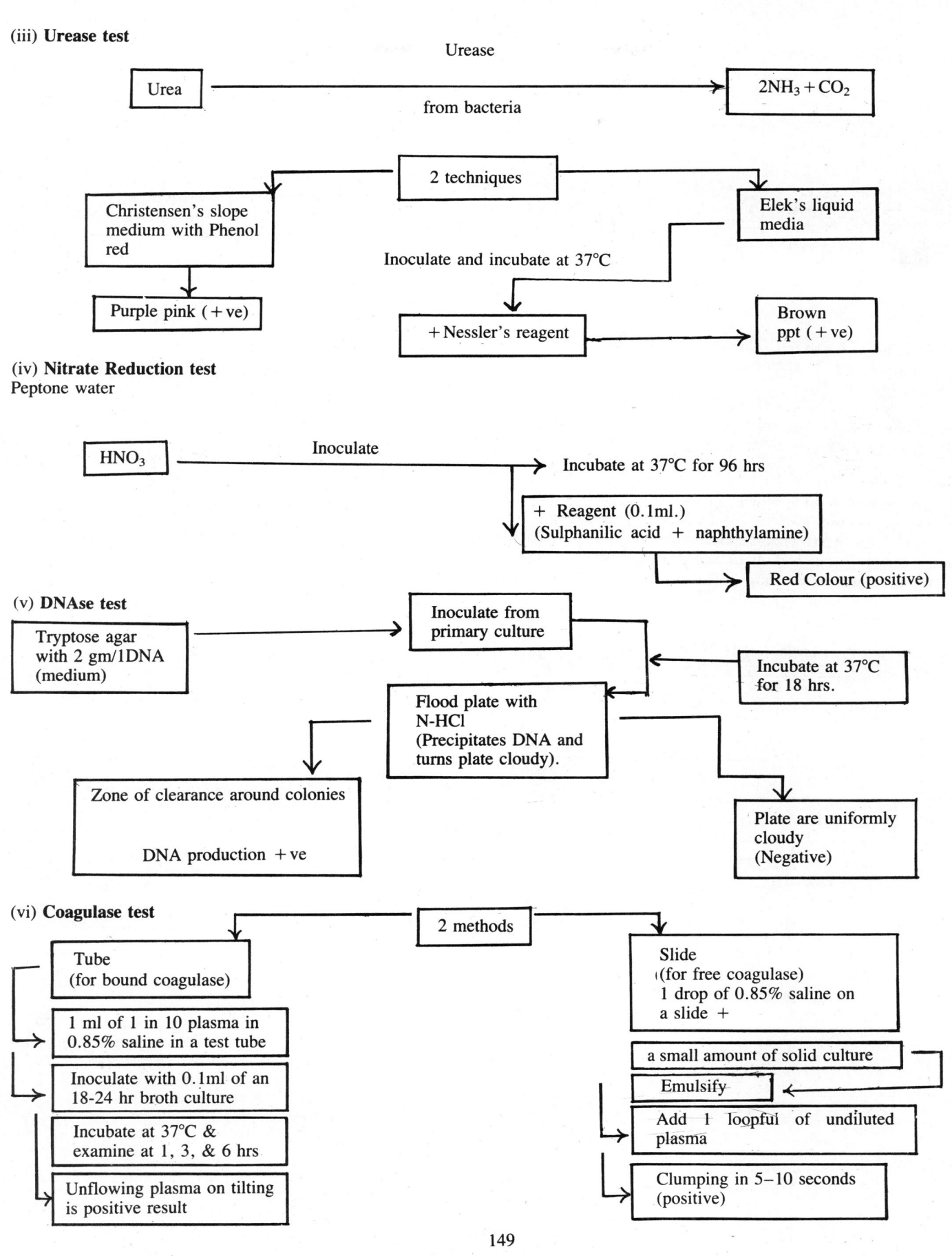

Urease

Urea $\xrightarrow{\hspace{3cm}}$ $2NH_3 + CO_2$

from bacteria

2 techniques

Christensen's slope medium with Phenol red

Elek's liquid media

Inoculate and incubate at 37°C

Purple pink (+ve)

+ Nessler's reagent $\longrightarrow$ Brown ppt (+ve)

(iv) Nitrate Reduction test

Peptone water

HNO₃ $\xrightarrow{\text{Inoculate}}$ Incubate at 37°C for 96 hrs

+ Reagent (0.1ml.) (Sulphanilic acid + naphthylamine)

Red Colour (positive)

(v) DNAse test

Tryptose agar with 2 gm/1DNA (medium) $\longrightarrow$ Inoculate from primary culture

Incubate at 37°C for 18 hrs.

Flood plate with N-HCl (Precipitates DNA and turns plate cloudy).

Zone of clearance around colonies

DNA production +ve

Plate are uniformly cloudy (Negative)

(vi) Coagulase test

2 methods

Tube (for bound coagulase)

1 ml of 1 in 10 plasma in 0.85% saline in a test tube

Inoculate with 0.1ml of an 18-24 hr broth culture

Incubate at 37°C & examine at 1, 3, & 6 hrs

Unflowing plasma on tilting is positive result

Slide (for free coagulase) 1 drop of 0.85% saline on a slide +

a small amount of solid culture

Emulsify

Add 1 loopful of undiluted plasma

Clumping in 5–10 seconds (positive)

149

(vii) Phenylalanine deaminase (PPA) test
PRINCIPLE :

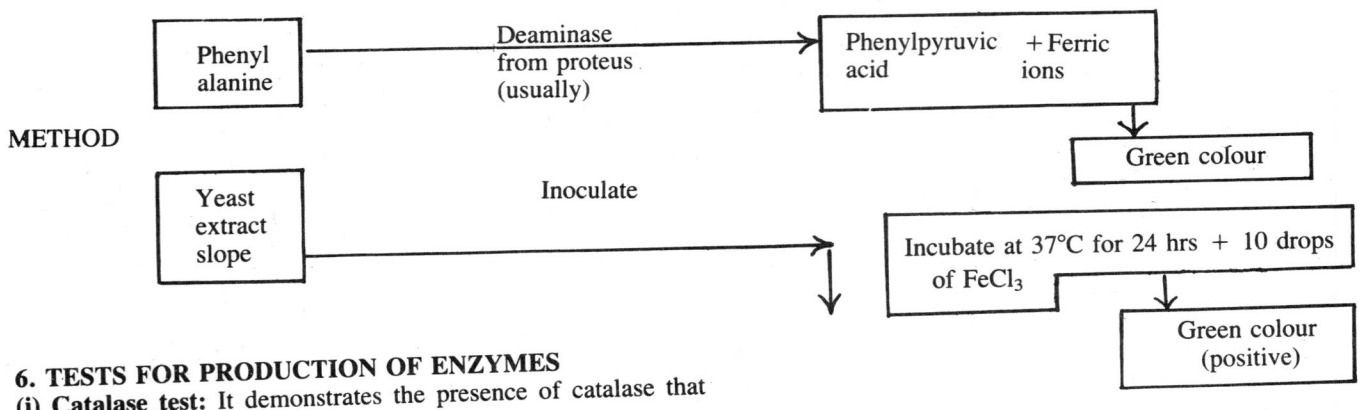

6. TESTS FOR PRODUCTION OF ENZYMES

(i) Catalase test: It demonstrates the presence of catalase that releases O_2 from H_2O_2.

Take 1–2 drops of H_2O_2 in a test tube. Put a small amount of solid culture from nutrient agar. Immediate production of gas signifies +ve test.

Precautions

1. Do not use blood agar which contains catalase
2. Do not use iron loop for inoculation.

(ii) Oxidase test: This demonstrates the presence of oxidase which catalyzes transport of electrons between electron donors & a redox dye (tetramethyl phenyldiamine)

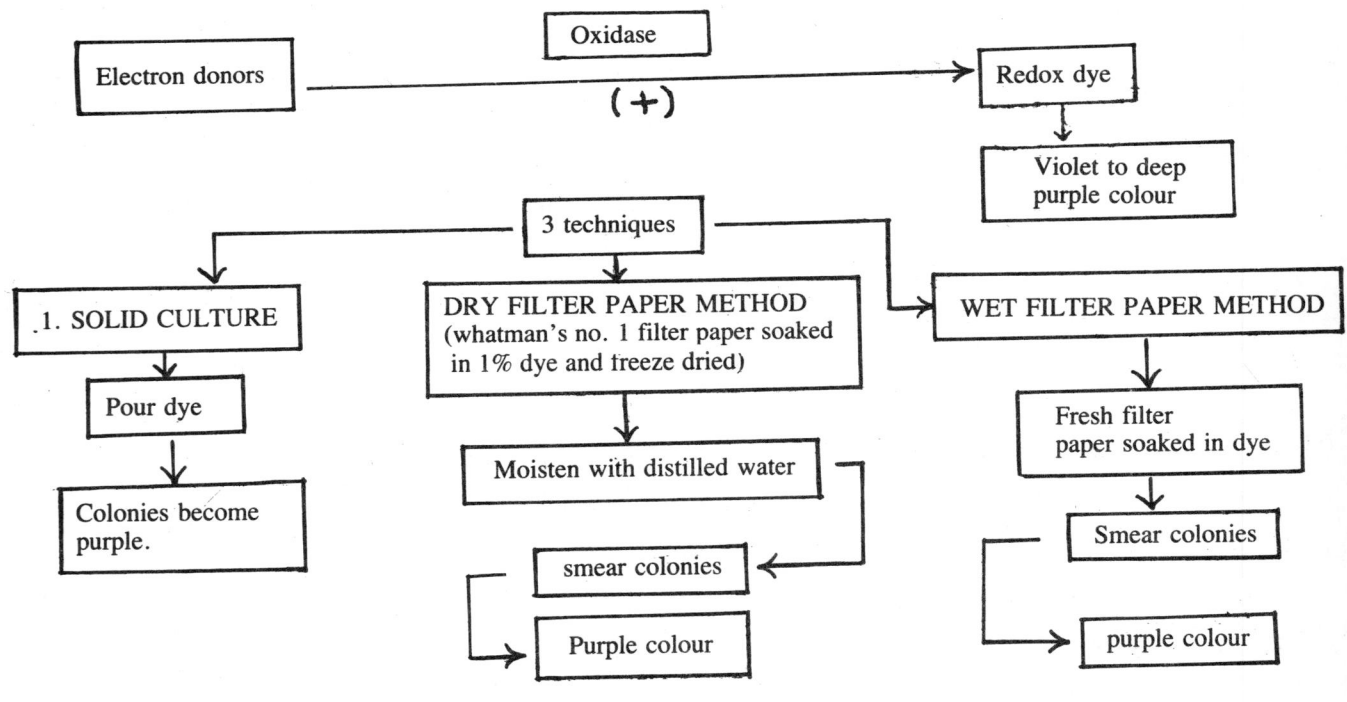

(iii) Lecithinase test (Naegler's test)

Some bacteria produce lecithinase or phospholipase that spilt lipoprotein complexes in human serum and hen egg yolk and produce opalescence or turbidity when grown in media containing these substrates.

Medium used — Nutrient broth with human serum or egg yolk suspension.

Test and control media are inoculated with a drop of liquid culture or a colony picked up from plate culture. A known lecithinase producing bacteria is placed in a control tube. Incubate under suitable conditions (aerobic/an aerobic) for 24–48 hrs, and lecithinase production is indicated by a pronounced turbidity with a yellowish curd on the surface of the test mixer.

Plate Test: Use a medium containing nutrient agar and sterile human serum with 5% fildes extract. Inoculate and incubate under suitable conditions (anaerobic for clostridia). Lecithinase producing colonies are surrounded by zones of opalescene (Naegler reaction).

In some cases an additional test is included by spreading a few drops of antitoxin to a specific lecithinase over half the plate before inoculation. Opalescence should be inhibited around colonies on antiloxin half, if the antitoxin is really specific.

7. Miscellaneous Tests

(i) **Potassium Cyanide test:** It tests the ability of an organism to grow in the presence of KCN. Basic Peptone water is utilized. Add 5% KCN soln to cold medium. Inoculate with the one loopful from a 24 hrs nutrient broth culture and incubate at 37°C. Observe after Inoculate Dubos and Davis slope medium.

(ii) **Niacin test:** Tubercle bacilli (hominis) produce niacin (Nicotnic acid) and this is detected with cyanogen bromide and aniline.
Inoculate Dubos and Davis slope medium
Incubate at 37°C for 72–96 hrs.
At regular intervals take a slope in a test tube
 +
1 ml of 10% cyanogen bromide
5 mins later add
1ml of 4% aniline in 96% ethanol.
Yellow color
(Positive)
Keep testing for 10 wks.
Then discard the culture.

SECTION VI
HISTOPATHOLOGY

CHAPTER 25

HISTOPATHOLOGY TECHNIQUES

Introduction:

The pathologist responsible for tissue diagnoses is heavily dependent on the competence of his histotechnologist. The ability to consistently turn out slides of high quality, well sectioned and well stained on a wide variety of tissue is indeed an art. To develop skill in this art requires not only training in basic principles, but also experience attention to detail, knowledge of the chemical rationale of the staining procedures carried out, and the ability to recognize quickly the probable cause of technical difficulties encountered in the daily work of the laboratory and to expediently remedy these difficulties.

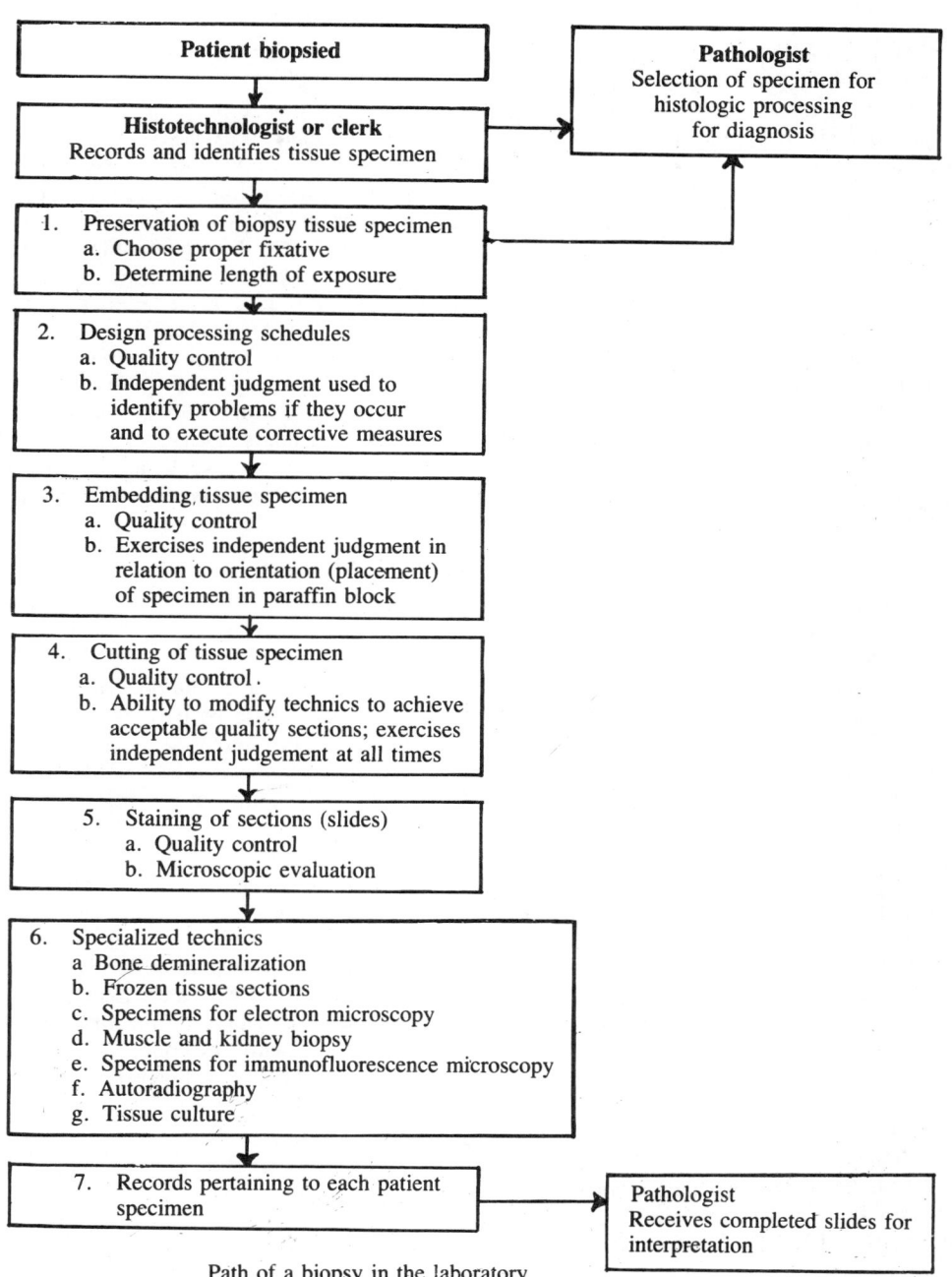

Path of a biopsy in the laboratory.

155

RECEPTION

Surgical pathology is that specialized branch of pathology that deals with the living. A requisition to the pathologist should be in the nature of a consultation request. It is not sufficient for the pathologist to merely say whether a lesion is benign or malignant. He must be able to tell the surgeon the extent of the disease, the adequacy of the excision and other pertinent information. He can do this only with the cooperation of the clinician who can give him all of the clinical and laboratory data.

It is for the technician posted at the reception to check whether the requisition form is duly filled. If inadequacies exist it may be brought to the notice of the pathologist who may contact the clinician to provide the missing information.

REGISTRATION:

The number of specimens received daily may be small or large depending on whether the laboratory caters to a small or large hospital. However, it is essential that accurate records are kept from the outset. This is best done by having a Reception Book in which all specimens are recorded, including all the relevant details. These consist of the name, age and sex of the patient; the OPD/MRD number; with ward and bed number of the inpatient; the name of the clinician and the organ biopsied or excised with the clinical diagnosis.

On arrival each specimen is given an accession number. This is followed by the year of entry, e.g. 1/85, continuing throughout the year and starting again as 1/86. The specimen will carry this number until it is processed, sectioned, reported and filed. It cannot be over-emphasized that whereas a specimen may change its place in a permanent collection, the initial accession number is final.

FIXATION OF SPECIMENS BEFORE GROSSING:

While every attempt is made to encourage the clinicians to send fresh specimens, often many specimens are received fixed in 10% formalin. The minimum amount of fixative required should be six to ten times the volume of the specimen. For any specimen containing inadequate quantity of fixative or which has been received in normal saline or in a dehydrated/autolysed state, a note should be made in the gross description and fixative added or replaced.

Hollow viscera like the stomach and intestine must be opened along the antimesenteric border. They should be pinned on paraffin trays of cork boards with the mucosal side up and fixed in 10% formalin in this state overnight.

FIXATIVES — THEIR MERITS AND DEMERITS

A good histological preparation requires immediate adequate and complete fixation. Fixation is required to (I) prevent post mortem changes such as putrefaction and autolysis (2) preserve various cell constituents in as life-like manner as possible (3) protect by hardening the soft tissues, allowing easy handling during processing; (4) Convert the normal semi-fluid consistency of cells to an irreversible semi-solid consistency (5) and in the visual differentiation of structure by using dyes and chemicals.

Ten percent buffered formalin is the most widely used fixative because it is compatible with most stains. The formaldehyde solution (approximately 40% formaldehyde gas in water) called formalin is treated as a 100% solution in making formalin percent solution (10 ml formalin and 90 ml H_2O = 10% formalin).

Formalin does not precipate proteins, it neither preserves destroys fat. It does not fix carbohydrates, it only preserves the proteins which in turn trap the glycogen so that it is not easily dissolved.

Formalin is buffered with sodium phosphate monobasic and dibasic to prevent its oxidation to formic acid.

Formalin Buffered

37–40% formalin-100 ml
Distilled Water — 900 ml.
Sodium phosphate monobasic — 4.0 gm.
Sodium phosphate diabasic
Annhydrous — 6.5 gm.

Formalin Neutral

Formalin (formaldehyde 40%) — 100 ml.
Tap water — 900ml.
Magnesium carbonate or
Calcium carbonate to excess.

Shake well and allow to stand several hours. Then decant off the volume of the clear fluid required for fixation.

Recommended for, particularly, nervous tissues. Also suitable for foezen sections. It is campatible with most stains.

Acetic Acid causes cell constituents to sweil. It does not fix carbohydrate or lipid. It gives excellent preservation of nuclei. It is used in combination with other fixatives having a shrinking effect.

Absolute alcohol is used for preservation of glycogen. It is the fixative of choice in cytology Carnoy's solution is rapid in action and may be used for urgent biopsy specimens for paraffin processing within five hours. Tissues can be directly transfered to absolute alcohol. It gives excellent nuclear fixation and preserves glycogen. Tissues should be directly transfered to 95% or absolute alcohol.

Carnoy's Solution

Absolute Alcohol	= 60.0 ml.
Chloroform	= 30.0 ml.
Glacial acetic acid	= 10.0 ml.

Picric Acid is used in a number of fixative mixtures. It requires damp storage because of its explosive nature. It colours tissue yellow. The yellow color is removed by washing in 50–70% alcohol. It preserves glycogen well. The tissues should be directly transferred to 80% alcohol for processing.

Bouin's Fluid

Saturated acqueous picric acid solution	= 75 ml.
40% formaldehyde	= 25 ml.
Glacial acetic acid	= 5 ml.

Mercuric chloride penetrates poorly and produces shrinkage of tissues. Tissues fixed with mercuric chloride containing fixatives contains black precipitates of mercury. These have to be removed from the sections with an alcoholic — iodine solution. The tissues stain more brilliantly, with most dyes following fixation with mercuric chloride.

Zenker's Solution

Distilled water	= 1000 ml
Mercuric chloride	= 50 gm
Potassium dichromate	= 25 gm
Sodium Sulfate	= 10gm

Add 5 ml. of glacial acetic acid to 95 ml of Zenker's solution before use. The tissues subsequently require through washing in tap water to remove traces of dichromate. (To further remove precipitates sections may be placed in 80% alcohol for 3 min. and rinsed in water. Next place in 3% aqueous sodium thiosulphate for 3 minute and wash in running water for 1–2 min.)

Glutaraldehyde penetrates large blocks poorly. However, it is the fixative of choice in electron microscopy where tissue blocks are one mm cubes in size. Post-fixation has to be done in osmium tetroxide solution otherwise certain components like membranes are extracted during dehydration.

The specimens should be covered with a layer of cotton after the formalin has been poured on the specimen. Large solid specimens should be bisected. The portion of the specimen being subjected to study may be serially cut at l cm intervals. For proper fixation insert layers of cotton soaked in formalin in between the cuts and fix the specimen in formalin.

Specimens like testicular biopies fixed in Bouin's solution may be transferred to 80% alcohol to facilitate removal of picric acid. Specimens fixed in potassium dichromate-containing fixative e.g. Zenker's fluid, require thorough washing in running tap water to remove traces of dichromate.

Specimens fixed in Carnoy's fluid should should be transferred to 95% or absolute alcohol directly.

GROSSING OF SPECIMENS:

Treat every specimen as infectious. Nothing other than the implements used for grossing and the specimen should be handled with the smeared gloves. The instrument as well as the board should be thoroughly washed in running water after grossing each specimen to prevent floaters from other specimens being introduced into the tissue blocks of the specimen being grossed.

It must be understood that the gross description as recorded on the requisition form is not being written to fulfill only a formality. It is a permanent record of what was received from the operating room. The general format of the gross descriptions should be as follows:

A. Number of pieces or general introductory statement about the specimen, such as "the specimen consists of a uterus with both tube and ovaries" or "received multiple pieces of".
B. Size in cms.,
C. Appearance,
D. Consistency,
E. Colour,
F. Contour, and
G. Tissues identified.

Blocks of specimen from the lesional areas are cut for processing. It is better to cut more blocks than few. The blocks should be thin, no greater than 4 mm in thickness and trimmed to a sufficiently small size to allow freedom of movement of the block within the capsule.

Specimens which consist of only very small pieces of tissue usually are processed in their entirety. Curettings when made up of larger pieces may require bisecting. Well preserved pieces with minimal areas of haemorrhage and necrosis should be processed.

For most tissue blocks, section are cut from the largest area of the tissue but there are many exceptions. Tissues of a tubular nature are frequently cut transversely. Skin is usually cut in a plane at right angles to the surface, as is tissue from the gastrointestinal tract, or any other epithelial surface. Muscle biopsies are sectioned in both transverse and longitudinal planes. When a particular feature is present on one surface only the opposite surface is nicked/marked with India Ink to ease difficulty in orientation during embedding later.

Nearly every bone specimen requires some decalcification. The preparation involves sawing the fragments of bone to demonstrate the lesion. 3 mm. thick sections from the lesional area is sawed from the specimen for decalcification. In case a bone biopsy contains soft uncalcified tissues, they may be processed separately (ensure there are no gritty areas as it will spoil the knife).

LABELLING OF TISSUES:

Once tissues have been selected for processing they are accompanied through all stages by a lable bearing the number given to the specimen. The lable is retained as a permanent record during sectioning and storage of tissue blocks.

Great care is to be taken to write the numbers of the blocks legibly and correctly on the labels before putting them into the capsules. The labels should indicate also the number of pieces being put into one casette. For example, if 2 pieces from a case with an accession number 802/85 are being put into one capsule the label should read 802/85 (2). In case, there are multiple pieces, (m) should indicate the number.

Very small biopsies like needle biopsies of kidney and liver, small curetting, etc. may be wrapped in filter paper soaked in formalin before being put in the capsules. Printed, graphite pencilled, type written or India Ink written labels are satisfactory. Ordinary ink should not be used as this may be dissolved in the reagents used during processing.

Remains of all specimens are preserved in formalin until the reported on are discarded. This may be indicated by writing SK(stock kept) at the end of grossing notes. In the event that no tissue is left, it may be indicated by writing NTL (No tissue left)

All specimens kept on the shelves are to be identified by legibly written numbers for future. All specimens of potential teaching value may be photographed and if considered worthy of display in the museum may be mounted.

DECALCIFICATION:

In order to obtain satisfactory paraffin or celloidin sections of bone or other calcified tissues it is necessary to remove the calcium salts to soften the tissues. This is carried out by treatment with reagents which react with calcium : acids to form soluble calcium salts or chelating agents to take up calcium ions.

Strong acid decalcifiers should only be used for urgent biopsy specimens with little mineralisations. 5–10 percent solutions of nitric and hydrochloric acids decalcify rapidly but when used more than 24–48 hours effect stainability of tissues.

5% Nitric Acid Solution

Nitric Acid, Concentrated (68–70%) = 5 ml.
Distilled water = 95 ml.

0.1% urea can be added to make nitric acid colourless as its yellow colour may interfere with staining reactions subsequently

Of the weak acids like formic, acetic and picric only formic acid is used extensively as a decalcifier in 5–10 percent solution. Decalcification should be complete in 1–10 days depending on the size and density of the specimens.

Aqueous Formic Acid

90% Formic Acid	= 5–10 ml
Distilled water	= to 100 ml.

The chelating agent widely employed for decalcification purpose is EDTA (Ethylene diamine tetracetic acid) in the form of its disodium salt. A simple solution upto 14 percent (approaching saturation) neutralised or with the addition of formalin is used.

Versenate (Ethylene diamine Tetra acetate) Solution:

EDTA	= 10 gm.
Distilled Water	= 100 ml.
(pH 5.5. to 6.5)	

Ion exchange resins, electrolysis and ultrasonics have been tried but any increase in acceleration in decalcification was negligible. To prevent "over decalcification" the tissue should be tested for completion of decalcification. The chemical and radiological tests are more reliable. Physical tests include "needling" or probing, cutting or trimming and palpation or bending and squeezing. While none of these are satisfactory and some actually destructive palpation can be a useful guide in experienced hands.

Blocks should be blotted or rapidly rinsed in tap water to remove excess acid before being routinely processed.

Processing of Tissue Specimens

Fixed tissues must be maintained in position by a firm medium so that thin, uniform sections can be cut. Media suitable for this purpose are paraffin, celloidin, and carbowax. Processing by the paraffin technic is accomplished most rapidly and gives the best results when thin sections of soft tissues are desired. Since paraffin is not miscible with water, the tissue must be dehydrated and then cleared in solutions miscible with paraffin before impregnation.

DEHYDRATION:

Some dehydrants used are ethanol, methylated spirit, methanol. acetone, isopropyl alcohol and dioxane. Alcohol is the most commonly used dehydrant usually starting with 80%. The dehydration process continues by upgrading the alcohols to absolute alcohol.

Ethanol due to high excise duty is too expensive for dehydration purposes. Commercial industrial methylated spirit has a more pronounced odour. It consist of ethanol to which has been added methanol to render the fluid unfit for consumption (making it cheaper by abolishing the liability to excise duty). It is easily available in strengths of 66–74 (OP) containing 95–99 per cent ethanol.

Methanol is poisonous and rarely, used as a dehydrant. Dioxane is a rapid dehydrant but the fumes are highly toxic. Acetone provides rapid dehydration and is cheap, but causes shrinkage and makes the tissue dry and hard making cutting difficult. Isopropyl alcohol can be used as a substitute for absolute alcohol, but absolute alcohol is always preferred.

CLEARING

The use of a clearing agent is necessary when the dehydrating agent, e.g. alcohol, is not miscible with the impregnating medium e.g. paraffin wax. As the dehydrant is removed, the tissue clears becoming translucent as many of these fluids have a similar refractive index as that of protein.

Xylene, toulene and benzene all clear well but are flammable and damaging on prolonged immersion of tissues. Chloroform is the clearing agent of choice in most laboratories. It is slower in action but causes less brittleness.

Carbon tetrachloride is toxic; amyl acetate and methyl benzoate have penetrating odour; cedarwood oil is slow in action; clove oil is expensive. Inhibisol (methyl chloroform) has been proposed as a replacement for existing clearing agents.

IMPREGNATION:

Although other media are available paraffin wax remains popular due to the ease with which large number of tissue blocks may be processed in comparatively short times with the minimum of supervision. In addition, sectioning and later staining presents fewer difficulties than other media.

Most histopathology departments have opted for the use of machines to process tissues. Superior results are possible by manual means but this may involve the changing of fluids at inconvenient times. Various schedule exist and can be modified by changing various processing fluids to suit individual laboratory needs.

MANUAL PROCESSING SCHEDULE: (Example)

1.	10% formalin overnight	
2.	80% alcohol	9.00 a.m. — 11.00 a.m.
3.	95% alcohol	11.00 a.m. — 1.00 p.m.
4.	Absolute alcohol	1.00 p.m. — 2.30 p.m.
5.	Absolute alcohol	2.30 p.m. — 4.00 p.m.
6.	Absolute alcohol overnight	
7.	Chloroform	9.00 a.m. — 11.00 a.m.
8.	Chloroform	11.00 a.m. — 1.00 p.m.
9.	Paraffin	1.00 p.m. — 3.00 p.m.
10.	Paraffin	3.00 p.m. — 4.00 p.m.
11.	Solidify	overnight
12.	Warm and then vacuum	9.00 a.m. — 11.00 a.m.
		embed and cool quickly.

AUTOMATIC TISSUE CHANGERS

The Autotechnicon, the oldest of the commercial tissue changers, is a valuable instrument in the histopathology laboratory. It is particularly so in large hospitals where an abundant volume of tissue is processed daily.

The Autotechnicon consists of a timing clock that is cut to determine immersion periods of the tissues; reagent beakers of glass or plastic which contain the reagents required by the particular technique being used; a beaker platform for precise alignment of breakers; a master shift carriage to automatically transfer tissues from one fluid to the next, in order, at time intervals predetermined by the timing clock; individual beaker covers, or a central cover to prevent evaporation of fluids; a displacer rotor, which provides constant rotation of the tissue basket during immersion in the fluids; receptacles, or cassettes, for carrying the tissue during the processing and paraffin baths.

The pathologist cuts the pieces of tissue and places them in the tissue receptacle with an identifying number. The receptacle basket is attached to the displacer rotor on an arm of the master shift carriage. The tissue basket rotates slowly during immersion and travels clockwise in an orbit, moving progressively from one reagent beaker to another through the various processing stages.

The sequence and duration of immersion periods are determined by the pathologist and are precisely maintained by the clock mechanism. The timing mechanism is an alternate-current electric clock controlled by a timing disc which permits a definite sequence of varying time intervals to be preset. The disc is calibrated over 24 hours and further subdivided into 5 minute intervals. When operating, it revolves on the clock face until a timing notch is encountered. At this point, a timing lever falls into the notch, starting the mechanism that raises the tissue basket from one fluid, shifts it, and immerses it into the next in line.

The basket is of stainless steel, with die-cut perforations. The firm closure of the cassette guards against the possibility of specimen loss or mix up. The snap-action opening facilitates removal of tissue when the receptacle is coated with paraffin from the paraffin bath. The cassettes are fully perforated at the top, bottom, and sides, permitting free passage and draining of fluids.

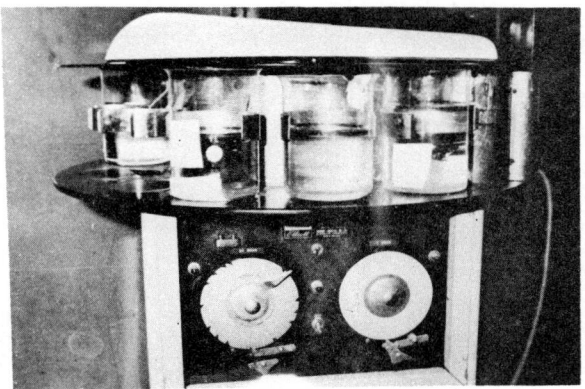

The care of the Autotechnicon is extremely important. Paraffin should be kept in the paraffin baths and removed from all other areas of the instrument with soft clothes soaked in xylene. The receptacles and basket should be soaked in xylene and washed in very hot soapy water to remove all residual paraffin. Individual lids or the large lid to cover beakers must be kept free of paraffin at all times.

AUTOTECHNICON PROCESSING SCHEDULE:
(Example)

1.	10% Formalin	— 2 hrs
2.	70% Alcohol	— 1 hr
3.	80% Alcohol	— 1 hr
4.	95% Aclohol	— 1 hr
5.	Absolute Alcohol	— 1 hr
6.	Absolute Alcohol	— 1 hr
7.	Absolute Alcohol	— 1 hr
8.	Acetone	— 1 hr
9.	Acetone	— 1 hr
10.	Chloroform	— 1 hr
11.	Chloroform	— 1 hr
12.	Paraffin (62°C)	— 2 hrs
13.	Paraffin (62°C)	—2 hrs

Embed and cool quickly.

REPLACEMENT OF PROCESSING FLUIDS

Solutions on the tissue processor should be changed once a week when an average of two basket loads of tissue are run each day. The solutions must be kept within one inch of the top of the beaker on the processor.

Any odour of the clearing agent in the final wax indicates that a change is required. Any spillage of fluid should be wiped away. Accumulation of wax must be removed particularly from beaker covers.

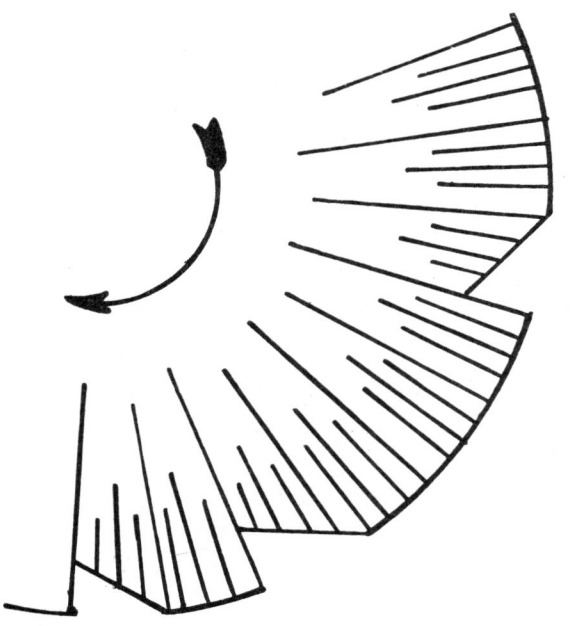

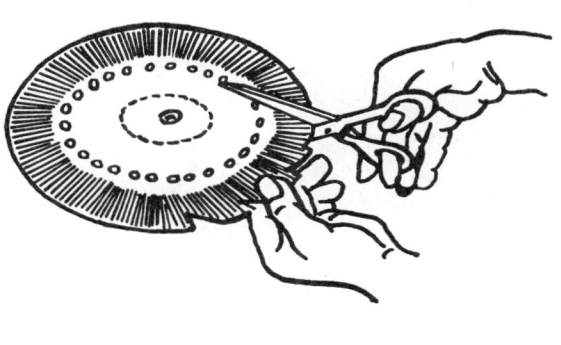

TIMING DISC
DIAGRAM: 5 A, Never cut straight along a line but rather angle back. as shown here. B, Timing notches are easily cut with ordinary scissors.

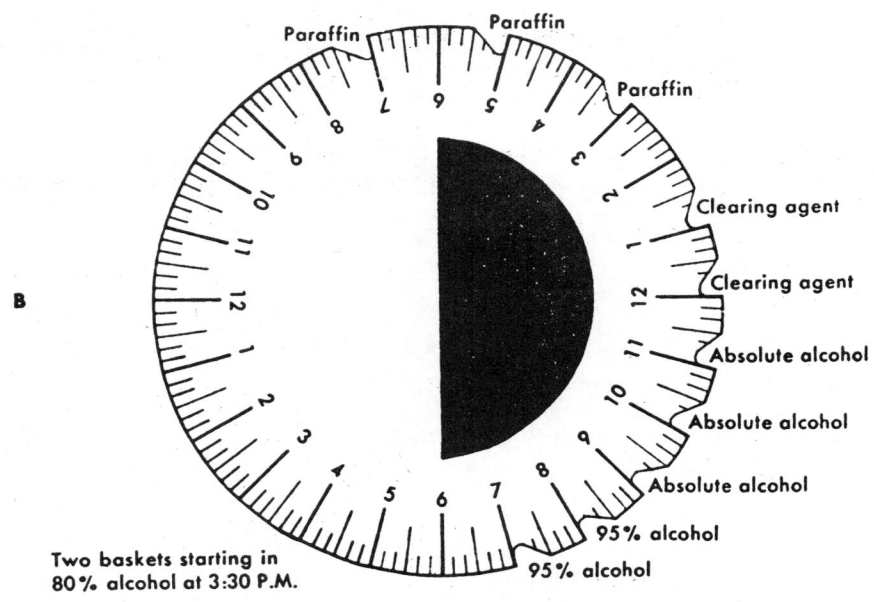

B

Paraffin
Paraffin
Paraffin
Clearing agent
Clearing agent
Absolute alcohol
Absolute alcohol
Absolute alcohol
95% alcohol
95% alcohol

Two baskets starting in
80% alcohol at 3:30 P.M.

DIAGRAM: 6 TIMING DISC FOR ROUTINE SPECIMENS.

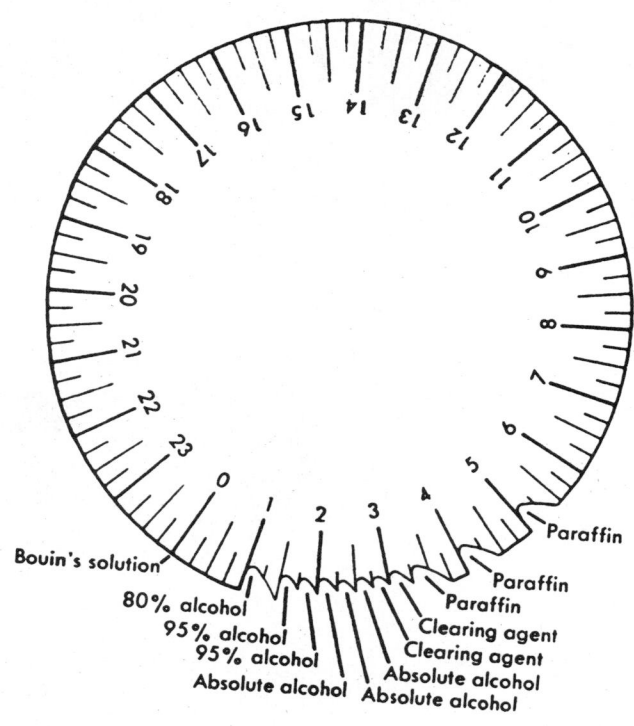

Bouin's solution
80% alcohol
95% alcohol
95% alcohol
Absolute alcohol
Absolute alcohol
Clearing agent
Clearing agent
Paraffin
Paraffin
Paraffin

DIAGRAM: 7 TIMING DISC FOR RUSH SPECIMENS

EMBEDDING OF TISSUE SPECIMENS

Embedding is the orientation of tissue in melted paraffin which when solidified, provides a firm medium for keeping intact all parts of the tissue when cut. For use as moulds in the production of wax blocks the most commonly preferred methods advocate the use of leuck hart's lead L's and the Tissue Tech embedding system.

Molten paraffin wax is dispensed into the mould to a depth more than adequate to cover the thickest tissue block. When a thin film of semi-solid wax has formed on the base of the mould, the tissue is introduced with warmed forceps, gently pressing the tissue flat into the semi-solid wax in the correctly orientated plane. Remember to "edge embed" the skin, cyst wall, mucosal or any other epithelial surface.

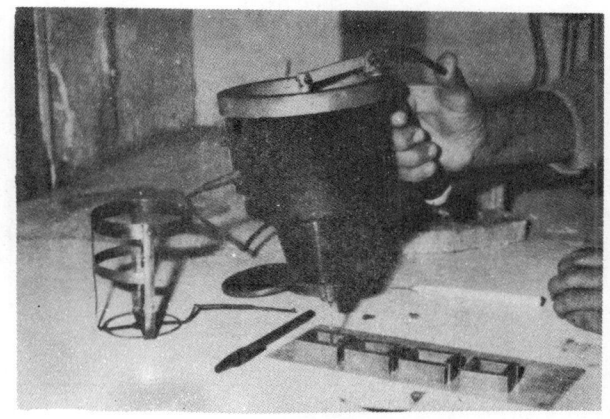

FIG: 68 : Showing Paraffin Embedding:

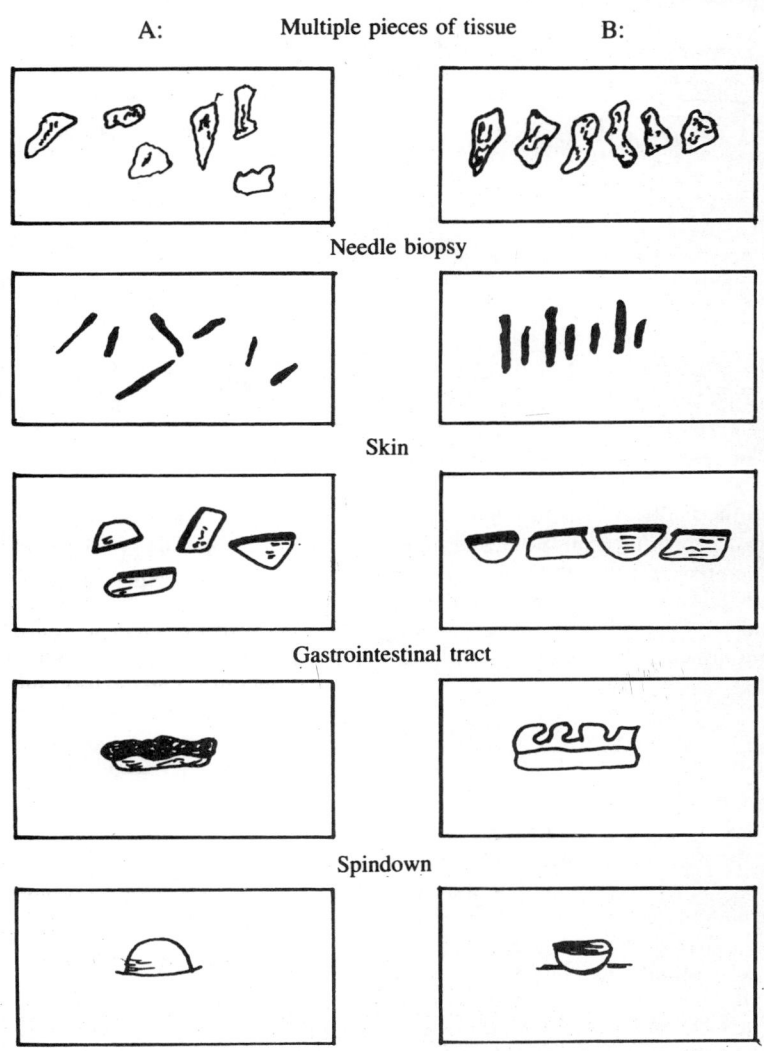

DIAGRAM: 8 : Showing A: Incorrect and B: Correct Embedding of different types of tissues.

161

Tubes

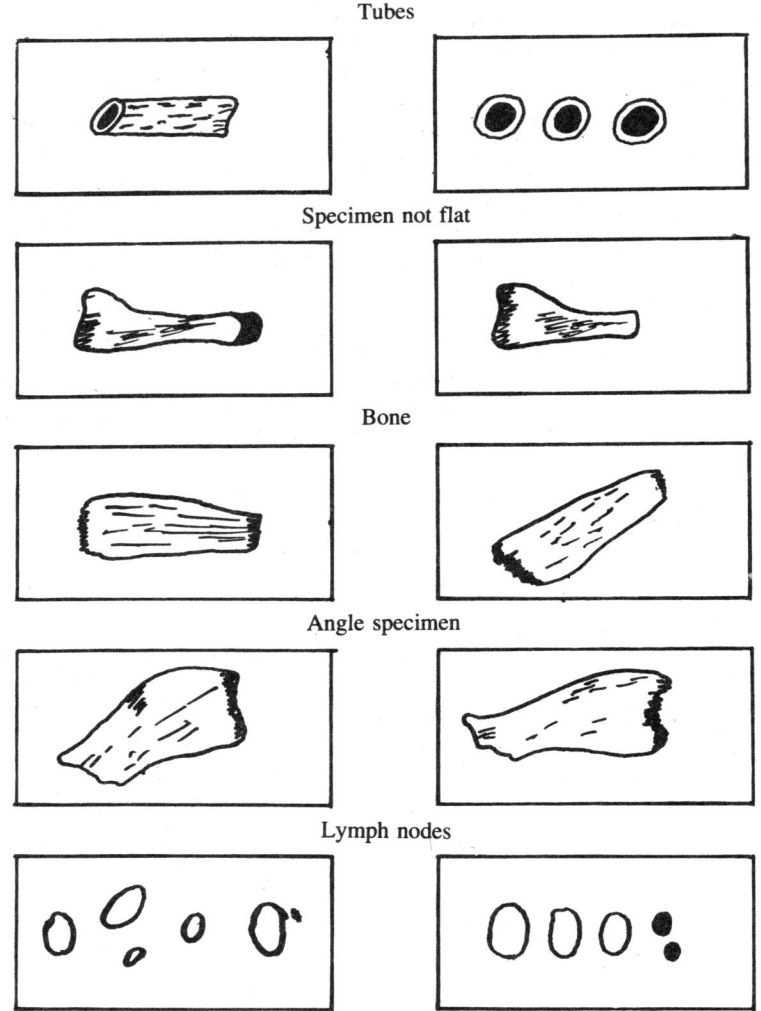

Specimen not flat

Bone

Angle specimen

Lymph nodes

When transferring tissue from the paraffin bath to embedding mould do not allow a thin layer of paraffin to solidify around the specimen. As soon as a film of semi-solid wax has formed on the surface the whole may be submerged beneath cold water to hasten solidification of the wax. This reduces the tendency to large crystal formation in the wax. Also trimming can be commenced without delay

TRIMMING OF BLOCKS:

The tissue surface towards the mould base is the one from which sections have to be cut. This surface may be lightly trimmed with a scalpel to expose the tissue. The opposite face, to be attached to the wooden block is trimmed flat and parallel to the first. The sides of the block which, in sectioning are to be parallel to the knife edge, are trimmed, leaving 2 to 3 millimetres of wax between the edge and the tissue for easy separation of sections later. The two remaining sides are trimmed leaving only a minimum of wax between edge and tissue to allow it to stretch on the water bath. Equal margins of paraffin should be left on all four sides of circular pieces of tissue.

The blocks are next attached to a wooden blocks, plastic type blocks or brass holders with the help of a heated spatula. In

attaching wax blocks to wood or metal blocks both are heated by means of the spatula and pressed together whilst molten.

Cutting of Tissue Specimens

MICROTOMES

All microtomes use the motion of a screw thread in order to advance the tissue block or knife a regulated number of microns. The most commonly used Rotary microtome has the advantage of producing large number of serial sections from tissues reasonable in size and hardness. Other are the Rocking, Freezing, Base sledge and Vibrating knife microtomes.

Knives can be divided into four basic profiles a) Wedge, b) Planoconcave, c) Biconcave and d) Tool edge.

The wedge is the most common knife profile type. Sharpening this profile is easier (either automated or manual) than with others.

SHARPENING OF KNIVES:

The sharpening of microtome knives may be carried out either by manual means or on automated machines. In hand honing good quality stones give the best results. The yellow Belgian and the Belgian black vein are the finest available. Synthetic slabs like carborundum are also used.

A liquid medium for sharpening with a hone is necessary

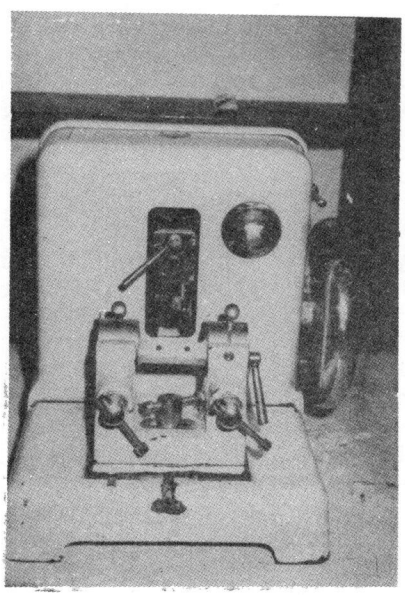

Fig: 69 : Showing Rotary Microtome

Lubricants act as coolants, allow fine metal particles to flow away from the knife, and fresh abrasive particles to contact the knife edge. A household 3 in 1 oil, mineral oil, vegetable oil, or a neutral soap solution may be used. The latter is easily prepared by dissolving household (bar) soap in water.

The majority of knives including the wedge type used in both rotary and base sledge microtomes, require handle and back to be attached for manual shapening. The purpose of the back is to lift the knife away from the sharpening surface in order to produce edge facets at a suitable angle. Backs should not be regarded as interchangeable. Each knife should have its own back, marked so that it may be fitted in the same position each time.

Microtome knives are dangerous instruments which should at all times be treated with respect. The transporting of a knife, even if the distance is only a few feet, should always be carried out with the knife in its box, with the lid fastened. Before commencing sharpening, the edge should be examined under a microscope. Any gross irregularities in the edge should be visible in the horizontal position, whilst in the vertical position any rounding of the edge is seen as a ribbon of reflected light.

The stone or glass plate to be used as the manual sharpening surface must be positioned on a non-slip surface on a firm bench, at comfortable working height and adequately lighted.

The surface may then be lightly charged with the chosen abrasive powder or paste. The action of sharpening is illustrated

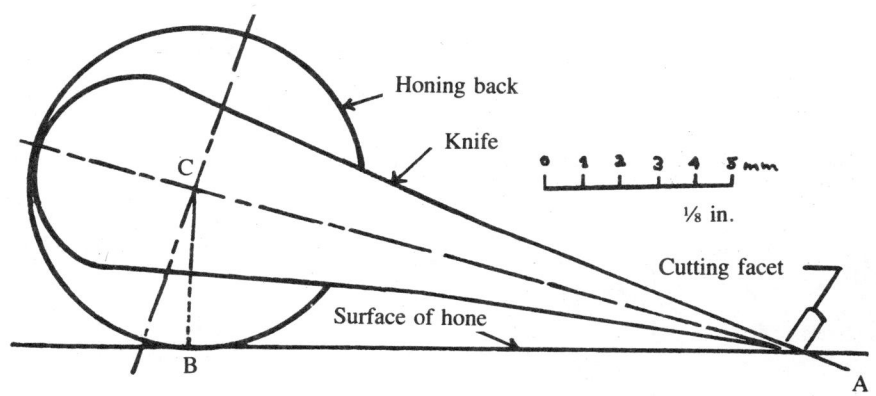

DIAGRAM: 9 : Knife and honing back drawn to scale to show extent and formation of cutting bevel and facets.

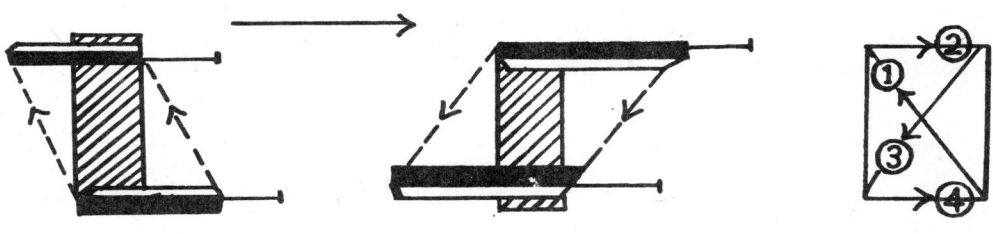

DIAGRAM: 10: Showing Sharpening procedure

It will be seen that the motion is rather similar to a figure of eight. The change over to the return stroke taking place by rocking and sliding the knife over on its back, never on its edge. While honing, the knife should be kept flat held to the hone by its own weight with its edge facing the direction of the 'heel to toe' motion, under continuous but light pressure speed is not essential. The aim is to maintain smooth even strokes. Any drying of the hone must be prevented by the addition of fresh lubricant.

The edge should be finished on a leather or linen strop to remove the microscopic knife serrations caused by the sharpening method. Traces of lubricant and debris must be removed with a cloth moistened with xylene.

Stropping should be performed so that all area of the knife edge are exposed to the strop surface equally, if possible. The movement of the knife should be from toe to heel for 8 to 12 times.

Excess stropping will round the edge and dull the knife. Six to 12 strokes on either side of the knife are usually sufficient.

Some strops are embedded with diamond particles. These strops are excellent but should be used cautiously. Five strokes on either side of the knife are recommended.

Strops are leather (horsehide, calfskin, and pigskin) or linen. Three are three types of strops: (1) the hanging strop (razor strop), (2) the saddleback strop, a strop stretched across a heavy frame and made taut by turning an extending screw at one end, (3) the block strop, a strop mounted on a felt-padded wood block. The block strop is recommended for better support of the knife.

Linen cloth, when fastened to a stropping frame and stretched to its maximum, serves as a fine finishing strop. The linen strop produces a sharp edge and is sometimes used alone to strop a knife that is slightly dull.

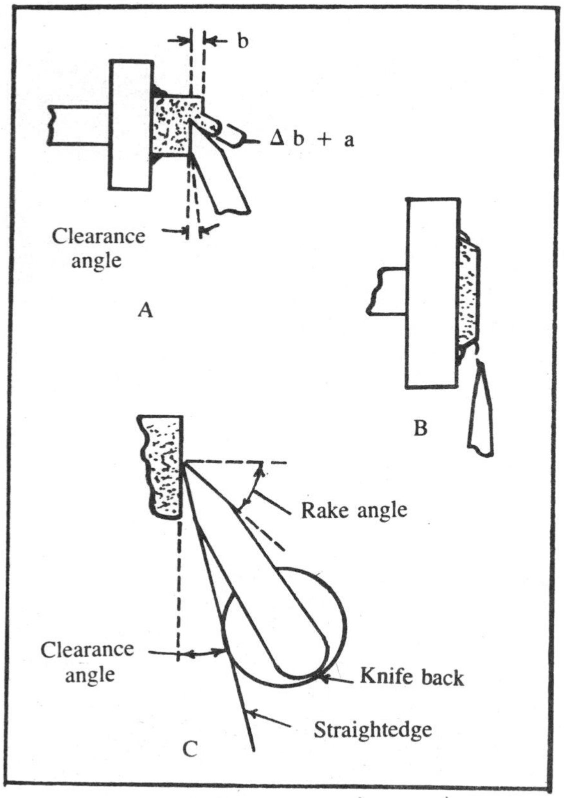

DIAGRAM: 11: A, showing clearance angle and increase in section thickness from compression. B. Wedging effect when there is no clearance angle. C, How to set clearance angle.

The knife should be cleaned after each use by removing the accumulated paraffin and sediment with a piece of gauze soaked with xylene

Store the knife in a safe, cool place in its own case. The care and use of the knife should never be minimized or neglected". "Remember, the tissue technician is only as good as his knife".

SECTION CUTTING

The rotary microtome is most commonly used as it is capable of producing large numbers of sections, particularly serial sections from anything other than the largest and hardest of tissues. A proper cutting angle between 5–10° is suitable for most tissues. Hard fibrous tissue such as uterus and bone may require a setting of 15°

The microtome is adjusted from 4 to 6 microns on the scale and oiled to ensure slow and even turn of the wheel. Apart from a microtome, several other items are required before sectioning is undertaken.

1. Water bath, kept at 10°C below melting point of wax. Any bubbles are removed by tapping the bath sides.
2. Hot plate, at the melting point of wax of a little lower temperature.
3. Fine pointed forceps.
4. Small squirrel hair brush and seekers. These instruments will help manipulation of sections during cutting and for the removal of folds and creases in sections after floating out.
6. Scalpel-
7. Clean cloth or paper towel.
8. Slide Rack
9. A supply of clean slides coated with adhesive.
10. Section adhesive like albumen, etc.
11. Blotting paper slightly moistened with clean water.
12. A supply of ice cubes to cool surface of block before cutting. In many laboratories paraffin blocks are cooled with ice before cutting. The need for this is dependent upon atmospheric temperature, melting point of wax and humidity. Any moisture introduced is removed by blotting.

Tissues impregnated in wax usually require a section adhesive for the tissue sections to remain adherent to the slides throughout most staining techniques. Albumin based adhesives are routinely used.

Mayer's egg albumin: Egg white — 50 ml. Glycerin — 50 ml. mix well and filter several thicknesses of gauze. Add a crystal of thymol to preserve.

Section cutting may be carried out with the operator standing or sitting. The bench height should suit the chosen attitude for sectioning in comfort, bearing in mind that several hours at a time may be spent in this occupation. Orientation of the block in the microtome should be correct. Long axis of block should be parallel to knife. Dense capsule or tough surfaces of tissue should be at the top. Before any movement of the microtome is attempted the tissue block must be brought forward until its surface is fractionally behind the knife level. In order to trim away any surplus wax and to expose a suitable area of tissue for sectioning, the section thickness adjuster is set at 15 um. or alternately the coarse feed mechanism is advanced manually before commencing each stroke. On exposing a suitable area of tissue, the section thickness is set to the appropriate level, for routine purposes 4 to 6 microns.

Sections should ribbon in a flat, unwrinkled fashion. This always indicates a properly sharpened knife. If sections are cut until the ribbon is several centimetres long, handling is greatly eased, the first section being held with the fingers or forceps and the last section being detached from the knife by means of a small brush or seeker. To obtain flat sections it is necessary to spend time in the cutting and the gentle stretching of the ribbon before floating on the water surface in the water bath. The action in floating out must be smooth. As the trailing end of the ribbon touches the water surface the slight drag produced is sufficient to produce tension in the ribbon and remove some folds from the sections. A heated scalpel or blade can be used to separate the sections from each other.

To pick up sections on the glass slides insert the slides smeared with adhesive, into the floatation bath perpendicularly to three quarters of its length and manoeuver the section into contact with the slide. On lifting the slide vertically from the water the section will flatten on to the slide. Care should be taken to orient sections so that it is placed centrally allowing free margins for subsequent cover-slipping and labelling.

Sections should be drained approximately one minute before final drying on a slide warming table or hot plate. The plate is regulated at the melting point of the wax, and the total drying and adhesion time is ten minutes.

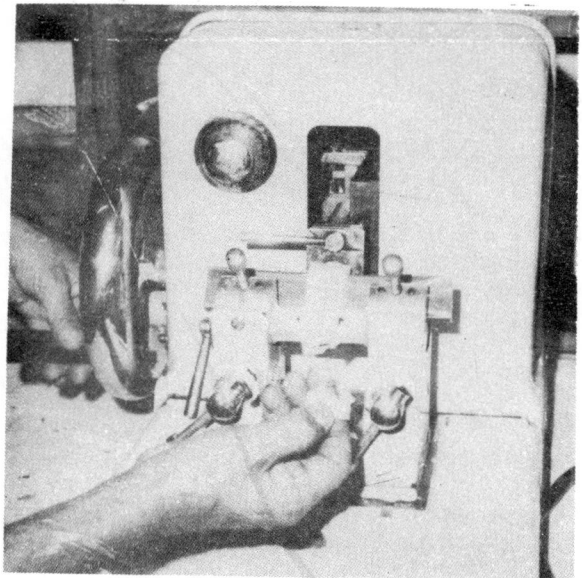

Fig: 70 : Showing method of ribbon formation

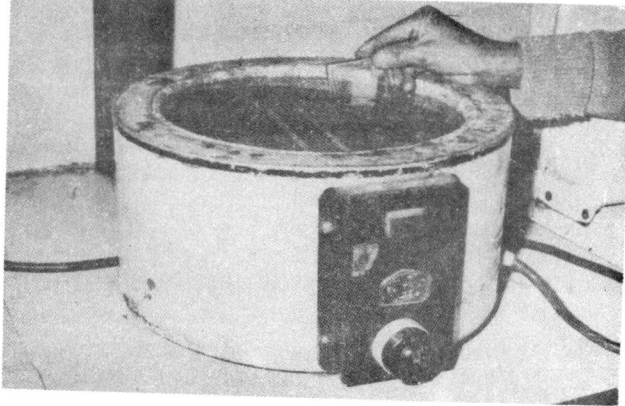

Fig. 71 : Showing Floatation bath

ROUTINE STAINING PROCEDURES

After sectioning and drying of paraffin sections, the general procedures outlined next are performed for most routine and special staining methods:
  Deparaffinization
  Hydration
  Staining
  Dehydration
  Clearing
  Coverslipping

Deparaffinization

The deparaffinization process functions to remove the paraffin wax from the tissue and surrounding area on the slide. Xylene is the usual reagent used for this purpose and three changes over a 10-minute period are desirable for complete removal of the paraffin wax. Sections should appear clear at this stage of the process. If while patches are seen. It most likely means that the slide has not been dried sufficiently and that water has been trapped under the paraffin. Put such sections in absolute alcohol for a few minutes: the water is soluble in this reagent. Then return the slide to xylene for completion of the deparaffinization process, and follow with the regular hydration sequence.

Slides that have just been removed from the drying oven should be allowed to cool to room temperature before being placed in the xylene. Slides should not be allowed to dry from the time hydration is begun until coverslipping is completed in most cases. An exception would be if celloidin-coating proved to be necessary.

All solutions used should adequately cover the tissue and slide itself during the deparaffinization and subsequent processes. Slides should be placed in the staining rack, basket, or other container, so that the side on which the tissue is mounted is facing the same direction for all the slides. This facilitates the coverslipping process.

Hydration

After deparaffinization, slides are hydrated. Hydration is a gradual process that uses a series of graded alcohols until water is used. The purpose of this process is to prepare the tissue to stain with a dye that has been dissolved in an aqueous solvent. The following procedure is suggested as a good guideline to proper hydration:

Reagent	Approximate time of immersion
Absolute (100%) ethanol	3 to 5 min
Absolute (100%) ethanol	3 to 5 min
95% ethanol	3 to 5 min
95% ethanol	3 to 5 min
80% ethanol	3 to 5 min
70% ethanol	3 to 5 min
60% ethanol	3 to 5 min
Tap water	until sections are clear

Comments on hydration process

1. Sections will turn from clear to slightly opaque when they are immersed in the absolute alcohol. If clear patches are visible after the tissue is immersed in the absolute alcohol, it means that all the paraffin has not been removed, and if this is the ease, the section or sections should be returned to xylene.

165

2. Drain sections as completely as possible before transferring to the next reagent.
3. Reagents used in the deparaffinization and hydration process should be changed at regular intervals depending on laboratory use. To economize, it is helpful to make the second change of each reagent (where applicable) the first change, and use fresh solutions to comprise the second change.

Dehydration and clearing

After staining, sections are commonly dehydrated by successive changes of graded alcohols and cleared in several changes of xylene. The following outline is a guide to proper dehydration and clearing, using ethanol and xylene as the principal reagents:

95% ethanol	15 sec to 1 min
95% ethanol	15 sec to 1 min
Absolute ethanol	15 sec to 1 min
Absolute ethanol	15 sec to 1 min
Xylene	15 sec to 1 min
Xylene	15 sec to 1 min
Xylene	15 sec to 1 min

Comments on dehydration and clearing.

Ethanol also functions to differentiate certain stains, notably eosin in the H & E technique. Besides ethanol, the following reagents may be used to dehydrate tissue: isopropanol, acetone, and tert-butanol. These other three dehydrants give better preservation of thiazin dye staining than does ethanol and are used in certain special staining technics. After the xylene treatment, sections should appear clear. If sections appear opaque either completely or in spots, it means that the dehydration process was inadequate and that water remains in the tissue. The inadequacy of the dehydration process is commonly caused by (1) insufficient time in the dehydrating fluids and (2) water contamination of the dehydrating fluids. If reason 1 is the cause, sections should be retreated with absolute alcohol for several minutes and then cleared again in xylene. If reason 2 is the cause, the contaminated alcohols should be changed and the sections dehydrated in the fresh absolute alcohol, followed by xylene clearing.

Xylene that is water-contaminated appears somewhat milky. Such xylene should be properly discarded in accrodance with safety pre cautions. If the same dish has to be reused, make sure it iswell-dried prior to filling it with fresh xylene It is preferable to fill a clean dry dish with fresh xylene.

A solution of carbol-xylene may be used in the dehydrating process to assist in removal of all water traces. This solution has the following composition: melted phenol crystals (carbolic acid), I part; xylene, 3 parts. Two quick dips are usually sufficient for 5μm paraffin sections.

Xylene that has been used for deparaffinizing slides should not be used for clearing after dehydration, since it contains paraffin in solution that will subsequently interfere with the proper hardening of the mounting medium.

Coverslipping

The purpose of coverslipping is to preserve the stained-tissue section for subsequent handling and microscopic examination. The cover slip (cover glass) is attached to the slide by a reagent called a mounting medium. There are numerous kinds of mounting media available.

MOUNTING MEDIA:

In order to provide the maximum degree of transparency to stained tissue sections the refractive index of the mounting media must be same as that of dried protein. Aqueous mountants are made up of gum arabic solutions in high concentration of sugars or solutions of gelatine in glycerol.

KAISER'S GLYCEROL JELLY:

Gelatine	=	10 gm
Distilled water	=	60 ml
Glycerol	=	70ml
Phenol	=	0.25 gm

Dissolve the gelatine in distilled water in incubator or water bath before adding the remaining ingredients. The medium sets solid and requires melting before use. Many aqueous mounting media remains permanently sticky with the possibility of the cover slips moving

Resinous mounting media dry quickly and fix the coverslips well in place permanently. DPX is the most commonly used routine mountant. It does not cause fading with the majority of stains. The coverslips provide protection of the section to abrasion.

Labels are placed at one end of the slide and the accession number inscribed on the label. The slides are placed serially on a despatch tray. The despatch trays of slides accompanied by their respective Requisition Forms are placed before the histopathologist for reporting. The reported slides are later permanently stored in the department. The Requisition forms are filed after the report has been typed. The slides and the forms will form a permanent collection.

Cover slips are purchased from laboratory supply companies in various sizes and are commonly used in laboratories in three different thicknesses.

Thickness number	Average thickness of cover slip
1	150μm
1½	180μm
2	210μm

The cover slip that provides an ideal range for photomicrography is number 1½.

Coverslipping should be done in a clean, well lighted area. Have a flat surface available for placing slides while the mounting medium dries. Have the necessary materials ready:
1. The mounting medium needed (the medium should be of a good consistency for rapid and even spreading)
2. Coverslipping forceps
3. Gauze or some lint-free cloth
4. Cover slips of various sizes

Methods

1. Drain the excess xylene from the slide to be cover slipped, and wipe the back of the slide using the lint-free cloth. Extraneous tissue or nonspecific stain may also be wiped off at this time. This wiping should be done quickly. Do not allow the tissue to dry or it will appear opaque when viewed microscopically. Reimmerse the tissue section in xylene if the section appears to be drying out.

2. The amount of mounting medium needed will vary depending on the size of the area to be cover slipped and the nature of the

medium itself. Too much mounting medium will result in a messy slide and will cause the section to appear cloudy when viewed microscopically. Too little mounting medium will cause air bubbles that can later enlarge and impair the quality of the section.

3. The correct amount of medium may be placed either on the slide or on the cover slip.

Slide method: Place the correct amount of medium over the section and angle the slide so that the medium flows down to the bottom edge of the slide. Then place the cover slip against the bottom edge of the slide at about a 45 degree angle and allow the medium to run along the bottom edge of the cover slip, Gently lower the cover slip, and the medium should spread over the section and slide. Allow the medium to harden.

Cover-slip method: Place the correct amount of medium in the center of the lower edge of the cover slip. Bring the slide up to the edge of the cover slip, position the slide so that the tissue will be adequately covered by the cover slip, and invert the slide over the cover slip. The medium should spread quickly under the cover slip and the slide is inverted again and allowed to dry.

Either of the above methods should take only 5 to 10 seconds to complete. When coverslipping by use of a synthetic resinous mounting medium and the coverslipped section shows that there are a few air bubbles present, gently remove them by applying pressure with the coverslipping forceps. If there are numerous air bubbles present it is a waste of time to try to chase them out and in addition, the tissue itself can be harmed. Instead, reimmerse the section with the cover slip in the xylene until the cover slip is removed. After the cover slip is removed, gently slosh the slide to remove traces of mounting medium, and remount the section. Never leave the removed cover slips in a jar of xylene. Cover slips become almost invisible in xylene (and other liquids) and can cause cuts. In addition, cover slips can break easily and will cut a finger even through heavy dishwashing gloves.

If there is excess synthetic resinous mounting medium present, it may be cleaned off immediately by gentle wiping of it with some xylene-moistened gauze. Do not disturb the cover slip during this process. Excess aqueous mounting medium may be cleaned off the slide using water-moistened gauze.

Removal of cover slips mounted with synthetic mounting medium: On occasion, it is necessary to remove a cover slip that has be come well adhered to the slide. One may do this as follows: (1) place the slide in a covered Coplin jar containing xylene and leave the slide immersed until the cover slip detaches. Do not force the cover slip off, since this can damage the tissue. (2) The removal process can be facilitated when the covered Coplin jar (screw-cap variety) containing the slide immersed in xylene is placed into the paraffin oven (56° to 58°C). Usually the cover slip detaches in about 30 miniutes with this process. CAUTION: This process is best done in a hood. There is a fire and explosion hazard if an improperly calibrated oven is used and the solution becomes too warm. (3) If liquid nitrogen is available, put the slide in a metal dish or hold the slide with long forceps. Dip in the liquid nitrogen and the cover slip will pop off. Dispose of all removed cover slips properly.

Destaining and restaining

If it is necessary to destain and restain a slide, first remove the cover slip with one of the methods described above and hydrate the slide to 70% alcohol. The section may then be treated with a 1%

solution of hydrochloric acid in 70% alcohol until it is fairly colorless. It is then washed well in tap water to remove traces of acid and rinsed in distilled water, and the new staining procedure is begun. Alternatively, weak ammonia alcohol or 5% oxalic acid may assist in removing color from any previously stained slide. Section previously stained with an iron hematoxylin stain should not be restained with the conventional Prussian blue reaction, since the iron-lake still present will react with the potassium ferrocyanide. The iron lake may be removed by treatment of the sections for 1 to 2 hours in 5% sodium dithionite ($Na_2S_2O_4$).

General Staining Consideration

Biological stains are dyes used for making microscopic object more clearly visible than they would be unstained. Dyes themselves can be classified into two groups the natural dyes and the synthetic dyes.

The most important of the natural dyes are haematoxylin, indigo, cochineal and carmine, orcein and Brazilin.

The synthetic dyes are referred to as acid or basic dyes. In an acid dye the chromophoric grouping is located in the anionic part of the molecule; the basic dye is a salt of a color base, that is the chromophoric groups are located in the cationic part of the molecule.

The staining processes allow a color to diffuse throughout the section and adhere to a particular structure in four main ways.

The first phenomenon is surface adsorption, a physical reaction dependent both on the charge of the ionized dye and the charge upon the materials on which the dye is precipitated. The second involves direct staining that employs a weak solution of a stain on the assumption that it will be differentially absorbed by various structures and tissues. Density of the tissue is a factor in controlling the absorption of the dye. The third way color may adhere involves indirect staining where the dye is applied from a relatively strong solution and is subsequently extracted from the unwanted structures either by a solvent or by some additional chemical reagent. The fourth type of staining employs mordants. A mordant is a salt or hydroxide of a divalent or trivalent metal and serves to strongly attach dye to a tissue. The compound formed by a dye radical with the mordant is called a lake, and these lakes may be unstable or insoluble depending on the exact nature of the combination and the solvents subsequently employed. There are three ways in which mordants may be used: mordant preceding dye; mordant and dye used together; mordant following dye. The use of mordants in dyeing technics has the advantage of making the dye relatively permanent in tissue (once the mordant-dye has combined with the tissue). It renders the dye insoluble in neutral solutions, enables other forms of staining to follow the mordant-dye technic, and will not decolorize on dehydration.

In action, stains may be classified as substantive, adjective, or impregnation stains. A substantive stain is one that acts immediately and directly upon the tissue without the intervention of any other substance. An adjective stain is one in which the tissue is first treated with some agent, which in turn attaches the stain to the tissue, such as is done in mordant staining. Impregnation stains involve the deposition of sensitive metallic substances over selected cells and tissue structures that are rendered visible by a subsequent reduction of the metal. Many neurologic methods employ impregnation. Actually this method is not staining in the true sense of the word, and it differs in that structures demonstrated are usually rendered opaque or black, the coloring matter is particulate, and the deposit is on or around, but not in, the element demonstrated.

In time, stains may be classified as progressive or regressive, Progressive staining is done by watching the degree of staining in sections under the microscope at various points during the staining process and stopping the process when the selective action of the stain has differentiated the desired parts.

When regressive staining technics are employed, all the stainable tissue components are completely saturated with dye. To have any value as a readable slide, some of this excess stain much be removed, and this process is called differentiation. Differentiation usually gives sharp staining contrasts because the hydronium and hydroxide ions in the solvents used to differentiate diffuse more rapidly than does any dye ion, and this accounts for the more even results obtained. The differentiation step is a relative one and removes the dye from certain tissue components more easily and rapidly than from others. A properly destained section will have the desired features retaining sufficient stain to make them clearly visible, and the other tissue components will be completely cleared from the dye. Some of the ways in which a section may be differentiated include the use of acidic or basic mediums, excess mordant, buffers, or oxidizers.

It is generally known that basic dyes are differentiated by a weakly acid medium, and acid dyes are differentiated by a weakly basic one. For example, when staining in alum hematoxylin, one may use a solution of acid alcohol to differentiate the section. If a section has been overstained in eosin (an acid dye), it can be differentiated in a basic medium composed of alcohol containing 0.1% to 0.5% concentrated ammonium hydroxide. Many of the acid and basic differentiators use alcoholic solutions rather than aqueous, since the alcoholic solutions usually give a better control of the differentiation process itself than do the aqueous ones. The reason is that the majority of dyes used in staining tissue are more soluble in water than in alcohol, and although staining should be done in a more soluble medium (aqueous), less of differentiation is desired. By use of this method, the whole tissue is completely stained and then differentiated to remove excess dye from the parts desired unstained.

The Haematoxylin and Eosin stain is probably the most widely used histological stain. It is popular for various reasons: It is simple to perform, it can stain different types of tissues fixed in different ways. The haematoxylin component stains the cell nuclei blue-black with good intranuclear detail whilst the eosin stains cell cytoplasm and most connective tissue fibres in varying shades and intensities of pink, orange and red.

Haematoxylin is extracted from the heart wood of the tree Haematoxylin compechianum found in Mexico and now mainly cultivated in the West Indies. Haematoxylin itself is not a stain. Haematein its oxidation product is the natural dye. Haematein can be produced from haematoxylin in two ways: (1) Natural oxidation by exposure to light and air. This takes 3–4 months but also lasts for a long time e.g. Ehrlich's and Delafield's haematoxylin solutions; (2) Chemical oxidation using sodium iodate (e.g. Mayer's haematoxylin) or mercuric oxide (e.g. Harris's haematoxylin). They are ready for use immediately after preparation but have a shortened shelf life.

Haematein requires a mordant to stain tissues. The most useful mordants for haematoxylin are salts of the metals aluminium, iron and tungsten.

EHRLICH'S Haematoxylin

Haematoxylin	= 2 g
Absolute Alcohol	= 100 ml
Glycerin	= 100 ml
Distilled Water	= 100 ml
Glacial Acetic acid	= 10 ml
Potassium Alum	= 15 g
(Aluminium Potassium Sulfate)	

Haematoxylin is dissolved in the alcohol and the alum in distilled water and mixed after these are in complete solution add the glycerin and acetic acid. It takes two months to ripen. It is particularly useful for staining sections from tissues which have been exposed to acid.

MAYER'S Haematoxylin

Haematoxylin	= 1 gm.
Distilled water	= 1000 ml.
Potassium or ammonium alum (Aluminium Ammonium sulfate)	= 50 gm.
Citric acid	= 1 gm.
Chloral hydrate	= 50 g.
Sodium Iodate	= 0.2 g.

The haematoxylin, potassium alum and sodium iodate are dissolved in the distilled water by warming and stirring. The chloral hydrate and citric acid are added and the mixture boiled for 5 min, then cooled and filtered. The stain is ready for use immediately.

Harris'S Haematoxylin

Haematoxylin	= 2.5 gm
Absolute alcohol	= 25 ml
Potassium alum	= 50 gm
Distilled water	= 500 ml
Mercuric oxide	= 1.25 gm
Glacial acetic acid	= 20 ml

The haematoxylin is dissolved in the absolute alcohol, and is then added to the alum dissolved in the warm distilled water in a 2 litre flask. The mixture is rapidly brought to boil and the mercuric oxide is added. The stain is rapidly cooled by plunging the flask into cold water. When the solution is cold the acetic acid is added and the stain is ready for use. A precipitate forms as the solution ages. The stain should be filtered before use and the staining time will have to be increased

Weigert's Iron Haematoxylin

A) **Haematoxylin Solution**

Haematoxylin	= 1g
Absolute Alcohol	= 100 ml

This is allowed to ripen naturally for four weeks before use.

B) **Iron Solution**

30% aqueous ferric chloride (anhydrous)	4ml
Hydrochloric acid (concentrated)	1 ml
Distilled water	95 m'

This solution is filtered and added to an equal volume of haematoxylin solution immediately before the stain is used. The mixture should be a violet black colour and must be discarded if it is brown.

The main use of Weigert's haematoxylin is as a nuclear stain where acid staining solutions are to be applied to the sections subsequently e.g. Van Gieson stain. Staining times with alum haematoxylins will vary according to:

1. Type of haematoxylin used e.g. Ehrlich's haematoxylin, 20–45 min., Mayer's haematoxylin 10–20 min (regressive and 5–10 min progressive).

2. Age of stain as the stain ages the staining time will increase.

3. Whether the stain is used progressively or regressively e.g. Harris's haematoxylin 4–30 sec (progressive in cytology) and 5–15 min. (regressive).

4 Pretreatment of tissues or sections e.g. in acid decalcifying solution or whether paraffin or frozen sections.

5. Post-treatment of sections e.g. subsequent acid stains such as Van Gieson. The optimal time must be determined for each batch by trial and error.

Eosin Y (Eosin Yellowish) C1, No 45380 is the most widely used type.

EOSIN

1% Stock alcoholic Eosin

Eosin Y	=	1gm
Distilled Water	=	20ml
Dissolve and add Alcohol 95%	=	80ml.

Working Solution:

Eosin stock solution (1 part) + 80% alcohol (3 parts)

Just before use add 0–.5 ml. of glacial acetic acid to each 100 ml of stan and stir.

ROUTINE HARRIS HAEMATOXYLIN AND EOSIN STAIN (REGRESSIVE)

Harris Haematoxylin
Acid Alcohol:
   Alcohol 70% = 1000 ml.
   Hydrochloric Acid = 10 ml.
   (Concen)
Ammonia Water
   Tap water = 1000 ml.
   Ammonium hydroxide = 2 to 3 ml.
   (28%)
Saturated lithioum Carbonate
   Lithium Carbonate = 1 gm.
   Distilled water = 100 ml.

Eosin Solution

STAINING PROCEDURE:

1. Deparaffinize in xylol hydrate through graded alcohols to water.

2. Remove fixation pigments if necessary.

3. Harris haematoxylin for 10–15 min.

4. Rinse in tap water until sections are 'Blue' -(5 min. or less)

5. Differentiate in 1% acid alcohol, three to ten dips. Check the differentiation with a microscope. Nuclei should be distinct and the background very light or colourless.

6. Wash briefly in tap water.

7. Dip in ammonia water or lithium carbonate water until sections are again blue (3 to 5 dips).

8. Wash in runing tapwater for 10 to 20 min.

9. Stain in Eosin for 15 secs to 2 min.

10. Dehydrate in 95% and absolute alcohols until excess eosin is removed. Check under microscope.

11. Clear in xylol and mount in DPX.

RESULTS

Nuclei	— blue black
Cytoplasm	– varying shades of pink
Muscle fibres	– deep pinky red.
Collagen	– pale pinky red.
Red blood cells	– orange — red
Fibrin	– deep pink

FROZEN SECTION

Frozen sections are normally produced by using a freezing microtome or a cryostat and can be cut either fixed or unfixed. Fixed tissues cut better on a freezing microtome while unfixed tissues cut more easily on a cryostat. The frozen tissue in this state is firm and the water in the tissue acts as an embedding medium. Therefore, it is possible to produce sections without the use of clearing agents and in some cases, embedding media, in the shortest possible time.

Frozen sections are commonly used for urgent surgical biopsies particularly, when a surgeon needs to confirm a suspicious area during operation also to decide the level of surgery in various resection or reconstruction surgery as in the treatment of various malignancies.

They are used for enzyme histochemistry, demonstration of lipids, in auto radiography and fluorescent antibody studies.

The tissues may be fixed in 10% for malin with the aid of heat Tissues may be frozen by using liquified gas like nitrogen (-190°C) solid carbondioxide (-70°C) carbon dioxide gas (-70°C) and aerosol sprays (-50°C).

Cryostat sections are generally cut at — 18°C to 20°C. To cut sections on a freezing mirotome place knife in its holder and near stage. Adjust the micron scale to approximately 30 microns place tissue on the stage of the microtome with a drop of water in between. Press gently with a slide and commence freezing by releasing CO_2 gas from the cylinder in short bursts of 1–2 seconds with a pause of 3–4 seconds. When the tissue is half frozen give a few cuts with a microtome knife to ensure good trimming. Now adjust the microtome scale to 5 microns and start cutting rapidly. The sections should be picked and immersed in a trough of water. Select suitable sections and transfer to albuminised surface of glass slides with the help of glass rods.

STAINING PROCEDURE

1. Fix sections in 10% neutral buffer formalin at room temperature for 20 secs. or give 1 dip in absolute alcohol followed by 1 dip in acid alcohol.

2. Rinse in tap water.

3. Place Harris haematoxylin on slide with dropper for 1 min.

4. Wash well in tap water.

5. Differentiate in acid-alcohol — 1 dip.

6. Rinse in tap water.

7. 'Blue' in lithium carbonate solution — 1 dip.

8. Rinse in tap water.

9. Stain in eosin for 10 secs.

10. Dehydrate in 95% alcohol and absolute alcohol.

11. Clear in xylene and mount in DPX.

RESULTS:

Nuclei — blue
Cytoplasm — pink

CHAPTER 26

CYTOLOGY

INTRODUCTION

Cytology is the study of cells. Cells may naturally exfoliate into various natural passages and their secretions like sputum and urine. They may be obtained directly from an epithelial or mucosal surface by direct scraping, by brush technique or by lavage. Cells may also be obtained by aspirating fluids from various body cavities like pleural and ascitic fluid, cerebrospinal, synovial and amniotic fluids.

Cells may be obtained for cytological studies from solid organs like thyroid and lymphnodes by aspirating with a fine needle. Similarly, any swelling, solid or cystic can be aspirated. The only contraindication for the technique is possible injury to vital organs, neurovascular structures in the vicinity of the mass or bleeding diathesis in the patient.

The cells obtained may be subjected to cytological examination. In addition, cytochemistry, cytogenetics, and electron microscopy may be performed easily on these materials. Exfoliative cytology is the study of cells, either naturally shed or collected from a tissue surface. The importance of exfoliative cytology as a diagnostic tool lies in the knowledge that any changes in these superficial cells can be a reflection of changes in the immediate underlying tissue.

Gynaecological cytology has three important applications:—
1. The detection of malignant lesions.
2. The assessment of hormone function.
3. The identification of vaginal infections.

Cytological examination of the sputum is of value in the diagnosis of
1. Malignant diseases of the lower respiratory tract.
2. Pulmonary asbestosis & pulmonary fungal infections.

Pleural and ascitic fluids, similarly, can be examined for the identification of malignant cells. Cellular patterns are sometimes associated with diseases like tuberculosis, leukaemias and nonmalignant conditions like cirrhosis of liver, cardiac and renal failure.

Examination of cells produced by gastric aspiration or brush technique; bronchoscopy or bronchial lavage can be valuable in the diagnosis of malignant conditions. CSF examination in both cases meningitis and leukaemias is another useful diagnostic exercise. Detection of malignancy by examination of breast cyst fluid or nipple discharge, and urine are other applications of cytology, in addition to synovial fluid examination in arthritis and amniotic fluid examination for foetal maturity.

FINE NEEDLE ASPIRATION CYTOLOGY (FNAC) has widened the scope of cytological examinations. Any swelling tumorous or inflammatory in nature, superficial and easily accessible can be aspirated with ease. The aspirated material can be examined to detect both malignant and benign conditions. Swellings associate with lymph nodes, thyroid and breast, soft tissue mass and lytic bone tumours are commonly aspirated as OPD procedures to screen these patients for any malignant disease.

The cytology material is received in the laboratory in the form of smears (fixed in absolute alcohol or by various aerosol/spray fixatives) and fluids (heparin 3 units/ml prevents clotting). All specimens accompanied by a properly filled requisition form are, on reception, duly numbered and entered in the register. The smears, already fixed, are ready for further processing. The fluids, however, need further centrifugation. The supernatant is discarded and the 'button' of deposit is smeared on a glass slide and fixed immediately. Sputum specimens need to be 'teased out' with a pair of forceps to select those portions likely to contain malignant cells. Translucent thread like structures, flecks of blood, edge of a blood clot, finer strands of a purulent material or fragments are looked for and smeared on a glass slide. Body fluids and watery exudates e.g. urine, spinal fluid, pleural and ascitic fluid will not adhere to the glass slides unless the slide is first coated with a layer of Mayer's egg albumen.

If the quantity of the fluid is small or very few cells are likely to be present the drops of fluid should be cytocentrifuged in a cytospin. Filter membranes can also be used to collect cells from a large sample like urine, ascitic or pleural fluid. The membranes are placed on glass slides and stained similarly. Any remaining sediment should be processed as a biopsy specimen for conventional histologic examination. Smears should be fixed in 95% alcohol for 15 minutes. Smears should be fixed immediately while still wet. Partial drying along the edge prevents the material from becoming detached from the slide. Papanicolaou technique is the routine method of choice giving dependable nuclear morphology with a clear translucent demonstration of the cytoplasm. The variability of the cytoplasmic staining is an advantage in hormone assessment.

PAPANICOLAOU METHOD FOR CYTOLOGIC SMEARS
SOLUTIONS
Harris's Haematoxylin
Acid Alcohol
    Ammonia
Orange G6 solution

Orange G6	— 0.5 gm.
Phosphotongstic Acid	0.015 gm.
95% Ethyl Alcohol	100 ml.

EA 50 solution:

Light green (0.1% in 95% ethyl alcohol	— 45 ml.
Bismark brown (0.5% in 95% ethyl alcohol)	— 10 ml.
Eosin yellowish 00.5% in 95% ethyl alcohol)	— 45 ml.
Phosphotungstic acid	— 0.2 gm.
Lithium carbonate (Saturated aqueous soln)	— 1 drop.

STAINING PROCEDURE:
1. Rinse in 95% alcohol.
2. Rinse in 70% alcohol.

3. Rinse in distilled water.
4. Stain in Harris' Haematoxylin 2 to 3 min.
5. Rinse in tap water.
6. Differentiate in acid-alcohol.
7. Place in gently running tap water for 5 min. to wash out acid and blue the nuclei.
8. Rinse in distilled water.
9. Rinse in 95% alcohol.
10. Treat with 0.1% ammonia in 95% alcohol for further blueing if necessary.
11. Rinse in 95% alcohol.
12. Stain in 0.6 for 90 sec.
13. Rinse in 95% alcohol two times.
14. Stain in EA 50 for 90 seconds.
15. Rinse in 95% alcohol two times.
16. Rinse in absolute alcohol.
17. Clear in Xylene.
18. Mount in DPX.

RESULTS

Nuclei — blue
Superficial cells cytoplasm — pink
Intermediate and parabasal cell cytoplasm — blue green.

Haematoxylin and Eosin: This technique cannot match the clarity and detail of papanicolaou. Many cytopathologists prefer this because they are already familiar with HEs on histological sections.

GIEMSA: This technique is preferred when Leukaemias or Lymphoma is suspected. It is also helpful when looking for eosinophils in allergic conditions. Feulgen reaction for DNA and special stains for sex chromation are also possible.

Klinger-Ludwig method for sex chromation

SOLUTION

Normal Hydrochloric Acid Thionin Solution (Stock)
  Thionin — 1 gm.
  Alcohol — 50%
Buffer solution (Stock):
  Sodium acetate — 9.7149 gm.
  Sodium barbiturate — 14.714 gm.
  Distilled water to make — 550 ml.
Thionin Working solution
  Hydrochloric acid IN = 32 ml.
  Buffer solution (Stock) = 28 ml.
  Thionin solution (Stock) = 40 ml.

STAINING PROCEDURE

1. Bring smears from 95% alcohol fixative to distilled water.
2. Hydrolyse in normal hydrochloric acid solution at 56°C for 5min.
3. Rinse well in distilled water for 5 minutes.
4. Working thionin solution for 5 min.
5. Differentiate in 70% alcohol, 95% alcohol and absolute alcohol for 1 min. each.
6. Clear in Xylene and mount in DPX.

RESULTS

Sex chromatin — Purplish red.
  Other cells structures — light blue
  Dried smears of the aspirated material can be kept aside and stained by any other special stains, similar to tissue sections, for glycogen, mucins, fat and various enzyme.

CHAPTER 27

SOME SPECIALIZED TECHNIQUES AND PROCEDURES
OF TISSUE PROCESSING

Plastic embedded sections and electron microscopy

The electron microscope has an increasing number of applications in diagnostic histopathology especially in renal biopsy work and in the identification of tumours whose histogenesis is uncertain by light microscopy. Even if an electron microscope is not available the study of 1 μ plastic embedded sections stained with toluidine blue, or even the more usual histological stains, can provide much useful information,

Fixation

For the ultrastructural histologist fixation is an exacting procedure which must be commenced within seconds of removal of the tissue from the body and he may even perfuse the vasculature with fixative during life. While it must be stressed that delayed and casual fixation must always be avoided where possible, these stringent requirements can seldom be adhered to when dealing with human material and are not always necessary for diagnostic purposes, for the ultrastructural features which are of clinical importance are often relatively durable and can sometimes be recognised even in material which has been fixed in formalin, embedded in paraffin and only re-processed for electron microscopy later.

Small biopsy specimens, such as needle biopsies, present no problem for part or all of the specimen may be fixed immediately after removal and, as the specimen is small, penetration of the fixative will be good. However, it must be realised that large surgical specimens will have been ischaemic for many minutes before they are actually removed so that immediate fixation of samples for electron microscopy does not prevent the production of artefacts due to early autolytic change. While it helps to collect the material in the operation room personally, even material transmitted to the laboratory fresh, e.g. for immediate frozen sections, can give good results.

The most generally used primary fixative is a buffered solution of glutaraldehyde.

Histochemistry

Many methods such as those for the identification of many pigments, inorganic materials and carbohydrates including mucins can be applied to paraffin embedded material. Paraffin sections cannot, for obvious reasons, be used for most lipids nor for the majority of enzymes. In general the detection of lipids requires the use of frozen sections and often some alteration in the fixative is desirable such as the use of formal calcium. Many techniques for the detection of enzymes preclude the use of most fixative so that fresh frozen sections are required or material may be fixed in cold formalin or cold acetone for a limited period of time. In some cases it is possible to allow the enzyme reaction to take place before fixation and embedding as in the tyrosinase (DOPA oxidase) reaction

The essential feature of using histochemical methods is to plan the procedure in advance in consultation with the clinicians so that sufficient fresh material is available and that it is handled in the way most appropriate for the individual problem.

Immunological investigations

Specific substances may be identified in tissue if there is available a specific artiserum for that substance and some method of detecting the sites where the specific antibody has been bound. This may be done by labelling the specific serum itself with a fluorescent dye but is more usually achieved by exposing the tissue to a second artiserum which is labelled with a fluorescent dye. This labelled serum is raised in another species, usually the rabbit, and absorbed so as to only react with the globulins of the species, i.e. man, under investigation. The entire procedure is usually carried out using unfixed fresh frozen sections so that the essential requirement is that some of the tissue should be removed and frozen before the main bulk of the specimen is fixed.

Morphometry

Morphometry may be applied to some pathological material prepared in a routine manner including material from the jejunum, bone, breast, lung and endometrium. Where the morphometry of whole organs is involved it is usually necessary to fix the organ intact and select the areas for histology in a pre-determined manner which ensures that they are truly representative.

Many of the methods employed depend upon the Delesse principle which states that the volume of a discrete component of a tissue can be estimated by measuring the area of a random section of the material that is occupied by that component. The area can be measured by the classical method of tracing a projected image on to a sheet of paper and estimating the areas of different components by planimetry or by cutting them out and weighing the pieces. Results may be achieved much more rapidly by point counting. A regular lattice of points is incorporated in the eyepiece of the microscope or an image of the section is projected on to a lattice drawn on a screen. By counting the number of points which fall on different components it is possible to calculate their relative volumes.

Tissue culture

In dealing with human tissues, tissue culture is not often required for diagnostic purposes. Exceptions are testicular biopsies when material may be required for meiotic studies but in the majority of cases such material is for research purposes only and prior arrangements should be made with those responsible for the culture procedures. The requirements are similar to those of the microbiologist in that the material must be fresh, unfixed, and free of bacterial contamination. The tissue required should be removed with sterile instruments and placed in a sterile container, preferably in some form of transport medium, for early transmission to the tissue culture laboratory. Should there be any delay the material should be kept cool in a 4°C refrigerator but not frozen.

Microbiology

It commonly happens that specimens arriving in the laboratory require bacteriological as well as histological investigation. In most cases of this sort, e.g. a tuberculous lymph node, the surgeon will have already sent some material to the microbiologist but if not, it is the histopathologist's duty to arrange this. There are two main requirements: procedures such as fixation, which will make culture impossible, must be delayed and secondly the specimen must not be contaminated with other organisms. Ideally, the micro-biologist and the pathologist should examine the specimen together and the microbiologist can then select his own samples. If this is impossible, then the pathologist should select the most likely areas, such as part of the wall of an abscess, remove them and place them in a labelled sterile container using sterile instruments. Any pus should also be sampled and a collection of sterile containers and swabs should always be available for investigations of this sort.

Chemistry

Chemical analysis of tissue is required less frequently than other investigations but the same principles apply. Material for analysis should be removed before fixation but should there be any delay then the material may be frozen with dry ice and kept in a deep freeze cabinet until required. Handling of such specimens is simplified if the precise requirements are known before the specimen is removed from the patient; this also gives the histopathologist an opportunity to choose the most appropriate methods for handling his own portion of the material. Where it is calculi that are needed for analysis these are simply removed before fixation and sent to the chemical laboratory in labelled containers.

CHAPTER 28

MUSEUM TECHNIQUES

A well organised pathology museum serves many purposes. It serves as:

1. A permanent exhibition of common pathological conditions for undergraduate and postgraduate education.
2. A collection of rare and interesting specimens.
3. A collection of specimens which can be used in medical exhibitions, examination vivas, lectures, demonstrations.
4. A permanent source of histologic and photographic material for teaching, research, exhibitions and publications.

RECEPTION OF SPECIMEN

Specimens, from operating theatres, post mortem room, research laboratories and histopathology laboratories is given an accession number and all relevant data recorded in the reception book. The label is tied to the specimen if a number of specimen are placed in one container. Liver specimens must be stored separately as the bile tends to discolour other specimens.

PREPARATION OF THE SPECIMEN

Ideally a specimen should be fresh and unfixed when it is received. Gross trimming and dissection must be carried out immediately to display the lesion as far as possible. The specimens must be washed in normal saline only and never in water as the resultant haemolysis will cause discoloration of the final mounting media. Specimens should be photographed in their natural color before fixation. Solid organs can be sliced and placed flat on paraffin trays or cork boards and covered with cotton soaked in a formalin based fixative. Cystic or hollow organs should be stuffed with cotton soaked in formalin to preserve their natural shape. Segments of intestine should be opened along the antimesenteric edge and placed flat on paraffin trays or pinned on cork baords and covered with cotton soaked in formalin.

FIXATION OF THE SPECIMEN

The fixatives most commonly used have been derived from Kaiserling and modified from laboratory to laboratory. The following solution has been found satisfactory and is based on Kaiserling's original formula. This solution is approximately pH 7 and is known as Kaiserling I (I).

Formalin	— 1 litre
Potassium Acetate	— 85 gm
Potassium Nitrate	— 45 gm
Water	— Make up to 10 litres

All containers should be lined by fixative-soaked lint or unfixed areas may remain at points where the specimen is in contact with the bottom of the container. Perfusion through arteries may be done to fix solid organs, limbs, brain and heart.

RESTORATION OF SPECIMEN

After fixation the natural color is lost. It is therefore, necessary to restore the specimen to as near its natural color as possible. Kaiserling method (Second stage) is highly recommended. The specimen is removed from the fixative washed in running water and transferred to 95% alcohol. The specimen is in alcohol for 1/2 hr. to 12hrs. during which time it is watched for development of color. When the color restoration is satisfactory it is removed and placed in the preserving or mounting solution. If the specimen is left too long in alcohol the color will fade permanently.

PRESERVATION OF SPECIMEN

The final preserving solution is the one in which the specimen will be mounted for display. The third solution of kaiserling, K-III is recommended. A 40% glycerine solution has the refractive index of perspex used in modern containers and produces a more solid effect to the final mount. The original solution contained sodium acetate in a 25% solution of glycerine.

Sodium acetate	— 1416 gm
Glycerine	— 4 litres
Water to make	— 10 litres

The specimen remains in this solution until it is well permeated. Initially it will float, later it will sink to the bottom of the container. Other method use addition of CO dithionite, pyridine and nicotine to improve colour of the specimens.

PRESENTATION OF THE SPECIMEN

Specimens may be mounted in glass jars available in various sizes or perspex jars which can be constructed to any specifica-

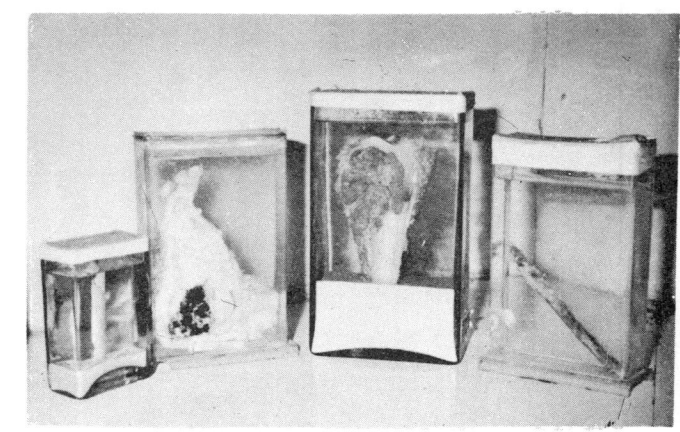

Fig. 72 Showing Mounted Specimens

tions. To support the specimen within the jar it is attached to the specimen plate or a frame made of glass rod by tying or stitching after orienting into its correct anatomical position. The frame may be fixed to side of a perspex jar or fixed to the base by filling the base with a layer of plaster of paris.

The container is filled with K-III solution to the brim to remove excess air. Various adhesives are available to seal the lid to the glass jars, like araldite and fevicol. Perspex lids may be sealed by touching with chloroform or polythene dissolved in chloroform/or plastics dissolved in chloroform.

ORGANISATION OF SPECIMENS

Specimens can either be classified by an anatomical system or by disease system. Having decided for example on an anatomical division a simple prefix letter is given to each organ followed by a serial number. The number is painted on the jar or labels are pasted on it. Simple loose-leaf catalogues or files containing all necessary in formation regarding the specimens should be provided for easy and ready reference.

CHAPTER 29

AUTOPSY TECHNIQUES

AUTOPSY PERFORMANCE

The autopsy is a scientific inquiry and should be regarded as constituting a postmortem examination of the body to determine the pathologic processes present and their relation to the clinical phenomenon and history to acquire knowledge concerning the disease from which the patient died.

PRE-INCISION DUTIES

Ensure that the autopsy permission is provided and duly counter-signed by the appropriate clinical staff. The identity of the body must be made sure from the name tag on the wrist. Restrictions on the autopsy stated in the autopsy permission, and the time by which the autopsy must be completed must be carefully noted. The pathologist on duty as well as the clinician should be informed. The mortuary attendant on duty is expected to be available on the premises and render active assistance. A proforma is provided for recording in rough the observations made in the autopsy room by prosectors which must be used.

External Examination.

All external marks, injuries and wounds must be noted. The sclera, pupils andirides are inspected as is the oral cavity. Dental status, dental prostheses, if any, and appearance of the tongue are recorded. Any abnormality in the external genitals, presence or absence of rigor or livor motis and discharge from the ear should also be noted. The body must be inspected from the back. A common incision permitted is a six inches long one on the abdomen or through a recent operative incision. The standard incision should be a Y shaped one on the trunk starting at the acromion processes on each side, converging at the lower end of the sternum and then extending in the middle of the abdominal wall, skirting the umbilicus and extending up to the symphysis pubis preferred by many. The chest wall is opened by a rib shear cutting along the costo chondral junctions of the ribs and the sternum with the attached anterior ends of the sectioned ribs is removed cultures from the heart's blood and lung tissue are obtained while the organs are still "In situ" pulmonary artery is nicked open to look for embolism.

The general relationship of the viscera in the thorax and abdomen is observed, and special features, if any, are noted. It is best to remove the intestines before evisceration. In order to avoid spilling of the intestinal contents, two sets of ligatures, about 1" apart, may be tied, one at the duodeno-jejunal junction, and the other at the lower end of the rectum. After the lower end of the rectum is dissected from the neighbouring viscera, the segment between the ligatures is cut by a long curved scissors. Similarly the duodeno-jejunal junction is cut between ligatures. The intestine separated from the mesentery by applying a sharp knife at the mesenteric attachment and putting the intestine against the direction, of the sharp edge. This is best done with the help of a second person. The intestines are then transferred to a pan and removed to the sink, where they may be opened under running water by means of cutting along the antimesenteric border.

Autopsy Dissection Procedure

The basic procedure of Rokitansky. Aschoff method is an en-masse evisceration followed by enblock dissection (1) Heart is removed weighed and opened chamber by chamber in the direction of blood flow. The coronary arteries are examined by multiple cross sections. (2) Lungs are weighed separately and divided into anterior and posterior halves by opening the branches at the hilum and slicing the lungs towards the pleural surface. (3) The liver is weighed by supporting the attached biliary duct, artery, veins, duodenum, pancreas and mesentery: The bile ducts and blood vessels are examined before the liver is sliced anteroposteriorly at the hilum (4) oesophagus, stomach, pyloros and first part of duodenum are dissected next. The oesophagus and duodenum are opened anteriorly. The stomach is cut along the greater curvature (5) Spleen is washed and cut into anterior and posterior halves through the hilum after washing (6) Small intestine is opened along the antimesenteric border. The appendix is oppened next. The caecum and colon are opened anteriorly (7) The abdominal aorta may be dissected with the genito urinary block. (8) The suprarenals are dissected and weighed. (9) The renal arteries, veins and ureters are identified and the kidneys after weighing are cut into anterior and posterior halves. (10) The bladder is opened anteriorly in the midline. (11) The prostate is cut in parallel slices at right angles to the prostatic urethra. (12) The vagina and uterus with adnexa are dissected together. (13) Brain is removed by an incision extending from ear to ear After the skin is reflected the skull is severed and the vault removed. The brain is removed weighed and suspended in formalin by means of a string under the basilar artery. Ten days are required for fixation; spinal cords are removed only where necessary (14) Periaortic, tracheobronchial and axillary lymph nodes may be removed and fixed if necessary. (15) Tissues from the thyroid, sternum, vertebrae, ribs may also be collected if required.

As soon as the viscera have been removed, the body should be carefully cleaned with wet sponges and cotton. The incision should be stitched after stuffing the cavities with adequate amounts of cotton. The body should be finally inspected before it is given over to the physicians or to the patient's relatives. It should be made sure that it does not appear to be mutilated or blood stained.

The blocks of tissue required for processing are trimmed and placed in labelled bottles and submitted to the laboratory. Slices of organs, of interest, for teaching purposes may be used for the museum, gross photographs of the lesions must be taken before the tissues are cut up. Cultures of heart, blood or any infective lesion may be sent to the microbiology department.

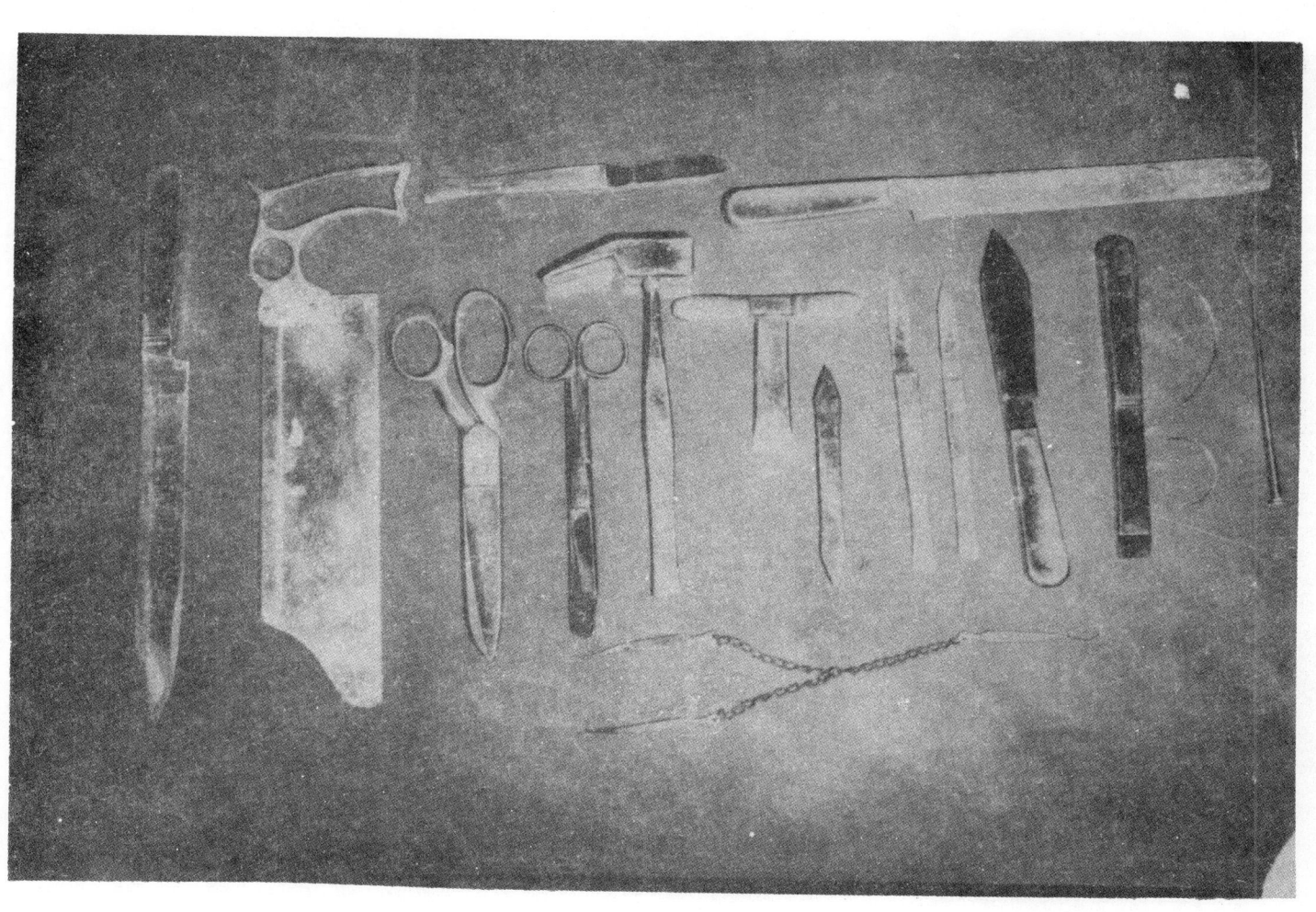

Fig: 73.   Showing surgical instruments used in Autopsy.

SECTION VII

BIOCHEMISTRY

CHAPTER 30

ANALYTICAL CHEMISTRY

(A) Definition of Solutions

1 Standard Solution

A standard solution is one in which exact concentration of solute is known.

2. Buffer Solution

Solutions which are capable of maintaining their hydrogen ion concentrations or pH, under all circumstances and situations.

3. Molar Solution

A solution which contains, one mol. of a solute in one litre of water. One mol. of solute is equal to the gram molecular weight. i.e. molecular weight expressed in grams.

4. Normal Solution

A normal solution is a solution which contains one gram. equivalent weight of the solute in one litre where

$$\text{equivalent weight} = \frac{\text{Molecular weight}}{\text{Valency}}$$

Normal solutions are the basis of all applied clinical chemistry. For monovalent atoms like Hydrogen, Sodium etc. molecular weight = Equivalent weight.

(B) Methods of expressing concentration

Concentration is defined as weight per unit volume.
It is expressed as:—
1. Percent
2. Molar
3. Normal

1. **Percent:** Garraway has expressed 'percent' in three ways.
(i) Weight/Unit weight–A 10% soln contains 10 gm. of solute in 100 gm. of solution or (90 gm. of solvent)
(ii) Weight/Unit Volume–A 10% soln. contains 10 gm. of solute dissolved in a final volume of 100 ml. of solution.
(iii) Volume/Unit volume–A 10% soln. contains 10 ml. of concentrate (solute). per 100 ml. of the solvent.

2. Molarity

1 mole of a substance = molecular weight of a compound expressed in grams.
   If 1 mole of a substance is dissolved in a final solution of 1 litre, the solution is called one molar or simply molar.
   For example: 1M solution of Sodium chloride or Common salt (NaCl).
   Molecular weight of NaCl is $23 + 35.5$. 1M soln. of NaCl will cotain 58.5gm. of NaCl in 1 litre of solution. Molarity of a solution is expressed as.

$$\frac{1}{\text{Molecular wt. of the substance}} \times \text{Concentration in the solution in gms/Litre}$$

3. Normal

Normality of solution is expressed as.
Normality = (Molarity) × (Valency)

For example

Normality of a 1M solution of $FeSO_4$
(Ferrous sulphate). Valency of Iron in the above compound is 2.
Normality = $M \times 2 = 2$.
   In case of a normal solution, concentration is expressed in terms of their combining weights. A gram equivalent contains same number of chemically active particles.
1 mEq (milliequivalent) is 1/1000 of an equivalent.

$$mEq = \frac{mg}{gm.eq. wt.}$$

To obtain mEq./Litre.

$$mEq/L = \frac{(mg./100ml) \times 10}{eq.wt.}$$

$$= \frac{(mg./100ml) \times 10 \times 2}{molecular\ wt.}$$

   or Conversely

$$mg./100ml. = \frac{(mEq/L) \times (molecular\ wt.)}{20}$$

(C) Dilution Problems

All volumetric solutions contain a definite amount of solute in a fixed volume of solution. Whenever a solution is diluted its volume increases and concentration decreases, but total amount of solute remains unchanged.

For example

If a 1:4 dilution of a solution A is to be made, 1ml. of a solution A is taken in a test tube and made to 4 ml. of solution with distilled water. Large dilutions can be carried out by doing a series of dilutions. For example A solution 'X' has to be diluted serially.
1:2, 1:4, 1:8, 1:16, 1:32 & so on.
1.   Take 1ml. of soln. X in a tube & make it to 2ml. with water.
2.   Take 1 ml. of soln. from tube 1, & make it to 2ml. with water.
3.   Take 1ml. of soln. from tube 2 & make it to 2 ml. with water.
4.   Continue similarly till last dilutional tube is reached from which 1 ml. of solution is discarded.

(D) Specific Gravity

Knowledge about specific gravity is useful in preparing normal solution of a liquid.
(Sp. gravity of soln.) × (Volume) × (%of material in soln.) = Wt. of solute in solution.
   To prepare a normal solution of a liquid of known specific gravity and percent conc. in soln.

$$ml.\ of\ liquid\ required\ per\ litre: = \frac{(Eq.wt) \times 100}{(sp.gr.) \times (conc)}$$

$$= \frac{(Mol.wt) \times)100}{(sp.gr) \times (Conc.) \times (valency)}$$

CHAPTER 31

INSTRUMENTS & ELEMENTARY COLORIMETRY

Colorimetric Analysis

Many methods for the quantitative analysis of blood, urine & other biological secretions are based upon the production of a coloured compound in solution, the intensity of which is used as a measure of the concentration of the dissolved material.

Determinations involving quantitative estimation of colour are known as *colorimetric Analysis.*

Advantages include

1. Complete isolation of the compound is not necessary and the constituents of a complex mixture like blood can be determined fairly accurately after treatment.
2. Many compounds are not coloured but can be made so by reaction with suitable reagents.

Principle

A substance X in a mixture such as blood is treated biochemically to produce a solution of a coloured compound. Light rays of a specific wave length (dependent on the colour of solution) are made to pass through the solution. The coloured solution absorbs some amount of the light in accordance with its concentration. This is called absorbance 'A'. The absorbance 'A' is directly proportional to the concentration of the substance being estimated in the solution.

Measurement of Light absorption by a soln.

There are two common methods of expressing the amount of light absorbed by a solution.

 (i) Percent transmittance (T%)
(ii) Optical Density. (O.D)

Optical Density is the negative logarithm of the percent transmittance. It is used for convenience in calculations. As the concentration of the coloured solution increases, optical density increases.

O.D. $= \text{Log } T\% = \text{Log } 100/T$
$\quad = \text{Log } 100 - \text{Log } T - \text{where}$
1. O.D. $-$ Optical density
2. T% $-$ Percent transmittance.
$\quad = 2 - \text{Log } T.$

Or Conversely
T $= \text{Antilog } (2 - \text{O.D})$

Absorbance, changes with the thickness of the solution and with the concentration of the absorbant in a manner characteristic for each absorbing material at a given wavelength. With all other conditions remaining constant, absorbance is directly proportional to the concentration of solute in a solution. A suitable standard curve can be obtained by plotting the absorbance of solutions of known concentration against the concentration of the solution at a given wavelength produced by a suitable filter.

Choice of wavelength

In general monochromatic (one colour) light is necessary if concentration — optical density relationship is to be linear. The correct wavelength to use is that of light which is most strongly absorbed by the coloured solution. The colour of the filter to be used is usually the colour complementary to the colour of solution under investigation.

Colour of soln	Filter
1. Red-Orange.	Blue-green. (380–570nm)
2. Blue	Red.
3. Green	Red.
4. Yellow	Violet.

Instruments For Measurement Of Absorbance

A. Colorimeters: instruments used for measuring light intensity, provided the thickness of the solution is constant. These may be calibrated in terms of percent transmittance or optical density or both. Two types of colorimeters are used.

DIAGRAM: 12 SCHEMATIC DIAGRAM OF A COLORIMETER

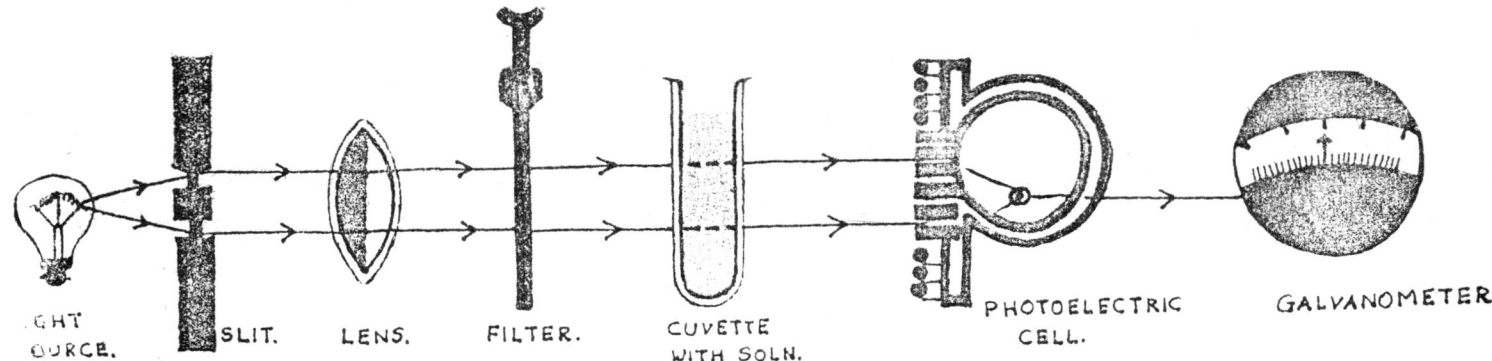

LIGHT SOURCE.　SLIT.　LENS.　FILTER.　CUVETTE WITH SOLN.　PHOTOELECTRIC CELL.　GALVANOMETER

1. Photoelectric colorimeters

In these, light passing through a colored solution is made to fall on photoelectric cells, which generates an electric current, which can be used to deflect a galvanometer needle. The deflection therefore is proportional to the light intensity transmitted which is inversely proportional to the concentration of the solution

This operates perfectly provided.
1. Cuvette is of uniform thickness.
2. Volume of solution remains constant.
3. Same filter is used.
   Certain colorimeters have a self generating photocell. They may be:
1. Direct reading single cell. or
2. Null point reading double cell instruments.

2. Visual colorimeter

1. Lovibond comparator. It consists of a box with compartments for tubes of blank and test solution, and it has a rotable disk which permits the superimposition of the coloured glass standards.
2. Dubosqy type
   It consists of 2 glass containers, each of which contains a solid plunger. Light traversing the 2 solutions is focussed in any eye piece. Each tube transmits light to one half of a circular field. Depth of soln. may be varied with the plunger unit. The 2 sides of the field are matched. Depth of the solns may be read on a scale.

DIAGRAM 13: LOVIBOND COMPARATOR

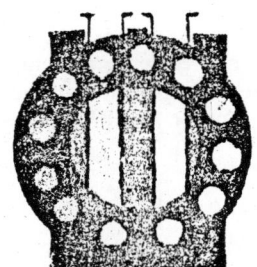

Spectrophotometers

These are essentially very similar to photoelectric colorimeters. Major difference is the method of producing monochromatic light which is provided by a diffraction grating or prism from which the desired wavelength may be chosen.

It can also be employed in UV & Infrared regions UV (360–400nm)IR (750–1000nm)

Table No. 37
Relation Between Optical density & Percent transmittance

T%	O.D.	T%	O.D.	T%	O.D.	T%	O D.
100	0.000	74	0.131	49	0.310	25	0.602
99	0.004	73	0.137	48	0.319	24	0.620
98	0.009	72	0.143	47	0.328	23	0.638
97	0.013	71	0.149	46	0.337	22	0.658
96	0.018	70	0.155	45	0.347	21	0.678
95	0.022	69	0.161	44	0.357	20	0.699
94	0.027	68	0.168	43	0.367	19	0.721
93	0.032	67	0.174	42	0.377	18	0.745
92	0.036	66	0.181	41	0.387	17	0.770
91	0.041	65	0.187	40	0.398	16	0.796
90	0.046	64	0.194	39	0.409	15	0.824
89	0.051	63	0.201	38	0.420	14	0.854
88	0.056	62	0.208	37	0.432	13	0.886
87	0.061	61	0.215	36	0.444	12	0.921
86	0.066	60	0.222	35	0.456	11	0.959
85	0.071	59	0.229	34	0.469	10	1.000
84	0.076	58	0.237	33	0.482	9	1.046
83	0.081	57	0.244	32	0.495	7	1.155
82	0.086	56	0.252	31	0.509	6	1.222
81	0.092	55	0.260	30	0.523	5	1.301
80	0.097	54	0.268	29	0.538	4	1.398
79	0.102	53	0.276	28	0.552	3	1.523
78	0.108	52	0.284	27	0.569	2	1.699
77	0.114	51	0.292	26	0.585	1	2.000
76	0.119	50	0.301				
75	0.125						

Standard Calibration Curve

Suppose we prepare it for a substance of known concentration in a standard mixture Y. Biochemical soln. used for conversion is B. Prepare following solutions.

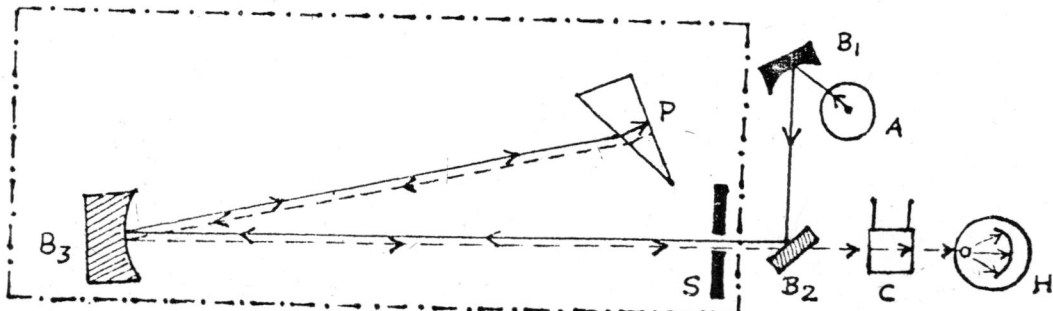

A: Light ; B₁ B₂ B₃ : Mirrors ; S-slit
P: Prism ; C: Cuvette ; H: Phototube

DIAGRAM 14: SCHAMATIC DIAGRAM OF A SPECTROPHOTOMETER

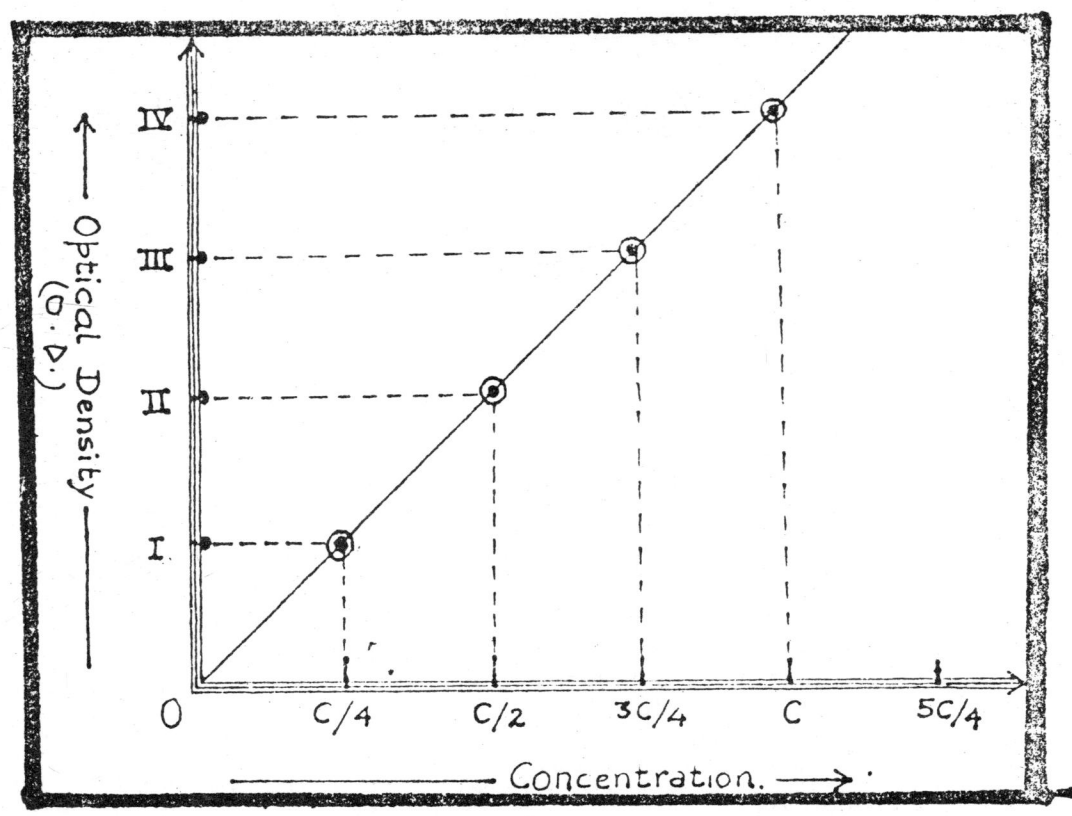

GRAPH NO 2 Showing relation of O.D. and Concentration of the solutions.

1. 4ml of soln. B (Blank)
2. 3ml of B + 1ml of Y.
3. 2ml of B + 2ml of Y.
4. 1ml of B + 3ml of Y
5. 4ml of soln. Y.
Suppose conc. of the substance in Y is C.

Find out the O.D. of each of the 5 solutions prepared beforehand adjusting the reading to 'O' with the blank solution and chart it as follows.

Soln.	O.D.	Conc.
1.	0	0
2.	I	C/4
3.	II	C/2
4.	III	3C/4
5.	IV	C

Now a curve is plotted with concentration along X. axis and O.D. against Y axis. With the help of this curve, concentration of the substance can now be found in any unknown mixture.

Though prepartion of a standard curve offers the possibility of dealing with many samples at a time, ideally each test sample should be put up in the colorimeter against a blank and a standard of known concentration, and calculations made as given below.

$$\text{Conc. of unknown} = \frac{\text{OD. of unknown}}{\text{O.D. of standard}} \times \text{Conc of standard.}$$

CHAPTER 32

PROTEINS ESTIMATION

I. Tests for the detection of proteins

Proteins are detected by colour reactions between one or more of the constituent radicals or groups of the complex protein molecule and the chemical reagent or reagents used in any given test.

(i) **Biuret test:** This test is given by substances containing two or more peptide linkages in the molecule. Proteins respond positively since there are pairs of –CO NH– groups in the molecule. This is a general test for the detection of proteins.

To 2 to 3 ml of protein solution in a test tube add an equal volume of 10% sodium hydroxide. Mix thoroughly and add a few drops of 0.5% copper sulphate solution. A purplish violet colour is obtained.

(ii) **Ninhydrin reaction:** When an amino acid is boiled with ninhydrin (triketohydrindene hydrate), a bluish violet colour is formed. However, the amino acids proline and hydroxy proline give a yellow colour. This a general test for proteins, peptides and amino acids.

To 1 ml of protein solution add 2 drops of 0.1% solution of ninhydrin and boil for 1 to 2 minutes. A bluish-violet colour is obtained.

iii) **Xanthoproteic reaction:** Compounds containing benzenoid radicals (e.g. phenyl group, $-C_6H_5$) react with nitric acid to form yellow nitro-derivatives which turn deep yellow in alkali, (tyrosine and tryptophan respond to the test). Phenylalanine does not respond to the test since, it is difficult to nitrate it under the above conditions.

To 2 to 3 ml of protein solution add 1 ml of concentrated nitric acid and heat. White precipitate is obtained which turns yellow later. It becomes orange on adding excess of 40% sodium hydroxide.

(iv) **Million-Nasse reaction:** This reaction is given by substances containing hydroxy phenyl group — C_6H_4 OH eg. tyrosine.

To 5ml of a dilute solution of protein add 1 ml of 15% solution of mercuric sulphate in 6 NH_2 SO_4. Place the tube in boiling water bath for 10 minutes; cool the contents in water for 5 to 10 minutes. Add 1 ml of 1% sodium nitrite. A deep red colour indicates positive test. Tyrosine or any other 3, 5 unsubstituted phenol answers this test.

(v) **Sakaguchi's arginine reaction:** To 5ml of protein solution add 5 drops of 5% sodium hydroxide and 4 drops of Molisch's reagent. Then add 10 drops of bromine water. A carmine red colour is obtained. Compare with blank.

This reaction is due to the presence of guanido group of arginine.

(vi) **Hopkins-Cole reaction for tryptophan:** To 1 ml of protein solution add 1 drop of 1:500 formalin and then 1 drop of 10% mercuric sulphate in 10% sulphuric acid. Mix well and add gently 30 ml of concentrated sulphuric acid along the sides of the test tube. Tap gently at the junction of the two layers. A violet ring develops.

This reaction is due to the presence of indole ring of the amino acid, tryptophan in the protein molecule.

(vii) **Sulphur reaction:** When proteins are heated in strongly basic solution, sulphur in the protein molecule will react to form sulphide. The sulphide can then be detected by the formation of lead sulphide upon the addition of lead acetate.

To 2ml of the protein solution, add an equal volume of 40% sodium hydroxide and boil for 2 minutes. Cool, and acidify with dilute HCl. Then add 1ml of 5% lead acetate solution and warm. A grey or black precipitate indicates a positive test. Cystine and cystine answer this, while methionine does not.

Precipitation of Proteins

Most of the proteins are lyophilic and hence can be precipitated by dehydration and neutralization of the electrical charges which they carry to bring them to their iso-electric point. Proteins like casein and metaprotein being practically lyophobic colloids require only neutralization of their charges for their precipitation.

The proteins can be precipitated from their solutions by

(1) salts of heavy metals(e.g. mercuric chloride, silver nitrate etc.)
(2) certain acids some of which are called alkaloidal reagents (eg. Picric acid, Phosphotungstic acid) (3) Conc. salt solutions (e.g. sodium sulphate etc.) and (4) by ethyl and methyl alcohol.

(a) precipitation by heavy metals

To 3 ml of the protein solution add 10% mercuric nitrate drop by drop till there is a maximum precipitation. Repeat the test with 5% zine sulphate solution.

(b) precipitation by alkaloidal reagent

To 8 ml of the protein solution add a few drops of 10% trichloracetic acid. A white precipitate is obtained.

Detection and separation of albumin and globulin

Albumins: Some of the native proteins present in serum, milk, egg white etc., belong to this class. They are soluble in water and dilute salt solution. They are coagulated by heating, and are precipitated only on full saturation with ammonium sulphate.

Globulins: These are also native proteins present in serum, milk, egg white, pulses, etc. They are insoluble in water but soluble in weak salt solutions. They are also heat coagulable and can be precipitated even by half saturation with ammonium sulphate, being less hydrated than the albumins.

(i) Denaturation and coagulation of proteins

Take 5 ml of egg white solution in a test tube, add 1 ml of 5% Na_2CO_3. Boil, cool, filter if necessary. The solution contains denatured albumin (Metaprotein). Add 2% acetic acid drop by drop, with mixing till maximum precipitate of metaprotein is obtained. Divide the mixture into two portions.

a) Boil one portion till a coagulum is obtained. To a portion of this coagulum 2% acetic acid is added in excess. Observe. To another portion of the coagulum 5% sodium carbonate is added, observe. The coagulum is insoluble.

b) The second portion of metaprotein solution is again divided into two. To one portion, add 2% acetic acid in excess dropwise. Observe. To second portion of metaprotein in solution, add 5% sodium carbonate solution dropwise. Observe. The metaprotein is soluble in both dilute acid and alkali.

(ii) Heat coagulation test

Take 5ml of the egg white solution in a test tube. If the solution is alkaline make it slightly acidic by adding a few drops of 2% acetic acid and heat the upper portion of the liquid. Coagulation taken place. The lower portion serves as control.

iii) Heller's test

To 2 ml of concentrated nitric acid in a test tube gently add along the sides 2 ml of egg white solution. A white ring is seen due to the formation of acid metaprotein. This is the most sensitive test for albumin and globulin.

(iv) Separation of albumin and globulin

Fractional precipitation with ammonium sulphate. To 5 ml of the egg white solution add an equal volume of saturated ammonium sulphate solution (half saturation). Globulin is precipitated. Filter. To the filtrate add solid ammonium sulphate till full saturation occurs. Albumin is now precipitated.

(v) Determination of the isoelectric point of a protein (casein).

You are provided with the solution of casein in 0.1 N sodium acetate.

Set up a series of nine tubes as follows:

Tube No	1	2	3	4	5	6	7	8
Distilled Water (mL)	8:38	7.75	8.75	8.50	8	7	5	1
.01N acetic acid (ml)	0.62	1.25	—	—	—	—	—	—
.1N acetic acid (ml)	—	—	0.25	0.50	1	2	4	8
.0N acetic acid (ml)	—	—	—	—	—	—	—	—

To each tube add 1.0 ml of the casein solution and shake the tubes immediately. Note the turbidities just after mixing and after 10 and 30 minutes. Record the results as below, indicating no turbidity by 0, degrees of turbidity by + signs and degrees of precipitation by x.

Tube No.	1	2	3	4	5	6	7	8	9
pH	5.9	5.6	5.3	5.0	4.7	4.4	4.1	3.8	3.5
Turbidity immediately	0	0	+	+++	++	++	+	+	0
Turbidity after 5 minutes	0	0	+	+	xxx	xx	++	++	0

The precipitation should be greatest in tube 5 which has a pH of 4.7, near the isoelectric point and point of least solubility of casein.

CHAPTER 33

ESTIMATION OF BLOOD UREA, SERUM CREATININE AND SERUM URIC ACID

BLOOD UREA ESTIMATION

Introduction

Urea is one of the main nitrogenous waste products excreted in the urine. It is the major excretion product of protein catabolism. Liver is the sole site of urea formation. Urea is formed from CO_2 and NH_3, passed to the blood & filtered at the glomeruli and partly reabsorbed in the tubules

Techniques for Blood Urea estimation

There are 2 major techniques. The initial step in both the techniques is same, involving liberating of ammonia from urea by urease.
1. Nesselerization (involves reaction of NH_3 with Nessler's reagent)
2. Berthelot's reaction — Liberated ammonia reacts with phenol and hypochlorite to give blue coloured Indophenol.

A third method involves urea directly.
3. Diacetyl monoxime method — Urea directly reacts with diacetyl compounds to give coloured compounds.
Here we will discuss in detail Nesselerization.

Principle

Blood sample is digested with urease and urea is converted to ammonia. After precipitating proteins, ammonia is made to react with Nesseler's reagent producing a coloured compound which can be compared against any of the following.
1. A std. $(NH_4)_2 SO_4$ solution
2. A urea solution

Reagents

(1) 10% Sod tungstate soln.
(2) 2/3 NH_2SO_4
(3) Urease solution
(5mg. Soyabean powder is shaken with 100ml of water. Prepare afresh daily. Alternatively urease tablet may be dissolved in 3 ml of 30% alcohol or urease powder can be used).
(4) Urea std. 0.5mg/ml.
(5) Nesseler's reagent

Procedure

	Blank	Test	Standard
Distilled water	3.4m	3.2ml	3.2ml
Blood	—	0.2ml	—
Urea Std. Solution (0.5mg/ml)	—	—	0.2ml

Add 20mgm. of urease powder to each tube and incubate all at 37°C for 20mins. Then add:

10%Sod. tungstate	0.3ml	0.3ml	0.3ml
2/3 NH_2SO_4	0.3ml	0.3ml	0.3ml

Mix well. Let it stand for few minutes, and centrifuge

Clear supernatant from above	2.0ml	2.0ml	2.0ml
Distilled water	5ml	5.0ml	5.0ml

Cool for 2 mins.
Add 1.0ml of Nessler's reagent to each tube and read at 480nm.

Calculations: $\text{Blood Urea} = \dfrac{O.D(T)}{O.D.(s)} \times 100 \text{mg/dl}.$

Interpretation

Normal blood urea level in adults is 10–20mg/dl.
Increase in Blood urea occurs with
1. Volume depletion — Loss of body fluids
2. Renal failure
3. Renal stasis
Only condition known to decrease blood urea is normal pregnancy.

SERUM CREATININE ESTIMATION

Introduction

Creatine is a nitrogenous substance found exclusively in muscle (98% of total body content). It is important for muscular contraction and is excreted as creatinine. It has advantages over urea as a renal function test because:—
1. It is inactive metabolically,
2. It is derived entirely from endogenous metabolism,
3. Its excretion is independent of diet,
4. It is quite constant in health and is not reabsorbed.

Technique

Folin & Wu's alkaline picrate method: It is a nonspecific technique, and other reducing substances also contribute upto 20% to the final colour.

Principle

It involves Jaffe's alkaline picrate reaction
Creatinine + Alkaline picrate = Creatinine picrate (Red in colour).
Nonspecificity due to other chromogens can be prevented by using Lloyd's reagent (Hydrated Aluminium Silicate) which absorbs creatinine specifically.

Reagents

0.04 M Picric Acid
Sod. Hydroxide
Working creatinine standard (0.04mg/ml or 4mg/dl)

Lloyd's reagent (optional)Not commonly used.
1. Prepare the following tubes

	B	S	T
Serum	2.0ml	—	—
Distilled water	2.0ml	3.0ml	4.0ml
std.			
(0.04mg/ml)	—	1.0ml	—

Add 2.0ml. of $2/3 NH_2SO_4$ and 2ml. sodium tungstate.
2. Contrifuge and remove supernantant
3. Proceed as follows.

	B	S	T
Supernatant	3.0ml	3.0ml	3.0ml
Picric acid	1.0ml	1.0ml	1.0ml
Water	1.0ml	1.0ml	1.0ml

4. Read at 520nm.
5. Calculation
Conc of creatinine $= (T/S) \times .015 \times 100/0.75$
$= T/S \times 2mg/dl.$

Interpretation

Normal serum creatinine values are
0.6–1.4mg/dl.
Serum creatinine is raised in Renal failure and obstruction to urine outflow.

SERUM URIC ACID ESTIMATION

Introduction

Uric acid is the end product of purine metabolism in man. Part of circulating uric acid is endogenous and part is from food metabolism. It may be secreted into as well as reabsorbed from tubules.

Techniques

1. Phosphotungstate reduction method, easier, more commonly used.

2. Uricase method — more specific and accurate.

Principle

Proteins of serum are precipitated by phosphotungstic acid reagent, which is simultaneously reduced by the uric acid of the sample to a scarcely known blue coloured product in an alkaline medium.

Reagents

Tungstic acid
Phosphotungstic acid (Dilute 1 in 10 for use),
Na_2CO_3 10%,
Standard working uric acid solution 0.002mg/ml or 0.2mg/dl.

Procedure

1. 0.1 ml serum + 3.5 ml water + 0.2ml sod. tungstate and 0.2 ml H_2SO_4 (Sulphuric acid).
2. Centrifuge
3. Proceed as follows

	B	S	T
— Supernatant	—	—	2.0 ml
— Distilled water	2.0 ml	—	—
— Standard	—	2.0 ml	—
(0.002 mg/ml)			
— Sodium cyanide	2 ml	2 ml	2.0 ml
(12%)			
— Phosphotungstic	2.0 ml	2.0 ml	2.0 ml
acid			

4. Compare in a colorimeter using 520nm
5. Calculations — $(T/S) \times .004 \times (100/0.05)$
$= (T/S) \times (4/1000) \times (100/5) \times 100$
$= (T/S) \times 8mg/dl.$

Interpretation

Normal values 2.3–7.0mg/dl in males and 1.3–6.0mg/dl in females.
Increased uric acid in serum (Hyperuricemia) may result from.
1. Renal impairment.
2. Urinary obstruction
3. Gout
4. Conditions characterized by rapid cell. destruction.

CHAPTER 34

CLINICAL ENZYMOLOGY

Common Serum Enzyme Studies

This is a heterogenous group of estimations concerned with various systems and diseases as will be mentioned during the course of the discussion.
These enzyme studies include
1. Serum Transaminases.
2. Serum Phosphatases.
3. Serum Amylase.
4. Serum Lipase.

1. Serum Transaminase Estimation

These enzymes catalyze the transfer of an amino (NH_2) group from an α-amino acid to an α-keto acid, forming a new amino acid and a new kero acid.
Important are
1. Glutamic Oxaloacetic transaminase (GOT).
2. Glutamic Pyrurate Transaminase (GPT).
Presently these enzymes have been renamed as Aspartate amino transferase for GOT & alanine aminotransferase for GPT.

A. Aspartate Amino Transferase (SGOT)

1. GOT catalyzes the following reaction.
Glutamic acid + Oxaloacetic acid = ketoglutaric acid + Aspartic acid.
2. Tissue sources are Heart, Liver, Skeletal muscle, Kidney & Pancreas (in descending order of concentration).

Principle

The Oxaloacetate formed in the above reaction decarboxylates spontaneously to pyruvate which reacts with 2, 4 dinitrophenylhydrazine (DNPH) to give a brown coloured hydrazone, which is measured in the colorimeter at 510 nm.

Reagents

2:4 Dinitrophenylhydrazine (DNPH)
0.4 N Sodium hydroxide,
Working oxaloacetate std.
GOT substrate.

Procedure

1. Mix 0.1ml of nonhemolyzed serum and 0.5ml of GOT substrate & incubate at 37°C for 1 hr. Add 0.5ml of 2, 4, DNPH Soln, & let stand for 15 mins. at room temp. Add 5.0 ml. of 0.4 N NaOH, Mix well & let stand at room temp. for 20 mins.
2. Prepare a standard curve by diluting in cuvettes the oxaloacetic acid working std. as follows.

ml. Std.	ml. water	Unit equivalent of
0.0	2.2	0
0.1	2.1	20
0.2	2.0	55
0.3	1.9	95
0.4	1.8	148
0.5	1.7	216

To each cuvette add 1 ml of 2, 4 DNPH, mix & let stand for 20 minutes. Read as before.
3. Plot the optical density versus unit equivalent on standard linear graph paper.
4. Determine the concentration of unknown from this curve.

3. Alternative technique for SGOT

S.No.		Test	Blank	S_1	S_2	S_3	S_4	S_5
1.	O.T. Substrate	1.0ml	1.0ml	0.9ml	0.8ml	0.7ml	0.6ml	0.5ml
2.	Standard	x	x	0.1ml	0.2ml	0.3ml	0.4ml	0.5ml
3.	Serum	0.2ml	x	x	x	x	x	x
4.	Water	x	0.2ml	0.2ml	0.2ml	0.2ml	0.2ml	0.2ml

Incubate test soln. at 37°C for 1hr.

| 5. INPH | 1.0ml | 1.0ml | 1.0ml | 1.0ml | 1.0ml | 1.0ml | 1.0ml |

Let it stand for 20 minutes at room temp.

| 6. NaOH | 1.0ml | 1.0ml | 1.0ml | 1.0ml | 1.ml | 1.0ml | 1.0ml |

Leave for 10 minutes
Read at 520nm (green filter) systronic 694.
Plot a calibration curve with the 5 standards plotting O.D. against SGOT Units.

4. Spectrophotometric methods

Reagents

1. Neutral phosphate buffer
2. 0.2 ml aspartic acid in 0.1 M phosphate buffer.
3. Reduced NAD.
4. Malate dehydrogenase (100 units/ml) prepare afresh.
5. X-oxghitarate (0.1M)

Technique

1. For test
0.2ml serum + 1.7ml buffer + 0.5ml aspartate + 0.3ml NADH$_2$ + 1.0ml malate dehydrogenase.

189

For Blank —

0.2ml Serum + 2ml buffer + 0.5ml aspartate and 1.0ml malate dehydrogenase.

2. Allow to stand for 15 minutes
3. Add 0.2ml oxglutarate to the test & mix well.
4. Read against blank at 1 min. intervals for 10 minutes.

Units/ml/min = decrease in extinction in 5 minutes x 1000

Interpretation

Normal values for serum glutamic oxaloacetic transaminase (SGOT) vary from 8–40 units per ml, values of 40–50 units are considered equivocal, and all values exceeding 50 units per ml. are considered elevated.

1. SGOT levels are elevated from damaged heart muscle within 6–12 hrs, after occlusion of coronary artery. Maximum value is reached within 48 hrs and returns to normal within 3–5 days. Values are usually ≤250 units/ml.
2. SGOT values greatly increase in acute liver damage. In viral & toxic hepatitis, values >500 units/ml are usually found (upto 1200 units/ml).
3. Moderate increases (≤300 units/ml) may occur in Chronic liver diseases.

B. **Alanine aminotransferase** (SGPT)

1. Reaction catalyzed by GPT is
Glutamic acid + Pyruvic acid = Ketoglutaric acid + Alamine
2. Tissue sources (in descending conc) are Liver, Kidney, Heart, Skeletal msl. & Pancreas.

Principle & Procedure

Same as for SGOT. except that the substrate contains alanine instead of aspartate.

Interpretation

Normal values for SGPT are 9–31 units per ml. Normal ratio of GOT/GPT is 1.3/1.0 SGPT values may be slightly elevated in myocardial damage, but this value is probably owing to secondary liver damage.

Serum Phosphatase Estimation

Normal blood serum contains several enzymes or groups of enzymes which catalyze the liberation of inorganic phosphate from phosphate esters such as glycerophosphate. The most active phosphatase, has an optimum pH of approximately 9.0; now known as alkaline phosphatase, to distinguish it from acid phosphatase. Acid phosphatase is of limited activity in normal serum but its activity is of significance in certain pathological conditions.

A. **Alkaline Phosphatase**

Phosphatases catalyze a variety of reactions. A wide range of organic phosphate esters are attacked. The phosphatases can also function as transferases, linking the released inorganic phosphate with a suitable acceptor substance. Alkaline phosphatase is found in the osteoblast cells of bone; Liver cells; intestine; kidney & placenta.

Principle

Estimation of phosphatase depends upon measuring the amount of hydrolysis which takes place when the enzyme is allowed to act on a suitable substrate, under standard. conditions. The amount of phenol so liberated is taken as a measure of the amount of enzyme present. Folin Ciocalteu's and phenol reagent precipitate the plasma proteins & produce a blue colour with phenol in the presence of Na_2CO_3.

Reagents

1. Bicarbonate buffer
2. Working phenol reagent.
3. Substrate soln. for phosphatases.
4. 15% Na_2CO_3.

Procedure

1. Take 2.0ml of HCO_3 buffer in a test tube marked as (T) & add 2.0ml of substrate. Incubate at 37°C for 3–5 mins. Add 0.2ml serum & continue heating further. Add 1.8ml. diluted phenol reagent & centrifuge. Take 4.0ml filtrate & add 2.0ml of Na_2CO_3.
2. Take 2.0ml HCO_3 buffer in a tube(C) & add 2.0ml substrate. Incubate as above. Add 1.8ml phenol reagent. Add 2.0ml of serum & centrifuge. Take 4.0ml of filtrate & add 2.0ml of 15% Na_2CO_3.
3. Take 4.0ml of working phenol soln. in a test tube marked (S) & add 2.0ml of 15% Na_2CO_3.
4. Take 3.2ml distilled water in a test tube 'B' & add 0.8 ml of phenol reagent. Incubate all the tubes at 37°C for 10mins. and read in a colorimeter with a green filter.

Calculation

$$\text{S. Alk. Phosph. activity} = \frac{OD(T) - O.D.(C)}{OD(S) - O.D.(B)} \times \frac{\text{Conc of Std.}}{1} \times \frac{6}{4} \times \frac{100}{0.2}$$
$$= \frac{T - C}{S - B} \times 30 \text{ K.A. Units.}$$

Alternative technique for calculations

Set up 6 tubes containing following volumes as stds. & design a calibration curve.

Tube No.	Working Std.	NaOH	Unit Value
1.	1.0ml	10.0ml	16.7
2.	2.0ml	9.0ml	33.4
3.	4.0ml	7.0ml	66.8
4.	6.0ml	5.0ml	100.2
5.	8.0ml	3.0ml	133.6
6.	10.0ml	1.0ml	167.0

Absorbance values are plotted against vertical axis and unit value against horizontal axis. Value of Alkaline phosphatase activity in serum may be determined from this curve.

Interpretation

KING ARMSTRONG UNIT

It is defined as the amount of the enzyme which will set free 1mg. of phenol in the given time under the conditions of the test. One I.U. = K.A. unit × 7.1.

Normal serum alkaline phosphatase activity is 3–13 K.A. units. These values are greatly increased in

1. Pagets disease (upto 50 times)
2. Rickets (Upto 20 times)
3. Hyperparathyroidism,
4. Obstructive jaundice. (except biliary atresia in newborn),
5. Cirrhosis,
6. Osteogenic sarcoma.

B. Acid Phosphatase

Apart from small amount in bone, liver, spleen & kidney, the 2 main normal sources are.

Prostate in males and Red cells (R.B. Cs.)

Acid phosphatase may also be found occasionally in women with cancer breast.

Technique & Procedure

It is exactly the same as with Ser. Alk. Phosphatase except that citrate buffer is employed in place of carbonate buffer.

Interpretation

Normal serum contains from 0.0 to 1.1 K.A. units of acid phosphatase. The serum level of acid phosphatase is usually elevated if a cancer of the prostate has spread to bone. The elevation may be considerable. Effect of hormonal therapy can be monitored by serial serum acid phosphatase estimations.

Serum Amylase Estimation

Amylase hydrolyzes a wide range of starches, polysaccharides and the liver storage polymer glycogen. The 2 main sources of amylase are:
1. Pancreas.
2. Salivary glands.
(The claim of liver being another source is still disputed)

Principle

A small amount of serum is incubated at 37°C with 0.4mg. starch and loss in blue colour which starch gives with Iodine solution is taken as a measure of the extent to which the starch has been digested.

Reagents

1. NaCl (Normal saline)
2. Neutral phosphate buffer.
3. Dilute iodine solution.
4. Standard starch soln (1mg/ml).

Procedure

1. TEST

(i) Dilute serum 1 in 10 with normal saline.
(ii) 0.5 ml buffer and 0.4ml starch soln. are taken in a tube & incubated at 37°C for 3–5 mins.
(iii) Add 0.1 ml of diluted serum (0.01ml serum) & mix.
(iv) Incubate further for 15 mins.
(v) Remove Add 8.6ml of distilled water & 0.4ml of iodine solution.

2. BLANK

In this, serum is added after incubating and putting distilled water and iodine solution.

Take readings in the colorimeter using a red filter.

Calculations

S. amylase activity in somogyi units/dl =

$$\frac{B - T}{0.01} \times \frac{100}{5} \times 0.4$$

$$= \frac{B - T}{B} \times 800 \text{ somogyi units/dl.}$$

Alternative method

Solution	Control	Test
Buffered starch	5 ml	5 ml
Serum	—	0.1 ml
Incubate for 7½ minutes exactly at 37°C		
Working iodine	5 ml	5 ml
Distilled Water	40 ml	40 ml

Take reading at 660 nm (using red filter).

One somogyi unit of amylase is defined as the quantity of amylase which digests 5 gms of starch at 37°C in 15 minutes:

$$\frac{\text{O.D. of control} - \text{O.D. of test}}{\text{O.D. of Control}} \times 800 \text{ somogyiunits/dl}$$

Interpretation

Normal values are 60–160 Somogyi units/dl. Serum amylase values rise within few hours after the onset of a/c pancreatitis, reaching peak value within 24 hrs. & returning to normal in 3–6 days. Increased values may also occur in a/c appendicitis (nonspecfic).

Note

Same technique may be employed for urine, substituting 0.1ml of undiluted urine in place of serum.

Serum Lipase Estimation

Lipases are of 2 kinds
1. Which catalyze hydrolysis of short chain fatty acid esters (Found in Liver, Kidney and Pancreas).
2. Which catalyze long chain fatty acid esters (Found only in pancreas).

Principle

Serum is incubated with an olive oil emulsion and fatty acids produced are titrated with NaOH.

Procedure

In each of 2 conical flasks, place 3 ml distilled water and serum. Place control flask into boiling water for 5 mins. & cool. Add 0.5ml buffer solution (phosphate — neutral) and 2ml of olive oil emulsion to both flasks, shake well & incubate at 37°C for 24 hrs. Then add 3ml of 95% alchohol & 2 drops of phenolphthalein & mix. Titrate each flask with 0.05 N NaOH until a permanent blue colour appears (pH — 10.0).

Calculation

ml. NaOH for (T) — ml.NaOH for (c) = units lipase activity per ml. serum.

Interpretation

Normal serum lipase activity by this method is upto 1.5 units. Determination of serum lipase is complementary to serum amylase in a/c pancreatitis because elevations of serum lipase disappear much more slowly.

191

CHAPTER 35

LIVER FUNCTION TESTS

Important liver function tests include

1. Serum Bilirubin estimation.
2. Serum enzymes (SGOT, SGPT & Alkaline phosphatase: have been discussed under clinical enzymology).
3. Serum proteins.
4. Prothrombin time (discussed under hematology)
5. Bromsulphalein (BSF) excretion test.
6. Blood ammonia levels.
7. Thymol turbidity test.
   The last three tests not in clinical use anymore.

Serum Bilirubin Estimation

Introduction

Bilirubin is synthesized in the reticuloendothelial cells from R.B.Cs & transported in conjungation with albumin (the normal indirect reacting bilirubin). On arrival at the sinusoidal surface of a hepatocyte, bilirubin separates from albumin and binds to a carrier protein. Within hepatocyte, bilirubin is conjugated and thereafter excreted in bile as bilirubin diglucuronide (normal direct reacting bilirubin when reacted with diozotized sulfacilic acid or Ehrlich's reagent). The azobilirubin formed thus is determined photometrically. There are 2 distinct forms of reaction.

1. FAST or DIRECT: Given by aqueous soluble conjugated bilirubin. Develops within 1 minute.
2. SLOW or INDIRECT: Given by insoluble albumin bound bilirubin. Reacts very slowly on long standing. Both forms of bilirubin are alcohol soluble in methyl alcohol.

Reagents

1. Freshly prepared diazo reagent — Mix 25 ml of diazo A with 0.75ml of diazo B.
2. Diazo blank soln. — 60ml of conc. HCl. diluted to 1 litre with water.
3. Methyl Alcohol.
4. Working bilirubin standard (0.04mg/ml of Methy Red) or (preferably bilirubin as such 0.01mg/ml.

Distilled water	4.3ml	4.3ml
Serum	0.2ml	0.2ml
Diazo (A + B)	0.5ml	—
Diazo (A)	—	0.5ml.

Mix well and keep for 5 minutes and take reading at 540nm. or an alford 645nm (Yellow green) filter for direct bilirubin by colorimeter. For total bilirubin 5 ml methanol is to be added to each tube and mix well. Read in colorimeter after 5 minutes Direct bilirubin.

$$\frac{T-B}{S-B} \times 10$$

Total bilirubin $\dfrac{T-B}{S-B} \times 20$

S − B is approximately 0.30. Hence,
Total bilirubin = (T − B) × 200 × (1/3)
& Direct bilirubin = (T − B) × 100/3

Precautions

1. Haemolyzed sample should not be used, because hemoglobin interferes with diazo reaction and also absorbs light at 540 nm.
2. Serum for bilirubin estimation must be kept away from bright light since bilirubin is destroyed in the U-V light. Same applies to azobilirubin.

Interpretation

Estimation of total and conjugated bilirubin in serum is of value in the differential diagnosis of jaundice.
The normal total bilirubin is usually less than 1mg/dl
Normal values for
direct bilirubin = 0.1–0.4 mg/dl
& indirect bilirubin = 0.2 — 0.7 mg/dl.
In pre-hepatic jaundice
— Indirect Serum bilirubin rises.
In Hepatocellular jaundice
— Both forms of bilirubin rise.
In Posthepatic or Obstructive jaundice
— Conjugated/Direct bilirubin rises.

Serum Protein Estimation

Introduction

Serum proteins represent a complex mixture containing a number of components which differ in properties and function. The major component of proteins include.

1. Albumin
2. Globulins
3. Conjugated proteins such as lipoproteins.
4. Fibrinogen (absent from serum). Liver is the organ mainly responsible for the formation of plasma — albumin and at least 30% globulins.

Techniques

1. Assay of nitrogen content by Kjeldahl digestion.
2. Lowrys' method for estimating tyrosine in protein.
3. Biuret method — most commonly employed clinically. Therefore here we will discuss in detail the BIURET METHOD.

Principle

The serum is treated with biuret reagent, which consists of copper alkali. Copper in alkaline soln. reacts with the peptide bonds of proteins, producing a violet colour proportional to the amount of protein present.

Reagents

1. Biuret reagent.
2. Std. protein soln. (0.5gm/dl).

Prepare following solutions.

Solution	Test	Blank	Std
Normal saline	2.9ml	3.0ml	2.9ml
Serum	0.1ml	—	—
Protein standard	—	—	0.1ml
Biuret reagent	3.0ml	3.0ml	3.0ml

Protein Conc = (T/S) × 0.005 × (100/0.1)
= (T/S) × 5gm/dl.

Interpretation

Normal Values

1 — Adults 6.3–8.2gm/dl.
2 — Infants 4.0–6.7 gm/dl.
(Adult levels are reached by about 3 yrs)

Estimation of total serum protein has value only when there is loss of every type of plasma protein which occurs for example as a result of burns or haemorrhage. Otherwise, the alterations in albumin and globulins are of clinical significance and their estimation should be done.

Determination of Serum albumin

1. Albumin is measured as above by analysis of the fluid remaining after precipitating the globulin fraction with 23% Na_2SO_4 solution.
2. Different fractions of plasma proteins in serum can be detected by electrophoresis (discussed elsewhere).

Interpretation of Serum Albumin

Normal serum albumin level is 3.7 to 5.2gm/dl. Oedema may develop when the level falls below 2.0–2.5gm/dl. A fall in the serum albumin concentration may be due to:

1. Low protein intake (malnutrition).
2. Protein losing enteropathies.
3. Chronic liver cirrhosis — defective production.
4. Increased loss in urine (Nephrotic Syndrome).
5. Increased protein catabolism (Diabetes and Chronic infection).
Increase of total plasma globulins is found in:
1. Most a/c or chr. infections
2. Metastatic carcinoma of liver.
3. Collagen diseases
4. Multiple mycloma etc.

CHAPTER 36

ESTIMATIONS OF BLOOD SUGAR
AND SERUM CHOLESTROL

BLOOD SUGAR ESTIMATION

Introduction

Determination of Blood sugar was one of the first biochemical estimations to be applied clinically. The abnormalities of blood glucose levels reflect disturbances in carbohydrate metabolism.

At room temperature, glycolysis in the RBCs reduces the blood glucose at a rate of 5% every hr. To prevent this loss, either the estimation should be performed within half an hr. after collection or an inhibitor of glycolysis such as NaF is added. More often, the sample is collected in a tube containing a fluoride-oxalate mixture. Blood glucose values are 10–15% lower than plasma values due to lower water content within R.B.Cs. Also, normal range for glucose in whole blood obviously varies with hematocrit.

Techniques

1. Glucose oxidase techniques — specific and represent true glucose.
2. Techniques dependent on the reducing property of glucose. These may over-estimate the blood glucose levels by as much as 5–20%. However since glucose oxidase method is not freely available in developing countries like India, we shall discuss in detail the reducing methods. Most commonly used is Folin Wu method.

Principle

A protein free blood filtrate is treated with alkaline copper solution, the cuprous oxide formed is treated with a phosphomolybdic acid solution, blue colour being obtained which is compared with that of a standard.

Reagents

1. Alkaline $CuSO_4$ solution.
2. Phosphomolybdic acid solution.
3. Standard glucose solution (0.1 mg/ml)
4. 10% sodium tungstate solution.
5. 2/3 N H_2SO_4

Procedure

	B	T	S
Distilled water	3.2ml	3.2ml	3.2ml
Blood	—	0.2ml	—
Standard	—	—	0.2ml
Distilled water	0.2ml	—	—
10% Sod. tungstate	0.3ml	0.3ml	0.3ml
2/3 N H_2SO_4	0.3ml	0.3ml	0.3ml

Mix well and centrifuge at 3000 r.p.m. for 5 mins.

clear filtrate from above	2.0ml	2.0ml	2.0ml
Alkaline Copper reagent	2.0ml	2.0ml	2.0ml

Mix & keep in boiling water baths for 6 minutes

Cool for 2–3 mins. Add. 2ml of phosphomolybdic acid to each one and dilute to 25ml with distilled water. Read in colorimeter

$$\frac{T - B}{S - B} \times 100 = \text{Sugar in mg/dl.}$$

Interpretation

The normal range of fasting venous blood sugar values by this method is 90–120 mg/dl of whole blood. Of this non-glucose reducing substances constitute 20–30 mg/dl. However this saccharoid fraction remains remarkably constant. Fasting hyper glycemia is highly suggestive of diabetes. On the other hand, diabetes can never be ruled out by a normal fasting blood sugar. A blood glucose below 40–60 mg/dl. occurs most frequently as a result of overdosage with insulin in treatment of diabetes mellitus.

Modifications of Folin Wu method

1. SOMOGYI — SHAFFER HARTMAN method:

Hemolyzed bood is deprotenized with $Zn(OH)_2$, giving a filtrate containing practically no reducing susbtances other than sugar.

2. NELSON SOMOGYI METHOD

Blood is deproternized by a $Zn(OH)_2$, – $BaSO_4$ procedure which gives a filtrate containing practically no reducing substance other than glucose.

Results of these methods are considerably lower than the classical. Folin Wu method.

Glucose oxidase method

It is based on the following reactions.

Glucose + $O_2 \xrightarrow{\text{Glucose Oxidase}}$ Gluconic acid + H_2O_2

H_2O_2 + Chromogen $\xrightarrow{\text{Peroxidase}}$ Chromogen
(Colourless) (coloured)

The colour of this chromogen is estimated colorimetrically. This method is highly specific for glucose.

GOP (Glucose oxidase peroxidase) method

The principle is similar to that of Glucose oxidase method except certain small differences in the reaction.

$$H_2O_2 \xrightarrow{\text{Peroxidase}} H_2 + O_2 \longrightarrow \text{oxidase phenol which}$$
combines with 4 aminophenazone to give a red coloured substance.

Intensity of the red colour is propotional to the concentration of glucose in the specimen under test.

Measure colorimetrically at 515nm. Ready made, ready to use, working glucose reagent is available as ETHNOTEST GLUCOSE WORKING reagent supplied by Ethnor Private Limited.

Procedure

	T	S	B
Set 3 tubes			
1. Trichloracelic acid	0.9ml	0.9ml	0.9ml
2. Blood	0.1ml	x	X

Mix and centrifuge test soln. at 3000rpm for 5–10mins.

3. Ethnotest glucose working reagent	5.0ml	5.0ml	5.0ml
4. Supernatant fluid pon above	0.25ml	x	x
5. Standard 1:10	x	0.25ml	x
6. Distilled water	x	x	0.25ml

Mix and place in water bath for 15 mins at 37°C. Measure O.D. at 515nm.

Glucose concentration = $(T/S) \times 100$ mgm/dl.

Glucose Tolerance Test

Introduction

Glucose tolerance test or GTT determines the ability of an individual to utilize a given quantity of glucose taken orally. The one disadvantage of this test is that it involves one factor unrelated to the insulin response — rate of absorption from GIT.

Preparation of Patient

1. Patient must be ambulatory, free from stress for at least 2 wks. prior to the test.
2. Drugs such as oral contraceptives, salicylates, diuretics and steroids must be discontinued 3 days prior to the test.
3. Hypoglycemic oral agents must be stopped 3 days before the test. Insulin should be discontinued on the day of the test.
4. Patient must have a diet containing 150 gm carbohydrate per day for 3 days prior to test.
5. Patient is asked to fast overnight, with an allowance of only plain water during the night.

Procedure

1. Obtain a fasting venous sample in a flouride-oxalate bottle.
2. Administer $40gm/m^2$ of glucose diluted to 300 ml and flavoured with lemon.
3. In addition to a fasting venous sample, obtain a fasting urine specimen.
4. Further blood samples and urine specimens are collected at 60mins, 120mins and 180mins.
5. Proceed with each sample as discussed in blood sugar estimation.
6. Plot the GTT curve.

Interpretation

(a) Normal response

Fasting value	60–80mg/dl.
1 hr. value	120–150mg/dl (<170mg/dl).
2 hr. value	— back to fasting.

No glycosuria occurs.

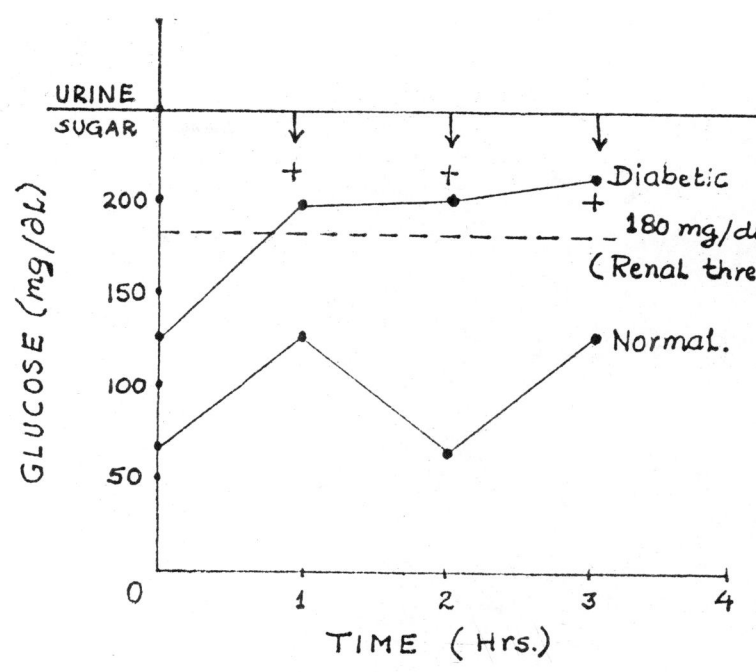

GRAPH 3: GTT Curve

(b) Impaired GTT: (Diabetic curve).
GTT curve is raised & prolonged
Glycosuria is normally seen.

(c) Renal glycocuria —
The curve is normal
One or more samples of urine contain glucose.

(d) Lag storage curve —
Fasting value-Normal.
Max. value at 30 mins — >180mg/dl. with glycosuria.
Hypoglycemic levels before 120 mins.

(e) Flat curve of enhanced GT —
Fasting value is ≤ normal & throughout the test, level does not vary by more than ± 20mg/dl.

Diagnostic glucose values for oral GTT.

Condition	Fasting	2hr. PP
1. Diabetes mellitus	≥120mg/dl.	≥180mg/dl.
2. Impaired GTT	<120mg/dl.	120–180mg/dl.
3. Normal	<120mg/dl.	<120mg/dl.

SERUM CHOLESTEROL ESTIMATION

Introduction

Cholesterol occurs in appreciable amounts in the body. Most of the cholesterol is synthesized by the liver from acetyl CoA, though all cells are capable of producing it. Cholesterol is concerned with the metabolism of lipids and is an important precursor for steroid hormones.

Colour reactions used in Cholesterol determinations

Majority of methods in routine use are variants of 2 basic reactions.
1. Liebermann Burchard (L-B) reaction.
2. Zak reaction.
Both these reactions are essentially oxidative.

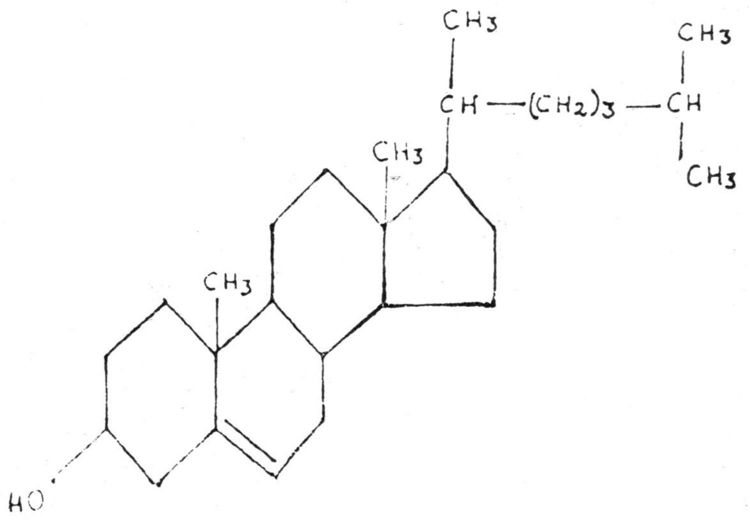

DIAGRAM 15 Structure of Cholesterol.

Principle

Fundamental chemistry on which all methods depend is basically identical. The 2 reaction centres in the cholesterol molecule are the double bond and the OH group. Cholesterol reacts with strongly acid reagents to produce coloured substances chiefly Cholestadiene sulfonic acids. Acetic acid and acetic anhydride are used as solvents and dehydrating agents while H_2SO_4 as dehydrating and oxidizing agent.

In the method, cholesterol in the serum is extracted into acetic anhydride in the presence of acetic acid. Addition of H_2SO_4 to cholesterol in the presence of acetic anhydride gives a green chromophore (Liebermann **Burchard** reaction).

Reagents

Acetic anhydride
Glacial acetic acid
Acid reagent — Glacial acetic acid + Conc. H_2SO_4 in a ratio of 1:1
Dehydrating agent — 10ml acid reagent + 10 ml of glacial acetic acid.
Standard (200mg/dl or 2mg/ml).

Procedure

1. Into a series of tubes, pipette the following

	B.	S.	T.
Std. Soln.	—	0.2ml.	—
Distilled water	0.2ml	0.2ml	—
Serum	—	—	0.2ml
Glacial acetic acid	0.8ml	0.6ml	0.8ml.

(In case of highly icteric or turbid sera, a serum blank is also necessary containing 0.2ml distilled water, 0.2ml serum and 0.6 ml glacial acetic acid).
2. Add 4 ml of acetic anhydride to each tube, letting it flow freely without touching the sides of tube. Mix gently by rotating.
3. Centrifuge the serum containing tubes and decant the supernatant into fresh tubes.
4. To all the tubes (except serum blank if there) add 1 drop dehydrating reagent & mix. If the solution does not become hot immediately add 1 more drop and mix.
5. Place in a 25°C water bath for 5–10 mins.
6. Add 1 ml. of acid reagent to each tube at 1 minute intervals and replace in water bath at 25° C for 20 mins.
7. Read against reagent blank at 630nm (red filter) at 1 minute intervals.

Calculations

Serum cholesterol (mg/dl) =
$$\frac{O.D. (Test) - O.D. (Serum\ blank)}{O.D.(Std) - O.D. (reagent\ blank)} \times 2 \times 20.2 \times (100/0.2)$$
$$= \frac{O.D.(T) - O.D(SB)}{O.D.(S) - O.D. (R)} \times 200\ (202)^*$$

* Factor of 202 is used instead of 200 to correct for the small amount of supernatant which remains after decanting.

Interpretation

Cholesterol in serum exists in 2 forms —
1. Free (comprises 20–40%)
2. Esterified with unsaturated fatty acids (65–75%)

Usually the total serum cholesterol is estimated. The normal adult value is 140–260mg/dl of serum, but age, sex and diet play an important role.
 i) Value increases with age.
 ii) Value is more in women.
 iii) Value increases during late pregnancy.
 iv) Values are higher with increased dietary intake of fats & cholesterol.

Most of the cholesterol is carried in the LDL fraction & increase in cholesterol generally reflects either increased LDL or VLDL or both.

Hypercholesterolemia increases risk of:
1. Myocardial infarction and CAD
2. Cerebrovascular accidents due to AS

Serum cholesterol

Increases in	Decreases in
1. Diabetes mellitus	1. Severe infection
2. Nephrosis	2. Severe anemia.
3. Biliary cirrhosis	3. Hyperthyroidism.
4. Lipoprotenemias	4. Malnutrition
5. Hypothyroidism	

CHAPTER 37

SERUM ELECTROLYTES & IONS

DETERMINATION OF SODIUM & POTASSIUM

Intoduction

Sodium and potassium of whole blood appear to be present entirely in the ionized state. Over 90% of blood sodium is found in the plasma whereas potassium is present primarily in the cells. Whole blood sodium or potassium have little significance, hence serum is ordinarily used for analysis. Separation of serum from cells should be carried out as soon as possible and precautions taken against hemolysis. Ideally a syringe should not be used for collecting blood for serum electrolytes. Blood should directly be collected via a needle into a test tube. It should be centrifuged after 20 minutes. Whole blood allowed to stand for 4 hrs causes serum potassium elevation by upto 4 meq per litre.

Techniques

Basically there are 2 techniques.
1. Chemical analysis based on precipitation of a metal complex.
2. Flame photometry has more or less replaced chemical analysis in most laboratories as chemical analysis is cumbersome and time consuming.

Flame photometry

Principle: Sample in solution is introduced in the form of a fine, continuous spray into a nonluminous gas flame. By the use of a colour filter or diffraction grating, the emitted light, of wavelength characteristic for the ion being analysed, is isolated and focussed on a photoelectric cell. Electrical response of the cell is measured on a suitable meter and then ion conc. is determined from a calibration curve, or by direct reading.

Procedure: A serum dilution of 1:100 is used for either sodium or potassium analysis unless otherwise specified by the instrument manufacturer. Standard solutions of both sodium (80 to 160) & potassium (3 to 8) are prepared beforehand and run through the photometer, thereby designing calibration curves which are utilized for determination of Na^+ & K^+ concentration.

Sodium Stds. — Prepare a stock std. by dissolving 5.85gm NaCl in water & diluting to 1 litre (eq. to 100meq Na/litre). Working stds. are prepared as follows.

Stock soln		Na^+ Conc. in meq/L. at a
1. 10ml		100 dilution of 1:100
2. 11ml	Dilute all to	110
3. 12ml	1 litre with	120
4. 13ml	distilled	130
5. 14ml	water	140
6. 15ml		150
7. 16ml		160

Potassium Stds: Std. solutions covering a range of 3–7 meq/L. at a dilution of 1:100 are enough for calibration. Stock std. is prepared by dissolving 746mg of KCl. in water and diluting it to 1 litre. Working stds. are prepared as follows.

Stock soln. (ml)		K^+ Conc in meq/L at a dilution of 1:100
1. 3.0		3.0
2. 4.0	Dilute all	4.0
3. 5.0	to 1 litre	5.0
4. 6.0	with distilled	6.0
5. 7.0	water.	7.0

A single standard may be used in determining Na^+ & K^+. It is prepared by diluting 10ml sodium stock solution & 3ml potassium stock solution to 1 litre. Thus final std. represents 100 meq Na^+ and 3 meq K^+ at a dilution 1:100.

Interpretation

1. **Sodium:** Normal serum sodium is 130–154 meq/L or 300–355 mg/dl. Decrease in Serum Na^+ occurs in pregnancy, pyloric stenosis, a/c Intestinal obstrn, pneumonia, severe nephritis & addison's disease.

Potassium: Normal serum K^+ is 3.6 — 5.6 meq/L or 14–22mg/dl. Pathologically serum K^+ increases in a/c bronchial asthma, uraemia & addison's disease. Serum potassium is very important because of the potential fatality of both hyperkalemia and hypokalemia.

DETERMINATION OF SERUM CHLORIDE

Chlorides of whole blood are distributed to the extent of about 1/3rd in RBCs and 2/3rd in the plasma. Serum is therefore ordinarily used for analysis.

Principle

The sample is titrated with std. mercuric nitrate soln. at proper acidity using diphenylcarbazone as indicator. Chlorides react with added mercuric ions to form soluble $HgCl_2$. When excess mercuric ions have been added, indicator turns purple.

Procedure

Transfer 2ml of tungsten serum filtrate to a small flask and add 4 drops of diphenylcarbazone indicator. Titrate with std. Hg $(NO_3)_2$ using a microburette. Stop as soon as soln. becomes deep purple.

Calculation

meq Cl/litre = ml Hg(NO$_3$)$_2$ soln used $\times$ (100/A)

where A equals no. of ml. of Hg $(NO_3)_2$ required for 2ml standard NaCl Soln. Now a days automatic chloride titrators are available. They are known as chloridometers.

Interpretation

Normal value of Cl^- varies from 98–108 meq/litre of serum. The values are indicative of hydration of the subject, increasing in dehydration and decreasing in hydremia. It is also indicative of CO_2 balance since Cl^- shifts to compensate for CO_2 changes in serum.

Acidosis ——>Low HCO_3^- ——>High Cl^-
Alkalosis ——>High HCO_3^- ——>Low Cl^-

Chloride changes also occur in vomiting (loss of gastric contents) and diarrhoea.

Serum Calcium Estimation
Procedure

	B	T	S
Naphthyl	5 ml	5 ml	5 ml
Hydroxamic acid			
Serum	—	0.2 ml	—
Ca standard	—	—	0.2ml
Distilled water	0.2ml	—	—

Keep it overnight and centrifuge for 1 hr. Discard the supernatant. To the residue add.

| EDTA | 0.1 ml | 0.1ml | 0.1ml |

Keep in boiling water and dissolve until there is no turbidity. Now allow it to cool. Add coloured reagent (60gms $Fe(NO_3)_3$ in 500 ml water + 5 ml Conc. HNO_3). Read at 400 nm (filter no. 623 systronic)

Serum calcium = $(T/S) \times 10$ mg/dl.

Interpretation

Normal human blood contains 9–11.5 mg of calcium per dl corresponding to 4.5–5.7 meq/L. Values for children are slightly higher than for adults. It is decreased in Parathyroidectomy — blood calcium is very low.

Infantile tetany — values are 3.5–7.0mg/dl.
Renal failure — Ca may be ≤ 7.0mg/dl.

Except in children and cases where calcium metabolism per se is abnormal, there is a definite relationship between serum calcium, phosphate, and protein.

$7 - 0.255$ P (mg/dl) + 0.566 protein (g/dl) = Ca(mg/dl).

SERUM PHOSPHORUS ESTIMATION

Introduction

Whole blood contains about 40 mgs of total phosphorus in 100 ml, present mainly as inorganic phosphate, organic acid soluble phosphate esters and lipid phosphorus. Cells contain mainly organic phosphate while inorganic phosphate is practically entirely in the plasma. What we determine is actually inorganic phosphate.

Principle

The proteins of blood are precipitated with trichloroacetic acid. The protein free filtrate is treated with an acid molybdate solution, which forms phosphomolybdic acid from any phosphate present. The phosphomolybdic acid is reduced by the addition of 1, 2, 4, aminoaphtholsulfonic acid reagent, to produce a blue colour whose intensity is proportional to the amount of phosphate present.

Procedure

Solution	B	T	S
10% trichloro acetic acid	4.8 ml	4.8 ml	4.8 ml
Serum	—	0.2 ml	—
Distilled water	0.2 ml	—	—
Standard	—	—	0.2 ml
Centrifuge at 3000 r.p.m. for 5 minutes			
Protein free filtrate	2.0 ml	2.0 ml	2.0 ml
Sod. molybdate	0.2 ml	0.2 ml	0.2 ml
Fresh ascorbic acid	0.1 ml	0.1 ml	0.1 ml
Distilled water	3.7 ml	3.7 ml	3.7 ml

Incubate at 37°C for 15 mins and take reading at 720nm (608 systronic filter).

Conc of inorganic Phosphates = $(T/S) \times 4$mg/dl

Interpretation

Normal inorganic phosphorus ranges of serum are 4–7mg/dl in infants & children and 2.5–5.0mg/dl in adults.
1. In rickets inorganic phosphorus may fall to ≤ 2mg/dl.
2. In severe renal failure (or nephritis), inorganic phosphorus may rise by 15–20mg/dl. and may bear a relation to the acidosis found in these cases.

SECTION VIII

BLOOD BANKING AND
BLOOD TRANSFUSION

CHAPTER 38

BASIC PRINCIPALS IN BLOOD BANKING — ORGANISATION, PLANNING AND DOCUMENTATION

Introduction

The idea that the blood of a healthy human or animal has rejuvenating properties, is probably as ancient as civilization. It is well known and hardly surprising that following the discovery of the circulation, attempts were made to transfuse blood directly from a healthy human donor or animal to a sick patient. Unhappily these dramatic operations, more often than not resulted in over-dramatic results, that is, tragedy for not only the patient but also occasionally for the donor. This resulted in the idea of blood transfusion or transfer as it was tried initially to be dropped though temporarily.

Ultimately the unquenchable thirst for knowledge of mankind led to the superlative discovery of blood groups by Landsteiner in 1900. It was this discovery and another addition later of Rh typing that really revolutionized the blood banking and transfusion.

What in essence is blood bank?

In literal terms it is the BANK for BLOOD. It is a compact unit where blood is accepted from donors, processed and stored and then issued to recepients in need as and when required. Infact nowadays even cheques are issued by Red Cross in the form of donor cards. Donor cards are issued to a person voluntarily donating blood. This donor card can be encashed for one unit of blood as and when the donor may require it for a period of one year.

Any blood bank has 2 distinct service setup.
1. DEBIT: Which deals with collection of blood and its storage.
2. CREDIT: which deals with issuing of blood to a deserving and needy recepient.

A very important point about blood banking that has to be kept in mind is that, the blood stock of the blood bank has to be replenished every time a unit of blood is issued for consumption. Thus encouragement should be given to the idea of donating blood for a patient before getting it issued for the patient. This implies deploring the practice of buying blood from private Blood banks if healthy donors are available at hand.

This brings us to another important point. People in developing countries, especially India have a false conception that blood donation is detrimental to health. It is the prime duty of one and all concerned with blood banking and transfusions including technicians, nurses and doctors to try and remove these misgivings by explaining that;
1. All required tests are beforehand and only healthy donors are selected for bleeding.
2. Human body (adult) contains 5.5 to 6 litres of blood and the amount withdrawn at a time (roughly 300 cc) is replenished in no time. Volume depletion is replenished in 48–72 hrs and Hamoglobin level in 3–4 wks time.

3. Blood from professional donors is of inferior quality in comparison to that from fresh donors. Moreover it is also likely to carry infection.

BLOOD BANK — ORGANIZATION & PLANNING

Location

The Blood Bank should be situated within the hospital premesis and should be run as independent unit for smooth functioning in respect of both technical and administrative matters.

Within a hospital, location of blood bank, should be such that it is at once easily annoying yet secluded enough to discourage unnecessary and annoying intrusions by attendants of patients and unconcerned hospital personnel, because interruptions during grouping and cross matching procedures may mean a mistake which may cost a life.

Designing

Design of the blood bank should be such that only three rooms are accessible to persons from outside the blood bank.
1. Reception Room. 2. Donation room. 3. Rest' room.

Reception Room

Careful attention is given to the planning of reception room. The room should be spacious enough to accommodate an unanticipated peak of donors. The room should be well ventilated and have following facilities.
It should have

1. 2 Registration counters
   (i) For donors where name of donors, age, sex and address of the donor is registered.
   (ii) For registering the name of patients whom the blood is delivered from the bank. At this counter the forms for the requisition of blood are checked and verified.
2. A doctors cabin where a qualified registered doctor examines the proposed donors and declares him fit or unfit for donation.
3. A small side lab for checking the haemoglobin concentration of the proposed donor, and checking of various laboratory parameters which may render the donor unfit for donation.
4. A proper seating arrangement for proposed donors.

Donation Room

This room must be comfortable and must be airconditioned. In some blood banks the doctors cabin and the side laboratory are part of this room.
This room must have
1. Comfortable beds for donors.

2. Sterile equipment for bleeding donors. Stacked away in a locked cupboard.
3. A refrigerator
4. Resuscitation equipment.

Donors rest cum refreshment room

This room should again be very comfortable and therefore air-conditioned. This room serves 3 purposes.
1. It provides rest to the donor.
2. It provides necessary space to the donor to have well deserved refreshment.
3. It provides the doctor a chance to keep the donor under observation for a few minutes before releasing him.

This room should contain a few comfortable beds and proper seating arrangement. It should also have a supply of healthy drinking water.

Laboratory

It is one of the most crucial part of a blood bank as it is the seat of the most indispensable event, the crossmatch. It has the following functions.
1. Grouping of would be recepients blood.
2. Grouping and proper labelling of the donated blood.
3. Crossmatching of the patients blood against stored/freshly donated blood.

This laboratory should be managed by an experienced technician adept at hematological techniques.

This lab should be spacious, must have a refrigerator and should preferably be airconditioned.

Room: For preservation and storage of blood.

Room: For deep freezing refrigerators to preserve and store plasma and other blood products.

Immunolaboratory for testing of various possible contaminants for example.
1. Australia antigen (HB$_s$Ag)
2. Malaria
3. Syphilis
4. AIDS (HTLV-III)

Working laboratory

For preparation of blood products. This should be secluded even within the blood bank. In it, complete sterility must be maintained at all costs and only restricted entry permitted.

Blood Bank Store

For storage of blood collection kits and other important equipment.

Sterilization section

For sterilization of needles, syringes, rubber gloves and blood collecting equipment. The need for this has now decreased with the availability of sterilised and disposal equipment at reasonale price.

Doctors premises   As per availability and within the
Technical staff premises   available limited resources.

Emergency power system: Containing a powerful generator time scheduled under direct supervision of Electrical Department.

EQUIPMENT REQUIRED

1. **Blood bank refrigerators** (walk-in-coolers)

2 types $\lbrace$ Cylindrical variety with rotating shelves
Conventional almirah shaped variety.

Each refrigerator should have
(1) Separate perforated shelves for the four groups. Each shelf is divided into 2 for Rh positive and negative blood respectively.
(2) An arrangement by which the oldest blood is at hand and first utilized.
(3) Been fitted with a safety light and an 8 day continuous temperature recording device.
(4) An alarm system which goes off if temp falls below 4°C or rises above 6°C.
(5) An automatic buzzer which blows of if refrigerator door is left open. Separate refrigerators should be available for storing Plasma, fibrinogen and other blood products respectively.

2. **Deep freezer**

Capable of maintaining a constant temperature of — 20°C to — 80°C necessary for storage of plasma and other blood products.

3. **Equipments for the immunological laboratory**
   (i) Electrophoresis apparatus
   (ii) An electric Balance
   (iii) Refrigerators
   (iv) Shakers (Rotators/agitators)
   (v) Centrifuges
   (vi) Microscope
   (vii) Kits (specialized testing such as Australia antigen and Syphillitic wasserman reaction).
   (viii) Water Baths
   (ix) Anciliary glass and plastic equipment.

4. **Equipment for Crossmatching laboratory:**
   (i) A microscope and slides
   (ii) Constant temp. water baths at 37°C, 56°C & 20°C.
   (iii) Opal glass tiles
   (iv) Racks
   (v) Pasteur pipettes:
   (vi) Glass test tubes in 3 sizes
        — 75 x 10 mm
        — 75 x 12 mm &
        — 100 x 12 mm
   (vii) Centrifuge

5. **Equipment for Donation room**
   (i) Beds or Tables-Cushioned and Bed side table
   (ii) Disposable, sterile needles, syringes and blood collection sets, Xylocaine vials 2%, spirit and iodine.
   (iii) Refrigerators maintaining temperature between 4–6°C
   (iv) Sphygmomanometer
   (v) CPD/ACD glass bottles
   (vi) CPD/CPD-A plastic bags

6. **Equipment for Doctors (examination chambers and side lab.**
   (i) Stethoscope
   (ii) Sphygmomanometer (B.P. Instrument)
   (iii) Weighing machine and Height measuring stand
   (iv) Colorimeter/Spectrophotometer
   (v) Refrigerator for storing Drabkin solution (when Cynameth Hb method is used for Hb estimation)

(vi) Otherwise- Sahlis Hb meter
(vii) Copper Sulphate solution, Specific gravity 1.052
(viii) Disposable sterile lancet.

7. **Equipment for working laboratory**

(i) Refrigerators
(ii) Centrifuge Machine and Ultra-centrifuges
(iii) Continuous flow centrifuges
(iv) Automatic cell washer
(v) Ultra filtration and filtration set ups
(vi) Anticoagulants
(vii) Fractionation and fractional distillation
(viii) Other necessary preservatives and chemicals
(ix) Rh. view box
(xi) Incubator
(xii) Sucksion pump
(xiii) Compound Microscope
(xiv) Hand Lens.
(All these should have a very high level of sterlity)

8. **Emergency Equipments**

(i) Small Oxygen Cylinder with mask
(ii) 5% Glucose or Normal Saline I. V. fluids
(iii) Sterile Syringe and needles
(iv) Sterile I.V. Infusion set
(v) Ampouls of Adernaline, Nor-adernaline, Mephantin, Betamethasonn or Dexa-methasone.
(vi) Aspirin and spirit of Ammonia Aromatice.

9. **Accessories**

(i) Blanket, Bed Sheets, basin, artery forceps, dressing jars, waste cans
(ii) Sterile Cotton balls, band aids
(iii) Denatured Spirit, Tincture Iodine
(iv) Towels

10. **Sera**

(i) Blood Grouping Sera — Anti A, Anti B, Anti AB and other anti sera for Sub-group and minor group.
(ii) Rho typing sera
(iii) Coomb's Serum
(iv) Albumine 20% –30%
(v) Anti H
(vi) R.P.H.A. or Elisa test kits for Hepatitis B Test
(vii) Reagent for tests for Syphilis.

DOCUMENTATION

Documentation or a precise and complete record system is absolutely indispensable for any blood banking for following reasons.
1. It is important in preventing mistakes
2. It provides an idea about the stores and availability of blood.
3. It provides legal documentary evidence in case of negligence on part of any laboratory personnel or doctor.
Documentation consists of 2 parts.

A. **MAINTENANCE OF BLOOD BANK RECORDS**

These include the following.

1. **Donors Registers**

2 in number

(i) for relative donors and
(ii) for voluntary donors
In this the following information is registered Name, Age. Sex, Occupation, Address, Date of last donation, reports of Australia antigen, malaria, syphillis & AIDS and medical examination reports

2. **Receipt registers**

This contains an every day account of the blood collected by the blood bank. These record donation number, Date/Year of collection, Blood group.

3. **Issue Register**

Contains almost same information as Receipt register. In addition it contains details of patient, ward and department for which blood has been issued. Serial no. of blood in this should coincide with that of Receipt register.

4. **Blood Stock Registers**

There should be separate registers for
1. Various groups of blood
2. Plasma
3. Other blood products

5. **Registers for requisitions**

Information entered in these includes Date & time of requisition, concerned department, ward & Unit, particulars of patient along with diagnosis, Hospital Registration number of patient, An explanatory note for urgency of blood, Date and time of compliance from the blood bank.

6. **Registers for**

1. Blood Grouping & Crossmatching
2. ABO and Rh typing of OPD and ward patients.
3. Australia antigen reports
4. Recording of all apparatus, equipments and chemicals of blood bank i.e. A blood bank general stock register.
It is of 2 types
1. Register for nonexpendable items
2. Register for expendable items.

7. **Attendence register for all blood bank personnel**

8. Proper colour labelling of blood collected by the blood bank as indicated below:—
(a) Blood group 'O' — Blue label
(b) Blood group 'A' — Yellow label
(c) Blood group 'B' — Pink label
(d) Blood group 'AB' — White label

B. **DOCUMENTS CONCERNED WITH BLOOD REQUISITION, DONATION & ISSUE**

1. **Blood Requisition**

A blood requisition from any Ward should be accompanied by the following documents and samples.
(a) A properly labelled sample of the patient in a plain vial.
(b) A Blood Requisition
(c) Sanction slip
(d) Blood Receipt slip

All the above forms must be signed by Senior Residents and above.

2. Blood Donation

Every donor is accompanied by donor slips filled in by qualified doctors and signed by the donors concerned in presence of the doctor.

3. Blood Issue

Every blood when issued must be accompanied by
1. A transfusion report.
2. Completion of the label indicated in column 8.

CHAPTER 39

BLOOD GROUPS

INTRODUCTION

Since Landsteiner's discovery in 1900 that human blood groups do exist, a vast number of antigens have been detected on human blood cells, of which about 10–15% form well defined systems and only 1–2% play a significant role in blood transfusion.
Human blood antigens may be

1. Erythrocyte related

At least 100 antigens have been recongnized on R.B.C. surface and almost 15 well defined blood group systems have been demonstrated in Europeans. Important among these are

Blood group

1. ABO		5 Kell
2. Rh. blood group		6 lewis
3. MNS's		7 Duffy
4. Lutheran		8 kidd

However out of the above only ABO & Rh. are important with relation to blood banking. Other are less important because the antigens are weak and/or because corresponding antibodies do not actually occur in serum.

2. Leukocyte related

These include
1. HLA typing
2. RBC grp. antigens in small amounts

3. Platelet antigens include

1. HLA typing
2. Platelet specific matching
3. ABO matching
4. Rh typing

(A) ABO BLOOD GROUPS

The ABO system consists of 4 main groups

(1)	AB	(2)	A
(3)	B &	(4)	O

which are determined by the presence or absence on the RBC of 2 antigens, A and B.

Inheritance of the ABO Groups

The A and B antigens, like other blood group antigens, are the expression of genes inherited from the previous generation. If an antigen is demonstrated, the gene controlling it must have been inherited from one or both of the parents, and this gene can be passed to the next generation.

The genes, *A*, *B* and *O* are *alleles*, i.e. any one of the three may occupy the ABO *locus* on each of the pair of *chromosomes* responsible for this system. (It is not known which chromosome pair it is.) If the chromosome inherited from the father carried the gene *A* and the chromosome from the mother carried the gene *B*, the child will be of the *genotype AB* and his or her red cells will have both *A* and *B* antigens. Persons who inherit *O* genes from both parents belong to group O. The *O* gene is an *amorph*, i.e., it does not produce a detectable antigen. Group O cells are recognized by the absence of A or B antigen. When the *O* gene is inherited with *A*, only the *A* gene expresses itself; red cells from an individual of the genotype *AO* will react in the same way as cells from someone of the genotype *AA* in tests with anti-A. Similarly, we cannot differentiate *BO* from *BB* in tests with anti-B. The symbols A and B denote *phenotypes*, whereas *AA*, *BO* etc are genotypes.

When the same gene has been inherited from each parent, for example *OO*, the individual is said to be *homozygous* for that gene. When different genes are inherited, as is evident in the case of *AB*, the individual is *heterozygous*. The genotype of someone of the phenotype A (or B) may be deduced from a study of his family; the person who is homozygous *AA* will pass an *A* gene to each of his children while the heterozygous *AO* individual may pass either an *A* or an *O* gene to his offspring. As for all chromosomes, chance alone determines which of the pair ends up in the *zygote* from which the new individual result. Figure 74 illustrates possible off-spring from various sets of parents.

Since each of the pair of chromosomes of an AB person carries either an *A* or a *B* gene, an AB parents cannot normally have a group O chiid. By the same reasoning, someone who is group O cannot have an AB child because the child must inherit one *O* gene of that parent, and the gene from the other parent could not transmit both *A* and *B*.

ABO Groups

The 4 groups are determined by the presence or absence on the RBCs of the blood groups, antigens A & B, therefore the blood group of the individual may be
1. Group A — presence of A antigen
2. Group B — presence of B antigen
3. Group AB — presence of both A & B antigen
4. Group O — Absence of both A & B antigen
In addition it has been shown that corresponding to the antigens A & B there are antibodies anti A (x) and anti — B, which occur as agglutinins in the sera of individuals whose RBCs lack the corresponding agglutinogen. These facts are known as Landsteiner's rules.

Agglutinogen & agglutinin content of RBSs & Sera of 4 blood groups.

BLOOD GROUP	Agglutinogen	Agglutinin
1. A	A	Anti B (μ)
2. B	B	Anti A (x)
3. AB	A and B	Neither
4. O	Neither	Both

Fig. 74: ABO Genotype Possible from Various Matings.

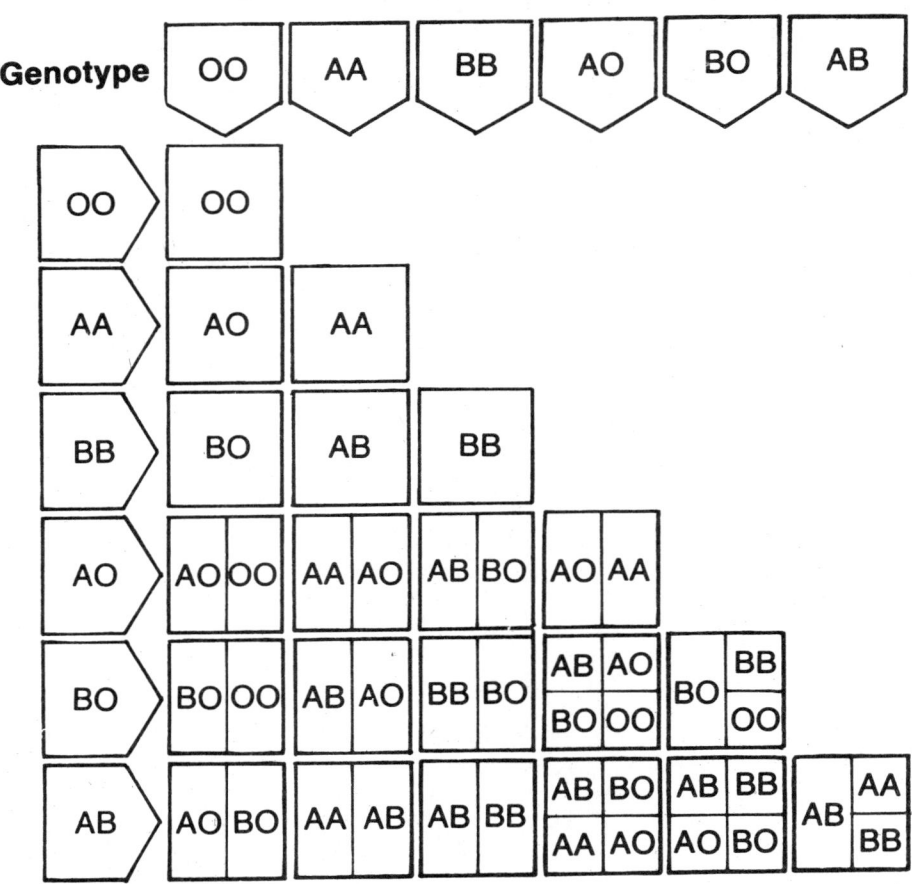

Frequency of various blood groups in the population

BLOOD GROUP	Frequency in British population	Frequency in Indian population)
1. A	41.7%	24.7%
2. B	8.6%	37.5%
3. AB	3.0%	5.3%
4. O	46.7%	32.5%

Principal of ABO Group Determination

It is by means of the agglutination reaction of red cells that the blood group of an individual is determined. It can be effected either by testing the individuals red cells with std. Anti — A & anti — B Sera or by testing his serum with standard red cells of Groups A and B. The most reliable grouping is achieved if both these methods are used.

Table 38 *Serological reactions in the ABO Blood Group system*

Blood Group	Agglutination with	
	Anti — A	Anti — B
A	+	0
B	0	+
AB	+	+
O	0	0

Table 39: *Reactions of serum from Different ABO Blood Groups with Reagent Cells*

Serum from Blood of Groups	Reagent Cells	
	A	B
A	O	+
B	+	O
AB	O	O
O	+	+

Direct blood grouping can be done on a slide or in a tube at room temperature. The usual procedure is to mix commercial reagent (antiserum of known specificity) with red cells (10 percent saline or serum suspension is used for slide tests; 2 percent is used for tube tests). Ingredients are mixed on the slide with a toothpick. The slide is tilted back and forth and observed over a two-minute period for agglutination. Longer periods of incubation should be avoided because the effects of drying may be interpreted as agglutination (pseudoagglutination). Strengths of reactions are graded on a scale from 0 (no reactivity) through +4 (massive agglutination). In the test tube, the ingredients are added, centrifuged, and examined macroscopically for agglutination. Centrifugation brings the cells together rapidly and facilitates the formation of large antigen-antibody complexes. Overcentrifugation should be avoided be-cause unagglutinated cells may become so tightly packed that only severe shaking can dislodge them from the bottom of the tube. Weak agglutinations may miss being detected when tubes are roughly shaken. By gentle rocking of the tube in an almost horizontal position, agglutination can readily be identified if it is present.

One of the most important controls on direct grouping is called reverse grouping or serum grouping. The patient's serum is tested with suspensions of known group A and B cells. These control cells can be purchased from several commercial sources. They should also be used to test the reactivity of anti-A and anti-B typing reagents. The expected reactions of serum from the four blood groups with these two reagent cells suspensions are given in Tables.

As an example, the serum from an individual of group A contains anti-B; therefore, this serum should agglutinate B reagent cells.

Why are these "natural" anti-A and anti-B antibodies regularly found in reciprocal relationship with B and A blood groups, respectively? In the early days of immunohaematology, it was hypothe-

sized that the gene responsible for the blood group antigen also determined the opposite antibody. For example, the gene specifying blood group factor A on the red cells was also responsible for that individual making anti-B in the serum.

TECHNIQUE OF BLOOD GROUPING

ABO Blood Grouping

ABO blood grouping can be performed by two techniques
1. Direct or Cell grouping
2. Indirect or Serum grouping
Each of these can be done in 2 ways
(i) Slide method
(ii) Tube method

I. Direct or Cell grouping

This consists in testing the patients R.B.Cs to detect the antigen on them by known antisera.

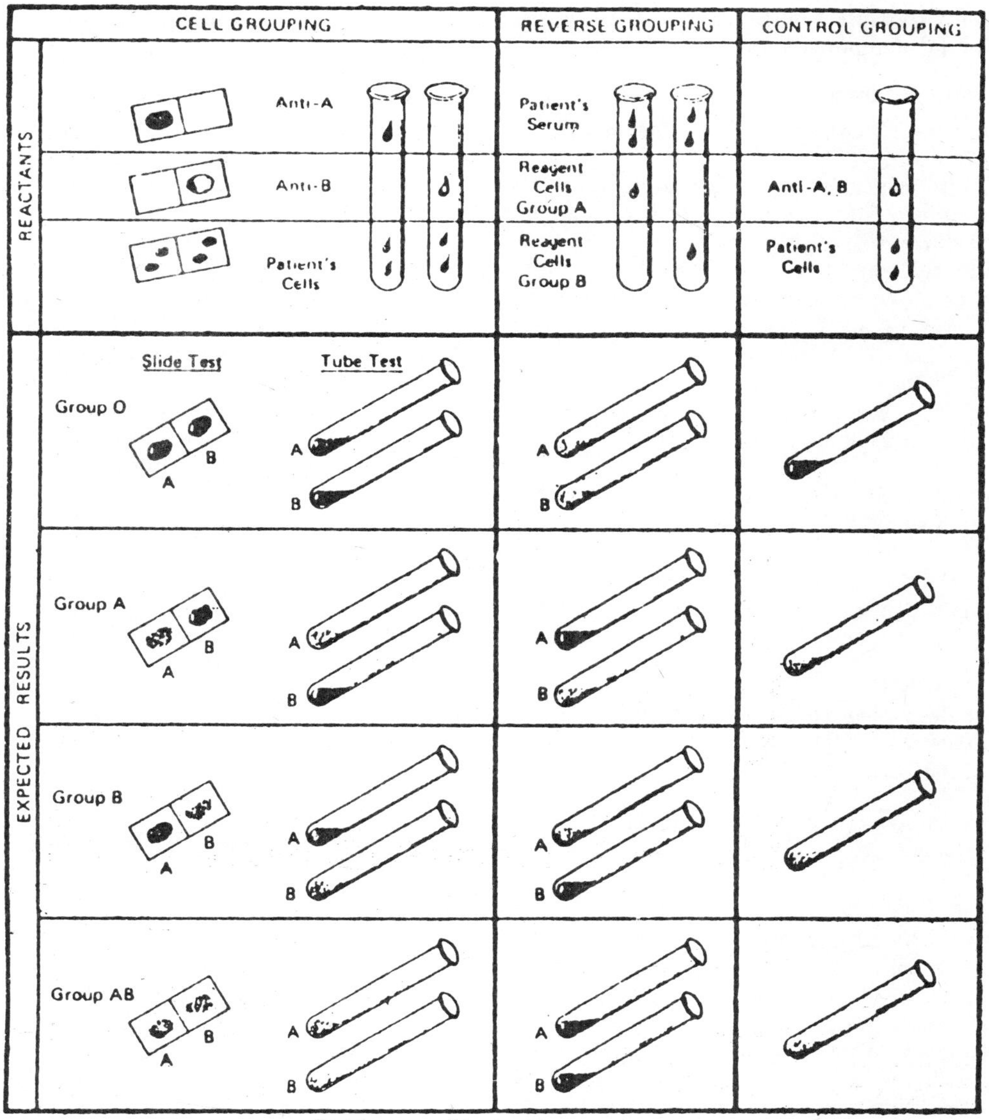

DIAGRAM: 16: Showing ABO blood grouping

207

1. SLIDE METHOD

1. Take 3 slides. A, B & C.
2. Take 1 drop of 10% saline suspension of patients (unknown) cells on each of the 3 slides.
3. Add 1 drop of Anti-A, 1 drop of Anti B, & one drop of anti AB (or Oserum) to slides A, B & C respectively.
4. Mix thoroughly with a toothpick
5. Tilt slides back and fourth
6. Observe for 2 minutes for agglutination

2. TUBE METHOD

1. Take 3 test tubes, A, B & C.
2. Take 2 drops of 2% saline suspension of patients' (unknown) R.B.Cs in each of the tubes.
3. Add 1 drop of Anti-A, Anti-B & Anti-AB (or O Group serum) to tubes A, B & C respectively.
4. Centrifuge at 1000 r.pm for 1 minute
5. Read macro-as well as microscopically for agglutination

* Overcentrifugation is to be avoided to prevent from getting false positive results, because centrifugation causes cells to pack tightly giving false impression of agglutination.

II. Indirect or Serum Grouping

1. Take 3 test tubes. Place 2 drops of patient's (unknown) sera into each of the 3 tubes.
2. Add 2 drops of 2–5% suspension of standard Group A Cells in tube 1 similar suspension of standard cells of B & O are put into the 2nd & 3rd tube respectively.
3. The tube is shaken and centrifuged at 1000 pm for 1 minute.
4. Read for agglutination both macro and microscopically.

Interpretation

1. DIRECT GROUPING

1. Agglutination in Slide 1 & Tube 1 and no agglutination in Slide 2 & Tube 2 — Blood Group is "A"
2. Agglutination in Slide 2 & Tube 2 and no agglutination in Slide 1 & Tube 1 — Blood Group is "B"
3. Agglutination in all Slides & Tubes — Blood Group is "AB"
4. Agglutination in none of the specimen — Blood Group is "O"

2. INDIRECT GROUPING

1. Agglutination in Tube 1. and No Agglutination in Tube 2 — Blood Group is "B"
2. Agglutination in Tube 2. and No Agglutination in Tube 1. — Blood Group is "A"
3. Agglutination in None of the Tubes — Blood Group is "AB"
4. Agglutination in 1 and 2 Tubes — Blood Group is "O"

Remarks

1. Ideally in all cases of Blood grouping and cross matching both direct & indirect grouping should be done.
2. Nowadays slides are available on which simultaneously 10 different samples can be tested.

Each of these slides is divided into 10 columns which are further divided into 8 rows each.

Each column is for one sample so that 10 samples can be tested at the same time.

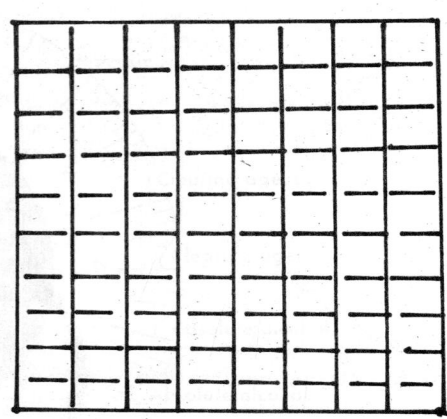

Each row of each column contains the following

Rows	1	2	3	4	5	6	7	8
	Anti A Serum	Anti B Serum	Gr. ABGro Cells	ABGro Cells	Ai Cells	A₂ Cells Standard suspension	B	O

Rows 1–4 are utilized for direct testing
Rows 5–8 are utilized for indirect testing

3. Most of the modern blood banks therefore utilize both 'A' & A₂ red cells suspensions for the indirect testing of blood samples. As shown above

The Bombay Phenotype

The first example of what has come to be known as the Bombay' phenotype was reported in 1952 by Bhande and his associates. Although the condition seems to be most common in the Marathi speaking people of India, about 30 such bloods have now been recognized in various parts of the World.

The red cells of a person with the 'Bombay' phenotype are (for all practical purpose) devoid of Antigens of the ABO system; in routine tests, the cells are agglutinated by Anti-A, Anti-B, or anti-H. The lack of reaction with Anti-A and Anti-B suggests that the red cells are a group 'O' individual; however, group O cells react strongly with anti-H and 'Bombay' cells do not react with anti-H. Serum samples from 'Bombay' individual contain anti-A, anti-B and anti-H. The presence of anti-H in the individual's serum is a further indication that his or her red cells are not group O. Because of the multiplicity of antibodies in the serum, the 'Bombay' transfusion recipient is incompatible with donors of group A, B. AB and O; only the blood of another 'Bombay' person could be compatible.

Discrepancies and Spurious Results

Any discrepancies between the cell and serum grouping or any peculiar reactions must be carefully checked. The more common causes are listed below,

1. Weak anti-B in group A. A weak or doubtful reaction with B cells is occasionally seen at 20°C.
2. Transfusions of another ABO group in the last two to four weeks may be the cause of a mixed-field picture.
3. A₂ and A₃ in the phenotype AB usually react very weakly with anti-A; if anti-A₁ is present, the sample may be called B in error. If sera from samples thought to be group B are tested

against A_2 cells as well as A_1 cells, those with an anti-A_1 but no anti-A (AB phenotype) will be noticed.

4. **Weak A or B variants.** If the reactions with grouping sera using a centrifugation method are not clear-cut, an absorption and elution should be carried out. Even though the cells appear to remove nothing from the serum, a strong, specific eluate can usually be obtained if a weak A or B antigen is persent. Confirmation of the group may be obtained if the person is a secretor of H and also secretes A or B substance.

5. **Hypogammaglobulinaemia.** Weak or "missing" iso-agglutinins may be the first warning of hypogammaglobulinaemia. Suspect sera should be submitted to immunoelectrophoretic analysis. One case of marked hypogammaglobulinaemia in a young, apparently healthy blood donor was discovered in this way.

6. Infected or polyagglutinable cells.

7. The concentration of group specific substances in the serum may be so high that anti-A or anti-B is neutralized when unwashed cells are used; three washes may be needed before accurate results are obtained. The patients in whom this rare phenomenon has been found have had ovarian cysts or carcinoma of the stomach or colon.

8. Additional iso-agglutinins.
   (a) Specific cold agglutinins such as anti-P_1 or anti-Le^a and even some saline-active Rh antibodies may be present in the donor serum and react with the test cells.
   (b) Anti-A_1 occurs as an extra iso-agglutinin in about 1% of A_2 and in up to 25% of A_2B people. It may also be found in the sera of weak A variants; see above.

Anti-H is found in the serum of all O_h persons and of occasional A_1 and A_1B persons as a saline agglutinin active at 20°C; it is found in persons of all ABO groups as a complement-binding cold incomplete antibody ("normal incomplete cold antibody"). Anti-H reacts stongly with group O and group A_2 cells and weakly with group A_1 and group A_1B cells.

Rh. Blood Groups:

Rhesus (Rh) system was so named because the original antibody was raised by injecting RBCs of rhesus monkey into rabbits and guinea pig.

Antigens

For most clinical purposes, it is sufficient to determine whether a subject is Rhesus positive or Rhesus negative. This division is made by testing the RBCs with the commonest type of Rhesus antibody, anti D. (In transfusion centres, ideally the R.B.Cs of Rhesus negative donors are further tested for presence of C & E antigens).

Inheritence

Like the ABO blood group system, the final antigens seem to be influenced by at least 2 pairs of gene complexes which are inherited independently. One pair is the CDE complex & the other is LW complex (discovered by Landsterner & Wiener).

Antibodies

According to Fisher's classification 7 different antigens are described. Antibodies against all the Rhesus antigens except 'd'

have been described eg. anti-D, anti-C & anti-E etc. D-negative individuals are relatively easily stimulated to form immune anti-D antibodies.

Antigens and Antibodies Other than D

In addition to the D antigen, which distinguishes Rh positive and Rh negative persons, there are other antigens in the Rh system. The major ones are C, c, E and e. Antibodies may be produced to any of these antigens by the person whose red cells lack them. As with anti-D, the antibodies to the other Rh antigens may cause transfusion reactions and hemolytic disease of the newborn. Although Rh antibodies other than anti-D are usually a response to red cells, they have been reported occasionally in patients who have had neither transfusions not pregnancies. Anti-C, anti-c, anti-E and anti-e are available as reagents to test red cells for the corresponding antigens.

Effects of Rh Antigen/Antibody Interaction *in vivo*

The presence of anti-D or any other atypical antibody in a patient's serum sets this person apart as one who must be given special care should transfusions be required. Every thing possible must be done in the laboratory to assure that a patient whose serum contains antibody is never transused with red cells which possess the corresponding antigen. Thus, tests for red cell antigens (grouping and typing) and tests for antibodies (screening and crossmatching) are vital procedures prior to transfusion. If antigen and antibody come into contact *in vivo* a transfusion reaction may result.

Transfussion Reactions

When antibody attaches to antigen on the surface of red cells *in vivo*, the red cells are no longer normal and they are labeled for destruction. Rh antibodies rarely cause lysis of the cells but they attach to the cells and sensitize them. Sensitized cells are recognized by the spleen as damaged cells which must be removed from the circulation. If a large number of cells, such as a unit of Rh positive blood, is accidentally transfused into an Rh negative patient who has anti-D, the spleen may be over-taxed. The toxic products of red cell destruction may also affect the functioning of the liver, kidneys and heart. The symptoms of a transfusion reaction experienced by the patient may be mild or the reaction may be of such severity as to cause death. Early symptoms are chills, fever, and low back pain. They may be followed by chest pain, fall in blood pressure and shock, thought to be caused by substances such as histamine released during the course of the reaction. The low back pain is indicative of renal damage. This may result from hemoglobin and other substances released when red cells are lysed.

These tragic consequences can usually be prevented by performing antibody detection tests to reveal the presence of antibody prior to transfusion. When antibody is detected in the serum of a patient it must be identified. The selected donor is then tested to confirm that the antigen corresponding to the patient's antibody is absent from his cells. The serum of the patient is crossmatched with the cells of the donor to assure that they are *compatible*.

Rh Groups and Hemolytic disease of the newborn

Hemolytic disease of the newborn (HDN) is an acquired hemolytic anemia of the newborn characterized by a severe anemia with erythroid hyperplasia, splenomegaly, and hyperbilirubinemia. It has various clinical degrees, based on the severity of the symptoms. These range from a mild anemia with little or no visible jaundice to a disease of more severe proportaions. Sometimes it can be severe enough to result in intrauterine death, with the subsequent delivery of a macerated fetus (hydrops fetalis). It has been shown that the greatest danger to the infant results from a deposition of bile pigments in the nuclei of the brain cells. This condition, known as *kernicterus* or, more recently, *bilirubin encephalophathy*, can result in permanent brain damage.

The first child is rarely if ever affected. Sometimes the second child has a very mild case and the severity then increases with each subsequent childbirth, eventually leading to hydrops.

The pathogenic mechanism operative in this syndrome is an immunologic one, the direct result of alloimmunization of pregnancy. The mother, lacking some blood group antigen, usually D of the Rh system, is immunized by fetal cells that carry the D antigen inherited from the father. The resulting alloantibodies of the IgG class cross the placental barrier and react with the fetal erythrocytes, leading to their destruction (Fig. 75)

Alloimmunization of pregnancy and hemolytic disease of the newborn are not confined to the Rh blood group system. The potential for alloimmunization of a mother can exist whenever any blood group incompatibility exists, and thus antibodies may be produced to almost any of the cell antigens or even the white cell antigens.

Not all blood group incompatible pregnanacies result in HDN. It has been estimated that within the Rh system alone, alloimmunization with subsequent harmful sequelae occurs only 5% of the time that a suitable incompatibility exists. The lack of immunization is due to several factors, one of which is the relatively weak immunogenic ability of the antigens involved. Another is that the immune response is somewhat suppressed during pregnancy because of the secretion of various natural hormones.

The observation that there was a greater incidence of Rh antibodies in the sera of mothers who were of the same ABO group as their infants than in the sera of those women who were ABO incompatible has led to the development of a unique prophylactic treatment for Rh hemolytic disease. This finding could possibly arise from rapid removal of the fetus red cells from the maternal circulation by naturally occurring alloantibodies. It was reasoned that the primary and by far the largest immunizing stimulus comes from a massive transfusion of the mother with fetal blood during the trauma of parturition. Therefore, if a mother could be passively immunized with Rh antibodies during a period shortly after delivery, the anti-Rh antibodies would act like anti-A or anti-B and help remove the fetal cells before they could exert an antigenic stimulus. Accordingly, Rh immuno globulin prepared from high titered anti-Rh sera is now administered prophylactically to all Rh_0-negative women who give birth to Rh_0-positive infants and who have no demonstrable antibodies. Since this practice was initiated there is a significantly lower incidence of anti-Rh antibodies in Rh_0-negative women at the time of their second pregnancy and the procedure is considered successful.

Although the mechanism by which this protection operates is still obscure, it is known that the procedure protects against primary immunization but is ineffectual against a secondary respone. The use of this substance has been extended to protect against immunization after transfusion of Rh_0-positive blood into an Rh_0-negative recipient. However, substantially larger doses must be given because of the relatively larger quantities of incompatible red cells involved.

Techniques of Rh Grouping

Rh. Grouping

1. Slide test
(A) 1 drop of 40% cell suspension of unknown cell + 1 drop Anti-D sera
(B) Cell suspension as in (A) + 1 drop 22% bovine alloumin (as control)
   Tilt back and forth and see for agglutination.
2. Tube test
(A) 1 drop of 5% unknown cell suspension + 1 drop Anti-D
(B) 1 drop 5% unknown cell suspension + 1 drop of 22% bovine albumin
   Centrifuge at 1000 pm for 1 minute look for agglutination both macro and microscopically.

Interpretation

1. If agglutination in (A) and no agglutination in (B) Test for Rhesus is positive
2. Agglutination in both (A) & (B) confirm again by retesting.
3. If agglutination is negative in both (A) & (B) Test for Rhesus is negative
   It should be confirmed as below.
   (i) Take 2 tubes
       (A) one drop of 5% RBC suspension of unknown cell + 1 drop Anti D
       (B) Same as in A + 1 drop of 22% bovine albumin
   (ii) Centrifuge at 1000 pm for 1 minute
   (iii) Incubate at 37°C for 15 minutes
   (iv) Fill with saline, centrifuge at 1500–2000 rpm for ½ minute Decant and repeat 3–4 times.
   (v) Add 1 drop AHG to both (A) & (B)
   (vi) Cetrifuge at 1000 pm for 1 minute
   (vii) See for agglutination.

Remarks

Ideally any blood negative for D antigen must also be tested for the presence of C & E antigens.

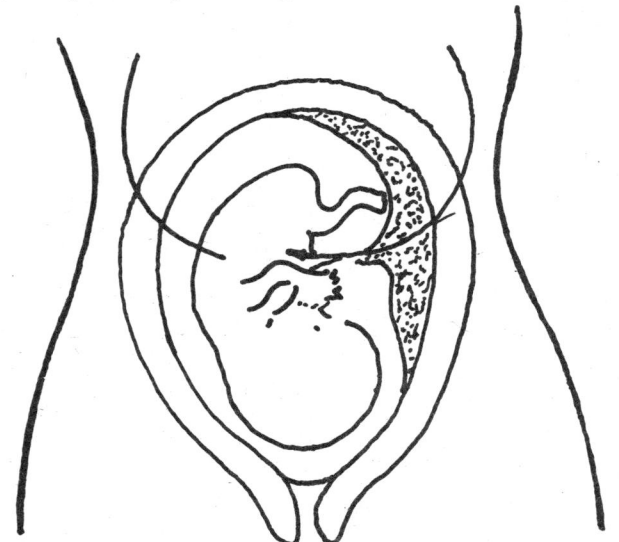

Fig. 75. Schematic representation of the pathogenic mechanism of hemolytic disease of the new born.

CHAPTER 40

SELECTION OF DONORS & COLLECTION OF BLOOD

CRITERIA FOR SELECTING DONORS

1. **Age** — 17–60 years

2. **Weight & height**
   1. For donors who are 5ft. tall. Above 45 kg (or 99 lbs.) can donate. For every inch increase in height the minimum necessary weight increses by 1 kg.
   2. Donors of and above 55 kg of any height can safely donate blood.

3. **Frequency of donation**
   Once in 3 months

4. **Hemoglobin level**
   $\geq$ 12.5 gm/dl.

5. **Blood pressure**
   Systolic:— 100–200 mm of Hg.
   Diastolic:— 50–100 mm of Hg.

6. **Pulse**
   50–100/minute

7. **Temperature**
   Normal 98–98.6°F (Afebrile)

8. **Vaccination**
   1. Those having received killed vaccines eg. cholera, Typhoid, diphtheria, influenza, tetanus, whooping cough should donate one week after vaccination.
   2. Those having received live vaccines eg. BCG, smallpox, yellow fever, rabies etc. must not donate for at least 3 wks. after vaccination.
   3. Those having received antisera such as ATS, Gas gangrene sera or Diphtheric sera should not donate for at least 4 weeks.

9. **Drug therapies**
   Avoid donation from patients receiving
   1. Anti-convulsants
   2. Anti-Coagulants
   3. Corticosteroids
   4. Hypotensives
   5. Analgesics/antipyretics
   6. Antihistaminics

10. **Medical ailments**
    1. (Severe) allergies — Permanently unfit
    2. (Severe) asthma — Permanently unfit
    3. Bronchiectasis — Permanently unfit
    4. Bronchitis — Fit after recovery
    5. Cardiovascular disorders — Permanently unfit
    6. Chickenpox — Fit 3 wks after recovery.
    7. Coronary artery disease — Refer to medical specialist for opinion
    8. Diabetics — Fit if well controlled
    9. Diphtheria — Fit 3 months after recovery
    10. Dysentry — Fit after recovery
    11. Eczema — Fit if not on drugs
    12. Embolism — Permanently unfit
    13. Emphysema — ,,
    14. Epilepsy — ,,
    15. Gout — Fit during remissions
    16. Gonorrhoea — Fit 2 months after recovery
    17. Hepatitis B — Permanently unfit
    18. Hyperthyroidism — Permanently unfit
    19. Hypothyroidism — ,,
    20. Infective hepatitis (A) — Fit 4 years after recovery
    21. Influenza — Fit after recovery
    22. Jaundice — Fit 3 months after recovery
    23. Malaria — Fit 6 months after recovery
    24. Measles — Fit 3 mths after recovery
    25. Mumps — Fit 3 wks after recovery
    26. Menstruation — Avoid during the period
    27. Pregnancy & Abortion — Fit 3 months later
    28. Polycythemia vera — Permanently unfit
    29. Psoriasis — Fit if not on drugs
    30. Syphillis — Fit if fully & properly treated
    31. Tetanus — Fit 6 months after recovery
    32. Tuberculcsis — Fit 2 yrs after recovery
    33. Typhoid — Fit 6 months after recovery

11. **Surgery**
    1. Tooth extraction — Fit after 7 days
    2. Appendicectomy — Fit after 6 wks.
    3. E.N.T. Operation — ,,
    4. Herniorrhaphy — Fit after 3 months
    5. Major operations — Fit after 6 months
    6. Gastrectomy — Permanently unfit
    7. Cancer Surgery — ,,
    8. Fractures (Major) — Fit after 6 months
    9. Minor/trivial fractures — Fit
    10. Minor Operations — Fit after 6 wks

Collection of Blood (Outline of Procedure)

Procedure for blood collection are of 2 types dependent on the presence or absence of vacuum in collecting bottles. Disposable equipment will have vacuum. Bottles prepared within blood bank will not have vacuum.

I. Tie a label on to the bottle that is going to have the blood. Write the donor's name on it, also his blood group, date of collection and date of expiry (3 wks later).

II. Ask patient to lie down on a bed. Put a towel under the arm to be bled.

III. Tie a sphygmomanometer cup around the patients upper arm, pump it up to 60 mm of Hg.

IV. Then proceed as follows.

If there is vacuum in the bottle

1. Choose a large straight vein.

2. Clean the place over the chosen vein with a swab soaked in spirit from middle outwards. Repeat the cleaning twice more with swab soaked in iodine and next with spirit.

3. Now inject Lignocaine to anesthetise locally near the proposed site of Veni-puncture.

4. Clamp the blood donor set with a forcep near the bottle and push the needle (meant for bottle) into the bottle. Next hold the needle meant for venipuncture, between your finger and thumb by the adaptor with bevel upward and push it through the skin and into vein.

5. As soon as blood is seen coming in the upper end of the tube, release the clamp.

6. Fix the needle to the patient's arm by means of sticking plaster.

7. If blood stops comming before the bottle is full, put in an air way to let the air out (probably the vacuum is not perfect).

8. Gently mix the blood and the ACD solution as the bottle fills by constant gentle shaking if shaker is not available otherwise put the bottle on mechanical shaker.

If there is no vacuum in the bottle

An air way is put into the collecting bottle before inserting the needle into the vein and there is no need to clamp the donor set as before.

Once the bottle is filled up to the measured mark, do the following

1. Clamp the tube of the blood taking set with an artery forcep to stop the flow of blood.

2. Release the pressure in the arm to 0 mm of Hg.

3. Put a piece of dry gauze piece over the needle and take it out of the donor's arm.

4. Put a cotton swab over the site of puncture and advise the donor to hold it tightly by holding the arm or by the help of other hand to stop the bleeding.

5. Take the collecting set out of the bottle and store away the bottle after collecting blood samples in two pilot tubes for test.

6. Put an adhesive tape over the site of Veni-puncture after the bleeding stops.

CHAPTER 41

THE COMPATIBILITY TEST, COOMBS TEST AND ANTI COAGULANTS

MAJOR AND MINOR CROSSMATCH

One of the most critical tests performed in the serological laboratory is the crossmatching of bloods for transfusion. If this test is improperly performed and/or interpreted, there is a risk of harming (or perhaps even killing) the patient by a transfusion incompatability. In this singular instance, the medical laboratory technologist is actually responsible for prescribing "medication" for a patient, as it is the technologist who selects the donor unit that will be transfused into the patient. Blood typing usually begins at the blood bank where agglutination tests are routinely made for antigens of the ABO and Rh blood group systems.

The technologist in the hospital where the blood will be used selects a unit of blood antigenically identical to that of the intended recipient in both the ABO and Rh systems. This requires the hospital technologist to take a sample of blood from the patient and perform direct blood-typing tests using antibody reagents of the ABO and Rh systems. A serological cross-match test is then performed, and if the donor and recipient bloods are found to be compatible, the technician releases the unit to the nurse or physician for transfusion. A compatibility test, when correctly performed and interpreted, should offer confirmation of the ABO groupings and detect the presence of atypical antibodies that could immediately react with cells of either the donor or the recipient. Some serological tests require heating of the serum to inactivate complement. This is never done for compatibility tests, however, because some antibodies may be tested only by their lytic activity in the presence of active complement (complement is destroyed by heating). Complement-mediated immune lysis also requires the presence of calcium and magnesium ions. Most anticoagulants used in blood banking function in the prevention of clotting by binding calcium (also required for coagulation). Therefore. anticoagulated specimens should not be used for crossmatching; serum is preferred.

A compatibility test actually consists of two parts. The major crossmatch involves mixing donor's cells with recipient's serum. It is designed to detect antibodies in the recipients's serum that could react with red cell antigens of the prospective donor. The minor crossmatch involves mixing recipient's cells with donor's serum for the reciprocal purpose. The major test is considered more important because of the possible destruction of the donor's cells by complement-mediated immune lysis. Furthermore, globulin-coated (opsonized) cells are usually recognized as foreign material by the reticuloendothelial system and may also be destroyed by this mechanism. Ruptured red blood cells release haemoglobin. Free haemoglobin is converted enzymatically into bilirubin and other products normally excreted as bile pigments. However, when massive red cell destruction occurs (as in an incompatible transfusion) excessive bile pigments may accumulate in the blood and produce a yellowish tinge in the skin known as jaundice. Bile pigments may be toxic in high concentration and result in lower nephron nephritis and, in severe cases, death. These phenomena are important parts of the **haemolytic transfusion reaction.** Agglutination is rarely a problem *in vivo* because of the destruction of incompatible donor cells. The major compatibility test is critical for the welfare of the patient. The minor test is usually considered less important because of the large dilution of donor antibodies that occurs when a unit of blood is transfused into an adult (approximately 5 liters of total blood is in a normal adult). However, if the donor antibodies are in high titer, even this large dilution factor may be insufficient to prevent widespread erythrocyte destruction. Thus, the minor test should not be considered trivial for the well-being of the patient.

There is considerable variation in the optimal conditions for reactivity of different blood group antibodies. In order to detect any of three major types of antibodies (saline, albumin, and AHG-reacting), the compatibility test should be performed in three phases.

1. The room temperature phase requires two tubes labeled I and II. Both tubes receive two drops of serum and two drops of an approximate 5 percent red blood cell suspension in their own serum or saline. In addition, tube I receives 22 percent bovine serum albumin (BSA) to enhance the reactivity of certain 7S antibodies. The tubes are spun immediately in a centrifuge and examined macroscopically (by naked eye) for agglutination and/or haemolysis. Saline agglutinins may be detected in either tube; albumin antibodies may be detected in tube I. If no reaction is seen in either tube, they should be shaken and tested in phase 2.

2. The warm (thermo) phase is designed to detect antibodies that react optimally at 37°C (normal human body temperature). Both tubes from phase I are incubated (either in a dry heating block or in a water bath) at 37°C for at least fifteen minutes, centrifuged, and examined macroscopically for agglutination and/or hemolysis. If there is still no reactivity, tube I should be tested in phase 3.

3. The Coombs phase (or antihuman globulin phase) should detect almost any blood group antibody that failed to react in phases 1 or 2. Tube I (containing BSA† from the thermo phase) should be shaken and then thoroughly washed by filling with physiological saline solution, mixing thoroughly, and centrifuging until all cells are at the bottom of the tube. Decant the wash saline disperse the cells by shaking, refill with fresh saline and repeat

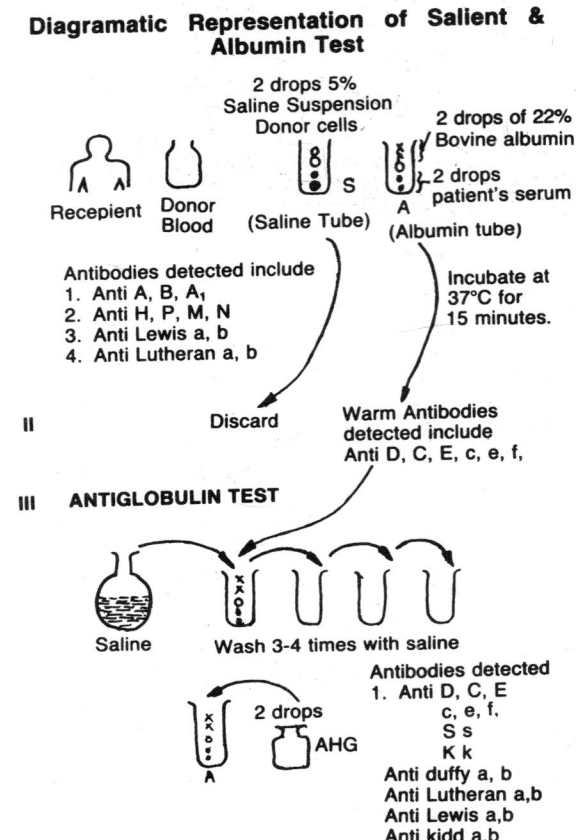

Diagramatic Representation of Salient & Albumin Test

2 drops 5%
Saline Suspension
Donor cells

2 drops of 22%
Bovine albumin

2 drops
patient's serum

Recepient Donor
Blood

(Saline Tube)   (Albumin tube)

Antibodies detected include
1. Anti A, B, A₁
2. Anti H, P, M, N
3. Anti Lewis a, b
4. Anti Lutheran a, b

Incubate at
37°C for
15 minutes.

II   Discard

Warm Antibodies
detected include
Anti D, C, E, c, e, f,

III **ANTIGLOBULIN TEST**

Saline   Wash 3-4 times with saline

Antibodies detected
1. Anti D, C, E
   c, e, f,
   S s
   K k
Anti duffy a, b
Anti Lutheran a,b
Anti Lewis a,b
Anti kidd a,b

2 drops
AHG

Diagramatic Representation of Saline & Albumin Test.

the wash cycle at least two more times (total washes three or four). Washing the cells thoroughly is extremely important to remove all unreacted globulins (antibodies). If any free globulins remain after the wash cycles, they may inactivate the Coombs reagent and result in a false negative reading. This inactivation involves a blocking antibody phenomenon. Soluble globulins can occupy the combining sites on the AHG reagent so that it fails to combine with globulins attached to the red blood cells. After the last wash solution is decanted, the remaining drop of cells is shaken, AHG is added, and the tube is centifuged and read both macroscopically and microscopically. If there is still no reactivity observed one final control must be made. Coombs control cells (also called Coombs check cells and a variety of other names) should be added to the tube, mixed, centrifuged, and read macroscopically. A truly negative compatibility test should leave the AHG reagent free to react with the globulin-coated 5 percent saline suspension of washed **Coombs control cells. Thus, agglutination of the control cells** confirms the fact that AHG was added to the test and that the washing of the cells was adequate.

In the performance of a compatibility test, four tubes will actually be needed—two for the major test and two for the minor test. No unit of blood should be transfused into a patient unless it has passed the compatibility test, i.e., without reacting in any of the three phases on either the major or minor sides. A negative-reacting pair of donor-recipient bloods in a compatibility test verifies that the ABO grouping was done correctly and ensures that the patient will not suffer an immediate transfusion reaction. The trasfused blood should survive for several weeks in the recipient. However, it should be realized that even though a donor and recipient have been determined to be compatible by this test the donor's blood may stimulate the patient to make antibodies against any foreign blood group antigens other than (Rh₀(D) factor and those of the ABO system.

Coombs Test

It is a test using an antiglobulin serum to detect the antibody coating the surface of Red Cells. For the principle of coomb's test refer to the chapter on crossmatching.

Indications

1. **Direct Coombs Test**
1. To detect whether Red cells have adsorbed the antibody in vivo. Such as in suspected cases of hemolytic disease of newborn.
2. To differentiate between acquired & congenital hemolytic anemias. In acquired it is positive while being negative in latter.
3. To detect incompatible transfusions. Cells of immediate post incompatible transfusions give positive results.

2. **Indirect coombs test**
1. To detect incomplete antibodies during pregnancy

2. To detect transfusions incompatibilities by Coombs compatibility test.
3. Antibody identifications.
4. To detect D u antigens (incomplete D antigen).
5. To detect some rare groups using certain antisera i.e. Anti Fya, Anti JKa, which work alongwith Coombs reagent.

Procedure

Direct Coombs Test

(A) Preparation of Cells for Testing:
1. Prepare 30–50% saline cells suspension.
2. Place 4 drops of the above suspensions in a test tube.
3. Fill with saline.
4. Centrifuge at 1000 rpm for 1 minute.
5. Decant completely
6. Repeat the washing 3–4 times.
7. Reconstitute to make 50% cell suspensions.

(B) Preparation of coombs reagent:
Dilute the A.H.G. serum as directed by the respective manufacturers.

(C) Preparation of Controls

Positive	Negative
1. Put 4 drops of known weak Anti-D sera in a test tube and add 2 drops of 30–50% susp. of known washed O Rh + Ve cells.	1. 4 drops of 30–50% suspension of non-sensitized human red cells, is washed 3 times & reconstitute to make 50% saline suspension.
2. Incubate at 37°C for 15 minutes	
3. Wash 3–4 times	
4. Reconstitute to make 50% saline suspension.	

(D) Test
1. Place 1 drop of 50% cell susp in tube 1, 1 drop of positive control in tube 2 & 1 drop of negative control in tube 3.
2. Add 1 drop of AHG sera to the 3 tubes.
3. Centrifuge for 1 minutes at 1000 rpm.
4. Read for agglutination.

Indirect Coomb's test
1. Put 5 drops of serum to be tested in a test tube. Also set up positive and negative controls.
2. Add 2 drops of washed O + ve saline cell suspension (50%) to the tube.

3. Mix properly by centrifuging.
4. Incubate at 37°C for 1½ hrs.
5. See for agglutination — If positive, presence of complete antibody.
6. Wash cells 3 times and reconstitute to make 50% susp.
7. Add 1 drop of AHG to all the 3 tubes as direct coombs test.
8. Centrifuge at 1000 rpm for 15 mins.
9. Read for agglutination.

Anticoagulants available:—

I. ACID CITRATE DEXTROSE (ACD) NIH formula A
Contains

citric acid	7.3 gm	per liter of soln
Na citrate	22.0 gm	(used as 15 ml/100 ml
Glucose	24.5 gm	of blood)

II. ACID CITRATE DEXTROSE (ACD) NIH formula B
Somewhat hypotonic

Citric acid	4.4 gm	per liter of soln
Na citrate	13.2 gm	(used as 25 ml/100 ml
Glucose	14.7 gm	of blood)

III. CITRATE PHOSPHATE DEXTROSE (CPD)

Citric acid	3.2 gm	per liter of soln
Na citrate	25.0 gm	(used as 14 ml/100 ml
Glucose	25.0 gm	of blood)
$NaH_2PO_4H_2O$	2.18 gm	

IV. CPD WITH ADENINE
Advantages of CPD
1. Better initial survival
2. Longer R.B.C. preservation
3. Net loss of intracellular K^+ is less
4. Blood is most alkaline. This results in better 2, 3 DPG preservation.

V. HEPARIN
Six ml of a heparin soln containing 75,000 units of heparin sodium/l of NaCl must be used for every 100 ml of blood.

DISADVANTAGES
1. Since anticoagulant lacks glucose, red cell ATP stores are rapidly depleted.
2. Heparinized blood must be utilised within 48 hrs because its effect is neutralized by anti heparin & thromboplastic materials released from cellular elements of blood.

Methods of preserving RBC, ATP
1. Addition of adenine at the beginning of storage.
2. Addition of inosine even after several wks of storage immediately boosts 2, 3 DPG & ATP levels (However inosine may cause dangerous hyperurecemia).

CHAPTER 42

BLOOD COMPONENTS

Blood can be fractionated into different components, such as Red cell, plasma, platelet, Granuloyte, Factor VIII, etc and the particular component as required by the patient can be transfused. Thus one unit of blood can be utilised for more than one patient. When the blood is drawn to the bottle/plastic bag containing anticoagulant and stored at 4°C, chemical and cellular changes occur which collectively are termed the "storage lesion", The pH decreases, 2, 3—DPG levels decline and the amounts of potassium, ammonia, and free acid increase in the plasma. Other changes occur which involve the procoagulants. After one-day storage, the granulocytes and platelets are no longer viable. Factors V as VIII are relatively unstable. Under the usual conditions of storage of whole blood, Factor V and Factor VIII have decreased to about 50% of their original activity by the end of 1–2 weeks. In view of this the components must be separated while the blood is quite fresh in order to retain maximal activity.

(1) PACKED CELL VOLUME & (2) PLASMA

Preparation: The blood collected in bottle/plastic bag is centrifuged or kept undisturbed overnight for sedimentation and thus the packed cell and plasma are separated by transfering the liquid portion (plasma) to second bottle/second bag (double bag) since the packed cell has the same cell mass as does whole blood, it provides the same oxygen-carrying capacity in smaller volume. This decrease in volume will minimise the possibility of circulatory overload and cardiovascular failure. The removal of plasma decreases the amount of Anti A and Anti B normally present in the blood of the individuals lacking the corresponding antigen. This is particularly of value when it is necessary to use group 'O' blood for recipients that are other than group 'O'.

(3) GRANULOCYTES:

Collection:— 3 techniques are available.
(a) CFC — Continuous flow centrifugation
(b) IFC — Intermittent flow centrifugation
(c) CFF — Continuous flow filteration

They allow processing of blood at 30–40 ml per minute with recovery of 25% of normal donor garnulocytes.

(4) FROZEN RED BLOOD CELL

An appropriate amount of Cryo-protective agent such as glycerol solution is added to red blood cells collected and stored at Ultra-low temperatures for long period of time. Prior to transfusion they are thawed and the glycerol is removed by a washing technique.

(5) PLATELETS

Preparation:—
TECHNIQUES: Platelets may be transfused as Platelet rich plasma (PRP).
Two methods of preparation of platelet concentrates.

1. Blood is collected in triple or quadruple pack units, centrifuge within 1 hr at 1000 rpm for 9 mins. Separate supernatant PRP. PRP is further processed to yield platelet concentrates (by centrifugation at 3000 rpm for 20 mins).
2. Plateletpheresis

STORAGE

Store at a PH of > 6.0 (about 6.5). Platelets are stored at room temperature (22°C)

They can be preserved in the frozen state with the help of cryoprotective agents (glycerol, DMSO — dimethyl sulfoxide, dimethyl/ethylacetemide & HO ethyl starch).

(6) CRYOPRECIPITATE: It is prepared by thawing a unit of fresh frozen plasma at 4°C and then recovering the cold-precipitated Factor VIII protein by Centrifugation. Each bag cryoprecipitate has about 30–50% of the Factor VIII activity of the original volume.

(7) FIBRINOGEN: It is available as a relatively pure coagulation factor which has been removed from pooled plasma by chemical fractionation.

CHAPTER 43

AIDS AND LABORATORY SAFETY

HIV infection is a relatively new disease which has reached a pandemic proportion. Over 10 million adults from 163 countries are estimated to be infected. There is a potential risk of transmission of the infection to health care workers unless they are extremely careful in observing the biosafety precautions.

Human Immunodeficiency Virus (HIV) infection was first recognized in 1981 in USA, and since then it has reached pandemic proportion in a span of barely a decade. There are an estimated 4,00,000 to 10,00,000 HIV infected cases in India. Till the discovery of an effective vaccine or a reliable curative treatment, prevention seems to be the only effective strategy to limit the spread of HIV infection. HIV is transmitted by the following routes :

(i) Sexual contact with an infected person homosexual and heterosexual.

(ii) Through use of nonsterile needles, syringes and other invasive instruments.

(iii) Through infected blood and blood products.

(iv) From infected mother to child in uterus.

Although the virus has been detected in practically all the body fluids only blood, semen, vaginal and cervical secretions have been implicated in the transmission so far.

Health Care Workers (HCW) are defined as persons (including students and trainees) whose activities involve contact with blood and other body fluids from hospitals, dispensaries, clinics or laboratories.

Recommendations for pathology laboratories

1. Avoid contact with skin and mucous membrane of blood or body secretions; use double gloves; wear goggles, mask and disposable water-proof gown; cover hair; minimize aerosolization of borne dust by using a vacuum attachment; prevent any abrasion or cut.

2. Decontaminate instruments containers, tissues and work area, decontaminate before discarding body fluids of contaminated water to sewage system.

3. Identify and limit potential risk for others: Affix warning labels, do not distribute organs for transplantation or to random researchers; put cadavers in impervious bags.

4. Limit access. Avoid pregnant, immunosuppressed or workers with abrasion/wounds, no other persons to be allowed in the laboratory.

A. General measures for HCW handling infected material/ work area/laboratory

(i) Entry should be restricted to the trained personnel only.

(ii) The laboratory door should be closed and have a 'Biohazard No Admittance' sign.

(iii) The laboratory should be clean, neat and free from extraneous materials and equipment.

(iv) Work surfaces should be disinfected with 0.1% hypochorite solutions at the end of each working day.

(v) Facilities for frequent handwashing should be available.

(vi) Eating, drinking, smoking and storing food should be prohibited.

(vii) The working staff should wear laboratory coats.

B. Hand washing

(i) Hand washing should be done before and after any patient care activity, with soap and water.

(ii) Before any invasive procedure, an antiseptic e.g. Povidone-iodine should be used for washing.

C. Protective attire

(i) Gloves.

(a) Gloves should be worn for all handling of infecticus material.

(b) Sterile surgical gloves of vinyl or latex or general purpose utility plastic gloves can be worn.

(c) Gloves should be worn for single use or those for re-use should be disinfected by rinsing the gloved hands in a hypochlorite solution followed by a rinse in soap and water.

(d) Gloves should be discarded if they are peeled, cracked or torn.

(e) Hands should be washed after removing the gloves.

(f) If gloves are not available in emergencies, another barrier e.g. a towel or a gauze soaked in sodium hypochlorite solution should be used to prevent direct contact with blood or body secretions.

(ii) Gowns

(a) Gowns should be disposable or worn with a plastic sheet beneath.

(b) Gowns should be used while conducting vaginal or cesarean deliveries, autopsies and cardiopulmonary resuscitation.

(iii) Masks
   (a) These are required when contact with oral mucous membrane is anticipated.
   (b) Masks should be used while suctioning, manipulating respiratory equipment or intubating. It should also be worn by endoscopists and dentists.
(iv) Eye goggles/glasses
   (a) They can either be disposable or re-sterilisable.
   (b) They should be used when blood or body fluid splatters to the eye are anticipated.

D. Precautions with needles and syringes

(a) Sharp instruments including needles, syringes, scalpels. IV tubing with attached needles, butterflies, angiocaths and blood tubes should be handled with extraordinary care.
(b) Wherever possible disposable instruments should be used.
(c) Reusable syringes should be decontaminated before re-processing.
(d) Needles should not be recapped, bent, broken, detached from syringes or manipulated with hand.
(e) Used instruments should be discarded puncture-proof containers sufficiently filled with hypochlorite solution by the HCW himself.

STERILIZATION AND DISINFECTION

Heat is the most effective method for inactivating HIV, thus autoclaving or boiling are the methods of choice. Chemical disinfectants are less reliable but useful in general laboratory decontamination. It is mandatory that all reusable instruments and equipments should be disinfected and cleaned thoroughly before they are preprocessed.

(i) Steam sterilization (Autoclaving) is the method of choice for reusable equipments, including needles and syringes. It is kept in operation for at least 20 minutes after a temperature of 121°C is reached.
(ii) Dry heat sterilization : Sterilization by dry heat is appropriate for instruments and equipments that can withstand a temperature of 170°C. Sterilization is accomplished at 160°C for a minimum of one hour.
(iii) Boiling : When an autoclave is not available, the simplest and most reliable method of inactivating most pathogenic microbes and HIV is by boiling. A high level of disinfection of instruments is achieved by continuous boiling for 20-30 minutes.

PRECAUTIONS TO BE OBSERVED BY THE HCW IN DIFFERENT SITUATIONS.

1. Invasive procedures

These include any surgical entry into tissues, cavities, organs or repair of traumatic injuries e.g. drawing of blood, injections, cardiac catheterization and angiographic procedures, vaginal and cesarean deliveries, and procedures in dentistry.

(a) Hands should be inspected for cuts, scratches or other breaks in skin.
(b) Gloves should be worn, if blood gets on gloves, these should be discarded.
(c) Laboratory gowns should be worn.
(d) Used syringes and needles should be kept in puncture-resistant containers.
(e) Specimen containers should be secured and the exterior should be wiped with a disinfectant.
(f) The hands should be washed with soap and water after removing the gloves.
(g) In the event of needlestick or other skin punctures, the wound should be washed with soap and water and bleeding should be encouraged.

2. Blood and body fluid spills

(a) All spills of blood and body fluid should be considered potentially infectious and should be immediately attended to.
(b) Gloves should be worn while handling spills.
(c) The spills should be covered with absorbent material (thick blotting paper).
(d) A disinfectant-hypochlorite solution with 1% available chorine or 3% hydrogen peroxide or 95% ethylalcohol, isopropyl alcohol or 3% lysol - should be poured around the spill area and kept for ten minutes.
(e) The spill area should be cleaned up with an absorbent material which should be disposed of along with contaminated wastes.
(f) The surface should be again wiped with the disinfectant.
(g) When the blood or body fluid spills occur on clothing, the article of clothing should be removed and laundered separately after decontamination.
(h) Needlestick and puncture wounds contaminated by spills should be washed with soap and water.
(i) The spills should be reported to the officer in charge of the laboratory/ward.

3. Resuscitation

(a) The need for emergency mouth-to-mouth resuscitation should be minimized and resuscitation bags or other ventilation devices should be used.
(b) Ambu bags should be regularly changed and sterilized twice a week.

4. Laboratory services

(a) Mouth pipetting should be avoided. Suitable mechanical devices for pipetting should be used.
(b) Laboratory coats should be worn by all personnel.
(c) Biological safety cabinet Class-II should be used for procedures that generate acrosol.
(d) Safety glasses, face sheilds or other protective devices should be worn during serological testing of infected material.

(e) Tissue or serum specimens should be stored after labelling as 'Potentially infectious'.

(f) Laboratory work surface should be cleaned with a disinfectant.

(g) Gloves should be worn to avoid contact with blood or other body fluids.

(h) The laboratory room doors should be closed.

(i) Public access to the laboratory should be restricted.

(j) An autoclave for decontamination of infectious laboratory material and wastes should be available nearby.

(k) Facilities for hand washing should be available.

5. Handling deceased persons

(a) Double gloves should be worn along with gown, mask and glasses.

(b) The body should be wrapped in polythene sheeting and placed in a tubular polythene bags and sealed at both ends.

(c) The words "Infectious Disease, Handle With Care" should be written on the covering before sending thebody for autopsy or to mortuary.

6. Autopsy

(a) Patients with HIV infection should be identified with appropriate tagging.

(b) Protective eye wear, mask cap, gown, foot coverings, waterproof apron and double gloves should be worn.

(c) Preferably a handsaw should be used on bone to minimize aerosol formation.

(d) After the autopsy, the table, instruments and equipment should be disinfected with 1 : 10 bleach.

(e) All the organs should be fixed in 100% buffered formalin before despatch.

(f) After the autopsy, the closed body should be washed with a detergent solution, then with dilute sodium hypochorite and rinsed with water. The body should be wrapped in a heavy plastic sheet.

7. Embalming

(a) All the universal precautions should be taken.

(b) Material to be disposed of e.g. body fluids, faeces, etc. should be decontaminated with 0.5% sodium hypochlorite.

8. Transport of specimens

(a) Transfer of blood, sera and other specimens have potential threat of spread of IHV infection.

(b) The specimen container should be labelled as "Infectious".

(c) Contamination outside the container should be washed off with a disinfectant.

(d) Specimen container should be placed in a secondary container either metal or plastic, during transportation.

9. Cleaning of instruments

(a) Instruments should be washed with soap, with water, wearing gloves.

(b) All equipment that can withstand heat should be autoclaved.

(c) Thermometers should be scrubbed with soap and water after use. They should then be disinfected with absolute alcohol, 2% glutaraldehyde or other disinfectant.

(d) Bronchoscopes, gastroscopes and other lensed equipment should be sterilized with ethylene oxide or 2% glutaraldehyde for 45 minutes. They should then be rinsed with water.

10. Linen and laundry

(a) Soiled linens of all patients should be placed in an impervious laundry bag which is not water soluble. This should be labelled as biohazard waste.

(b) Gloves and masks should be worn while handling such linen.

(c) Bleach or lysol should be added while laundering after the linen is washed with detergent in hot water (71°C).

11. Infective waste disposal

Infective wastes include needles, syringes, instruments, containers, laboratory wastes, culture stocks of infective agents tissues, body parts and infected human fetuses.

(a) They should be collected and stored separately in containers, preferably closed.

(b) Hospital wastes should be burnt in the incinerator.

(c) Blood and body fluids should be safely flushed down a toilet or drain connected to a sanitary sewer.

12. Laboratory research involving animal subjects

(a) Animal cages should be decontaminated by autoclaving before they are cleaned and washed.

(b) Laboratory coats, gowns or uniforms should be worn by personnel entering the rooms.

(c) All activities should be done after wearing gloves.

(d) Necropsy of animals should be done after wearing gloves and gowns and attempts should be made to decrease aerosolization.

Precautions for HCW under special conditions

(a) HCW with open skin lesions:
   (i) The skin lesions should be covered with waterproof dressings.
   (ii) Double gloves should be worn.
   (iii) Those with weeping skin lesions should refrain from direct patient care and handling patient equipment.

(b) Pregnant HCW.

Prevention of AIDS

1. Universal precautions to be taken in operation theatre, dentistry, autopsy, dialysis, and so on.
2. Avoid contact with blood/body secretions of AIDS and pre-AIDS.
3. Environmental considerations for sterilization and disinfection of contaminated reusable items and polluted work surfaces. Any spill of blood/body fluid should be carefully cleaned.
4. Satisfactory house keeping while handling/transporting bags containing AIDS-related materials. Education courses should be given to members of housekeeping department.
5. Precaution to be observed in pathological laboratories; use disposable and impervious caps, goggles, gowns etc.
6. Proper labeling (Precaution-AIDS/KS) of all AIDS-related materials, which should be placed in special plastic bags with zip.
7. Careful disposal of infected waste and disposable items after proper disinfection; avoid any accidental reuse.
8. In indoors, isolate the patient in a single room but give him/her adequate moral courage.
9. Control of blood and blood-product is essential; donors should accordingly be screened; discourage unauthorised blood banks.
10. Avoid non-essential use of blood/blood products.
11. Plasma processing also requires certain prerequisites including reduction of number of donors contributing to a certain product; use specified donor material for a certain patient to prevent multiple donors exposures to him.
12. Precautions for health care personnel including those who have had exposures or have developed the disease.
13. Survillance of high-risk groups at fairly regular intervals.
14. HTLV-III testing for high-risk population, exposures, blood donors and suspected AIDS patient; and instructing them to observe precautions should they be positive for it.
15. Keep random researchers with inadequate facilities at bay.
16. Mass health education of the populations by the media such as newspapers, radio and television, highlighting means of prevention under different headings, like :
    — Avoid sex outside marriage.
    — Avoid numerous sex partners.
    — Avoid homosexual practices.
    — Avoid drug abuse, and so on.

THE ROLE OF SEROLOGIC TESTING

The serologic test for HIV antibody is potentially an important tool for prevention.

Infected persons

If all infected (antibody-positive) individuals could be identified through voluntary and confidential testing programs and if these individuals could be counseled on ways to prevent exposure to others, then a major step toward decreasing AIDS could be achieved. Infected men and women could be advised of their risk to sexual partners or those exposed to their blood. Infected women could be advised to avoid pregnancy.

Susceptible persons

If uninfected (antibody-negative) individuals at increased risk of infection could be identified and counseled, their risk-taking behaviour might decrease substantially.

In summary, serologic testing allows for knowledgeable clinical and preventive counseling of patients, including medical evaluation and early intervention, personal counseling regarding decreasing transmission, contact tracing/notification, and counseling to prevent perinatal transmission.

WASH AND WEAR

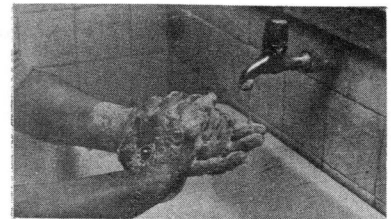

Fig. 76. Wash your hands thoroughly with soap and water.

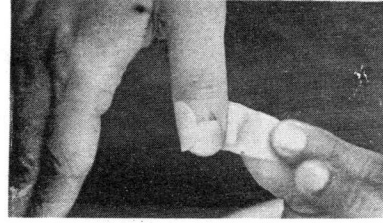

Fig. 77. Check your hands for any cuts, sores or rashes. Cover any cuts etc. with water proof adhesive plaster.

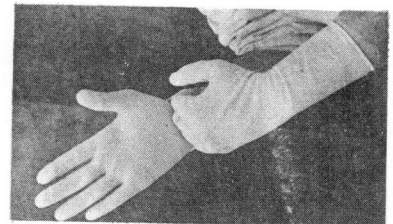

Fig. 78. Always wear gloves on both hands.

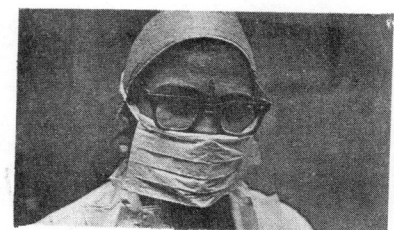

Fig. 79. Remember to wear protectives if you anticipate splashes or sprays of blood/amniotic or body fluids.

MAKE SAFETY A HABIT

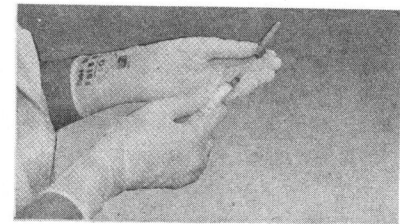

Fig. 80. Never re-cap, bend manipulate or remove needles from syringes.

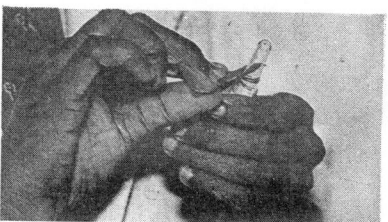

Fig. 81. Break ampoules with an opener or file. Never pipette the blood or any other body fluid by mouth. Always carry sharps, needles etc. in a kidney tray before and after use.

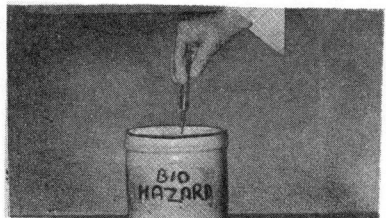

Fig. 82. Dispose sharps etc. carefully.

STERILISE PROPERLY

By using any of the following methods :

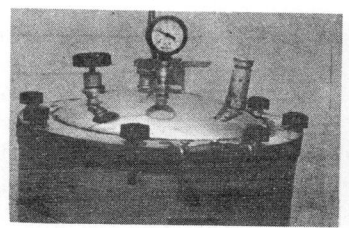
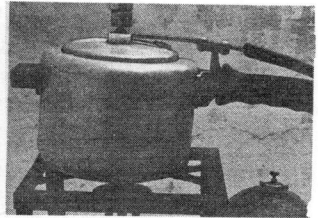

Fig. 83. Cover any spills of blood or body fluids with absorbent material like cotton etc. and pour plenty of disinfectant. Leave it as such for 20 minutes.

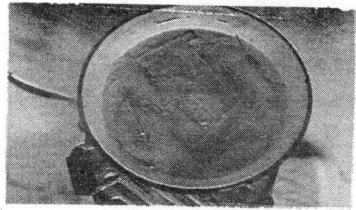

Fig. 84. Disinfect instruments, reusable syringes, needles etc. after use.

CHAPTER 44

ELISA, EIA, PCR, FCM — PRINCIPLES AND USES

A. ENZYME IMMUNO ASSAY (EIA)/ENZYME LINKED IMMUNOSORBENT ASSAY (ELISA)

Enzyme Immuno Assay is attracting a great deal of interest as a diagnostic tool and the literature on the subject is overwhelming. Enzyme Immunoassay has proved to be a power tool in many years and it has almost replaced Radio Immuno Assay RIA as the regulations on the handling of radioactive isotopes became tighter and the disposal of radioactive waste becomes more difficult.

Now a days, when almost everybody is producing monoclonal antibodies, demands on rapid, simple, specific and sensitive Immunoassays for screening of these antibodies are high.

PRINCIPLE OF ENZYME IMMUNO ASSAY (EIA)

It is an assay that depends on Ag and Ab reaction as a base and the enzyme reaction as a marker.

SEVERAL GROUPS OF EIAs

1. EIAs in which the substances to be assayed are antigens (or haptens) or antibodies.
2. EIAs in which reactions are competitive or non competitive.
3. EIAs in which the bound and free forms are separated or not separated (homogenous EIA).
4. EIAs in which the heptens used as antigen to produce the antibody are different from the haptens used for labelling with enzyme (heterologous EIA) or the same as the latter (homologous EIA).

Determination of antigens

Competitive method

(i) Solid phase method
(ii) Double antibody method
(iii) Homogenous EIA
(iv) Enzyme inhibitor Immuno assay

Non-competitive (direct) method

(i) Sandwich method
(ii) Immuno enzymometric assay

Determination of antibodies

Competitive method

(i) Solid phase

Non-competitive method

(i) Immunoenzynometric assay
(ii) Indirect enzyme linked immunosorbant assay
(iii) Enzyme antienzyme method

Enzyme immunoassays (EIA) can be subdivided into two groups :

1. *Homogeneous enzyme immunoassays* : In this kind of assay the enzyme activity is altered by the immunological reaction between enzyme-labelled antigen and antibody. These assays do not require a separation step and, therefore, are very rapid. A drawback of homogeneous enzyme immunoassays is that in general only small molecules like drugs can be measured.
2. *Heterogeneous enzyme immunoassays* : In this kind of assay the enzymatic activity is unaltered by the immunological reaction between antigen and antibody. Heterogeneous assays require a separation step to separate reacted from unreacted antigens or antibodies. Heterogeneous assays, therefore, are less rapid than homogeneous assays. However, both small and large molecules can be measured.

ELISA FOR ANTIBODY DETECTION

Generally three kinds of assays are used for detection of antibodies : competitive ELISA, indirect or sandwich ELISA and antibody class captive ELISA.

A. Competitive ELISA

In competitive ELISA, microtitre plates are coated with antigen. Enzyme-labelled antigen-specific antibodies are incubated together with the test sample in the wells of the antigen-coated microtitre plate. If the test sample contains antibodies specific for the coated antigen, the antibodies will compete with the enzyme-labelled antibodies for binding to the solid phase, resulting in a reducing absorbance value compared with a negative control. The reduction in absorbance value is a measure of the amount of antigen-specific antibodies in the test sample.

B. Indirect or sandwich ELISA

In indirect or sandwich ELISA, first described by Engvall and Perlmann (1972) and van Weemen and Schuurs (1971), antigen is passively absorbed to a solid phase.

The various steps in indirect ELISA, exemplified for detection of IgM antibodies against *Toxoplasma gondii*, are schematically shown in Fig 44.1. Patient serum, diluted 1 to 100, is added to the wells of the microtitre plate, coated with *Toxoplasma* antigen. After a 1-hour incubation at 37°C, the microtitre plate is washed three times with PBS containing 0.05% (v/v) Tween-20. *Toxoplasma*-specific IgG, IgM or IgA is subsequently detected by incubation with class-specific enzyme-labelled antisera, followed by a second washing and addition of a suitable substrate.

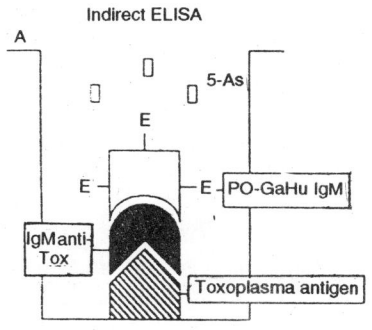

Indirect ELISA

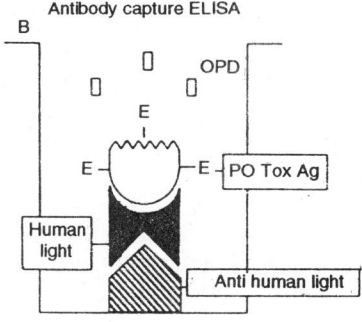

Antibody capture ELISA

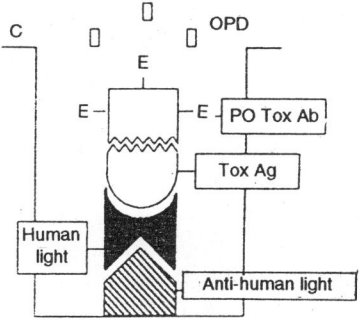

Antibody capture ELISA

Fig. 85. Characteristics of indirect ELISA (A) and antibody class capture ELISA with peroxidase-labelled Toxoplasma *antigen (B) or peroxidase-labelled anti-*Toxoplasma *serum (C).*

Indirect or sandwich ELISAs have found broad application in the serodiagnosis of infectious diseases and in clinical immunology. For most applications in infectious diseases and clinical immunology, partially purified antigens can be used for coating the solid phase.

C. Antibody class capture ELISA

In antibody class capture ELISA, affinity-purified antibodies, specific for human IgM or IgA, are coated to the solid phase. After addition of human serum, IgM or IgA will be bound at random. Antigen-specific IgM or IgA is then detected by addition of unlabelled antigen, followed by addition of an enzyme-labelled antibody specific for the antigen.

B. PCR (POLYMERASE CHAIN REACTION) TECHNOLOGY - USES AND APPLICATIONS

Mechanics of PCR

The same enzymatic process used by dividing cells in nature is applied to the PCR process to procure copies of specific segments of DNA.

In dividing cells, as the individual strands of DNA double helix separate, the enzyme DNA polymerase reads along each strand, using it as a template to synthesize a new complementary strand of DNA. The nucleotides are placed one by one along the new strand, matching adenine to thyamine and guanine to cytosine likewise in PCR, template or target DNA is added to a tube with DNA. Polymerase and deoxynucleotides, subjected to an elevated temperature that renders it singlestranded and the polymerase synthesizes a new strand of complementary DNA. The newly synthesized DNA in turn becomes the template for the next synthesis. This process repeated many times and continually producing more DNA in termed "amplification."

In theory, starting with one double stranded copy after one complete cycle of synthesis, there will be two double-stranded or four stranded copies. As these denature and are replicated there will be eight copies then sixteen, then thirty two. After 30 cycles of completely efficient reaction, potentially over a million copies of one original target sequencecould be generated for a Schedule representation of PCR amplication.

Performance of PCR is a complex process. Specific DNA sequence are amplified from among the thousands of different genes in a human sample. Specificity is accomplished by employing a pair of oligonucleotides referred as "Primers" to define the boundaries of the intended sequence. These short stretches of synthetic DNA are approximately 20 nucleotides in length. The nucleotide sequence of one premier is complementary to one of the sequences flanking the segment of target DNA and the other premier is complementary to the other flanking over the target DNA so that the denaturation by heat, when the temperature is lowered to approximately 55-65°C annealing of premiers to the template is favoured over the reassociation of the two original target strand. After the premiers have annealed and defined the section to be amplified, the DNA polymerase attaches and begins synthesis.

223

Taq DNA polymerase synthesis by Cetus Corporation is a breakthrough in the utility of PCR at DNA extreme denaturation temperature. Specific DNA replication and amplification used to take weeks and very high labor now with PCR only in hours.

Diagnostic application

PCR for human diagnostic purposes has been developed. The main areas where PCR is currently being applied.

1. Infectious diseases

When pathogens conventionally havebeen too scarce to be detected by antigen tests or difficult, impossible and dangerous to grow.

(i) HIV DNA in AIDs

(ii) CMV cytomegalovirus antibody levels

(iii) Cold agglutinin for Mycoplasma Pneumoniae

Various diseases where PCR has been successfully used in clinical laboratories :

1. Bacterial and fungal respiratory diseases.
2. Gastro intestinal diseases, bacterial, viral, protozoal.
3. Genital/STD group of diseases - syphilis, cervical cancer.
4. Cerebrospinal diseases caused by bacterial, viral, fungal and Protozoal (amoebic meningo encephalitis).
5. Sense organs - viral (deafness).
6. Systemic and other diseases - Bacterial (Lyme, Leprosy, Sepsis, Rocky mountain spotted fever), AIDS, Acute T-cell leukemias, Tropical Spastic, Paraperesis, Hepatitis, Protozoal (Sleeping sickness, chagas disease, Toxoplasmosis; malaria etc.).

2. Genetic diseases

1. PCR is currently most useful in detecting those genetic mutations for which no other test is conclusive.
2. Combination of PCR and DNA Hybridization increases discrimination, discernment between the homozygons and heterozygous (carrier) state can be resolved.
3. Prenatal testing early in gestation.
4. Haemoglobinopathies - Hbs, Hbc, thalassemias.
5. Disorders such as cystic fibrosis (autosomal Recessive Disorder).

3. Cancer diagnostics

Detection of mutation of gene associated with cancer including mutation which is expressed in RNA examination of genetic message is best examination tool, Applications :

1. Large solid tumors and blast crises in leukemias, enough material for DNA is no problem but when the patient is in remission or small biopsies, FNAC are used PCR provides distinct advantage.
2. To monitor patients in remission is distinct advantage to detect relapse before it is clinically evident.

3. Since PCR can detect one malignant cell in thousands, early detection of cancer is added advantage.
4. PCR helps in identification of atiological agent/associated viral pathogens.
   — HPV (Human Pallioma virus)
   — HTLV (I) Human T Leucocyte virus
5. PCR will add in understanding cancer pathogenesis furnishing chiesas to where the malignant process might be interrupted.

4. Transplantation

1. HLA antigens of the major histocompatibility complex (MHC) has been examined extensively specifically HLA Class II in transplant rejection and graft verses host disease.

FLOW CYTOMETRY (FCM)

FCM is a technology that allows simultaneous measurement of multiple physical characteristics of a single cell. These measurements are made on a per cell basis at rates approaching 10,000 cells per second in a moving fluid stream.

Basic principles of flow cytometry

FCM gives information about the relative size of a cell, its relative granularity and its fluorescence intensity. These characteristics are detected and recorded when the cell interacts with a focussed laser beam in the flow cell.

The advent of flow cytometry has brought new hopes for haematologic, Immunologic, neoplastic, Chr. Renal failure and AIDS patients by adding new dimensions to diagnosis/prognosis/treatment of these fatal diseases.

Summary of the basic uses FCM

— Determination of cell population heterogeniety for diagnosis of neoplasia.
— Correlated multi parametric analysis at the single cell level especially for immunophenotyping of neoplastic cell.
— Cell size and internal structure analysis especially for neoplastic cells.
— Total DNA content especially for prognosis in neoplasia.
— DNA within chromosomes for prognosis in neoplasia.
— Total RNA content in neoplastic and immunologic conditions.
— DNA composition - Research application.
— Total cell proteins for genetic disorders.
— Enzyme activities - Cell toxicity.
— Membrance potentials - Cell activity.
— Cell sorting - Cell selection under electromagnetic field.

The advent of bench top, easy to use FCM which can routinely perform five parameter analysis on thousand of cells per second coupled with the explosive increase in monoclonal antibody availability has resulted in diverse clinical applications in every discipline of Medicine.

CHAPTER 45

COMPUTERS IN THE LABORATORY

There is a tremendous explosion of the information technology in the field of Laboratory Medicine. The advances in computer technology are well utilized by other technical branches like engineering and design etc. Most doctors in India are not aware of the tremendous potential computers have in the field of patient care, medical research and education. Many instruments used in the laboratories today have a built in microprocessor to do many of the functions automatically. Hence the knowledge about computers, their use and its application in interpretive diagnosis in a laboratory is a must for every one involved in medical services.

Today, the doctor's familiarity with computers is mainly with computerized machines like CT scan etc. which is just one of the many uses of computers in medicine. Few doctors aretrying to use data base managements for patient records. There is a great need to make doctors conversant with the other applications of computers in hospital practice.

It is a general feeling that computers are associated with mathematical calculations and engineering field. As doctors have left this field long back, most are apprehensive about learning anything about computers. There is also a feeling that computers need bright young brains and one is too old to even try to understand this new field of Medical Informatics. It is true that computer programming needs a good brain and dedication and training early in life. But just as many of us are not mechanical engineers but drive the car without fear and get all the benefits of a car, without being an expert programmer or knowing any computer language proficiently, one can still learn a few basic skills and become a "trained user" and can use of computer in the field of modern medicine. There are numerous "user friendly" packages (which give precise instructions to the user at every step) in the market, which really bring the "world of Medicine to your finger tips (meaning using the computer key board)"

Computers are becoming a common sight in the laboratories now-a-days. The computers are in use at every level of the laboratory work like:

Doing the actual experiment, collecting data, processing data, interpreting the data, representing the data graphically and preparing the laboratory test reports.

The extensive laboratory technology development in the past 3 decades led to the need for interpretive diagnosis, so that the laboratory specialist could play a more active role in the patient care.

There are enough computer brains in our country and excellent expert hands who could develop indigenous computer programming tools for expert system which can be very powerful for interpretive diagnosis. The expert systems are here to stay and it will be prudent for the future pathologist to be both a laboratory expert and information specialist by being computer literate.

COMPUTER ASSISTED MEDICAL DECISION-MAKING (CADM) AND EXPERT SYSTEMS

The inability of the physician to use optimally the medical knowledge explosion of the last 20 to 30 years is evidenced by several studies, for less than 5% of the laboratory data requisitioned is actually used. Computer assisted decision making system may be a solution to this problem, as their use has actually resulted in tangible improvement in performance.

The potential benefits of the CADM systems in the laboratory are :

1. Improved speed and consistency in data interpretation.
2. Separate uninteresting from a few interesting cases.
3. Facilitate a better presentation of the latter.
4. Improve the consultative role of the laboratory.
5. Improve the teaching capability of the laboratory.
6. Improve patient care by enhancement of diagnostic capabilities of the laboratory.

However there are a few pit falls too :

1. The danger that the reasoning behind the recommendations of a CADM will not be available to the user.
2. CADM system may lend authority to shallow knowledge and prejudice.
3. In fact what used to be easy may become difficult if CADM is used for simple problems.
4. Poorly conceived commercial systems may be flooded by the industry creating problems rather than solving them.
5. There may be a temptation to retain outdated systems to cut costs, in the fast expanding world of medical science today, when they become obsolete in the developed world and sell them in the third world markets.

The medical informatics has a great potential, for the new software and hardware tools in medicine, especially in the laboratory. It is for this reason that informatics training should be made desirable for all pathology courses and training programs. Research and training in the so-called field of medical informatics be encouraged, to create computer literacy among the pathologists and the clinicians. If the clinical pathologist is in fact an "information specialist" there will be optimal and rational use of CADM systems. Many pathologists should be able to fill the role of both knowledge engineer and domain expert.

Finally, since computers and computer technology are stated to play an increasingly large role in the laboratory, we need to ensure that this technology is understood and properly applied, and that the laboratory is aware of its potential pitfalls. We must keep our expectations in line with reality and remember that machines are just tools, and can not be full substitute for sound heuristic knowledge and human experts. They should be made to work for the humans and not the other way around.

CHAPTER 46

QUALITY CONTROL IN LABORATORY MEDICINE

What is quality control

A test wrongly done is worst than a test not done. Quality control is the process to ensure a test from being done wrongly.

Aims of quality control

The primary aim of QC is to see that the very purpose for which a test is performed is not defeated due to unreliability of the result. The broad aim of QC is to fulfil the aim that results from one lab should be comparable to that from any lab in the world provided the same method is followed.

Technique of quality control

Quality control is implemented under two broad heads :

1. Internal QC (Intra-laboratory) : Performed by individual labs at their own levels. Forms the basis of day to day work quality assurance.
2. External (inter-laboratory) : Performed by many labs at the same time, monitored by one. Periodic monitoring of the lab's performance.
   Internal QC : It is implemented in two phases viz. Prospective (preventive) and Retrospective (corrective).

1. Prospective phase QC

All precautions that go into the preoperational period of any lab's working are covered in this phase. These involve planning of lab environment including layout electric installations, plumbing, waste disposal, computer terminal and scope for future expansion. The equipments require careful weighing of all aspects like cost, requirements, reputation, spares, after sales service, active life and job requirements against resources. The laboratory staff has to be selected carefully and a positive management staff relationship always pays. The workload has to be optimum, neither too much nor too little. The methods for analysis have to be selected after considering all aspects. All laboratory procedures should be documented. Lab equipment has to be preventively maintained, reagents and kits and standards have to be assured against deterioration. Desired QC material should be procured in advance.

2. Retrospective phase QC

The approach here differs in case of quantitative procedures and others.

RETROSPECTIVE QC FOR QUANTITATIVE PROCEDURES

1. Optimum condition variance (OCV)

This is the lowest variance a lab can get on a known value QC material by a defined method. For this under the best available conditions for the lab, a QC sample is analysed consecutively 20 times and results plotted. Mean and SD are also calculated. A satisfactory performance is denoted by not more than 1/20 results falling outside 2SD and an almost equal scatter on both sides of the mean.

2. Routine conditions variance known value (RCVK)

For this the same QC material as used for OCV is analysed 20 times under 'routine' conditions, with no preferential treatment. The results are plotted like in OCV and mean and SD calculated. A satisfactory performance is reflected by a SD about twice of OCV with the rest remaining the same.

3. Modified levey

Jening's graph : QC material of values not known to analyst is introduced within the daily batches of analyses and results plotted against recommended values (mean and range). It is a very helpful visual guide for day to day monitoring of performance.

4. Routine conditions variance, unknown values (RCV-D)

QC material of different levels of analytes is used. The values are unknown to the analyst. The rest is same as in RCV-K. Results are plotted as % variance (V).

$$\frac{\text{Observed value} - \text{correct value}}{\text{Correct value}} \times 100$$

and are analysed both visually and statistically.

5. Composite and long term records

Each day's performance on RCV-U can be plotted and/or fed into computer for review and future reference. Thus a monthly or yearly record become available. 2SD is taken as 'Warning limits' and 3SD as 'Action limits' for purpose of QC.

6. RETROSPECTIVE QC USING PATIENTS' MATERIAL

Under this the following methods are used :

(a) Randomised duplicate analysis using patient's specimen measures precision.

(b) Daily mean of all the cases for a particular test would be an index of accuracy.

Cumulative sum (CUSUM) : It is calculated from daily mean values and is even more sensitive index.

7. Computer aided checks

When large amount of data in quantitative tests QC becomes available, it can be put to better use through computer programmes like Delta check, absurd value check and pattern identification based upon various established norms.

ACCURACY AND PRECISION

The terms accuracy and precision are used to define the quality of an analysis. Accuracy of a test result is its closeness to the true value. Precision of a result is its reproducibility. Precision is possible without accuracy, but accuracy is not possible without a certain degree of precision.

A method is said to be repeatable if it is capable of giving one specific value again and again for a test sample when the analysis is repeated by the same technician using the same lots of reagents and the same instruments. A method is said to be reproducible if it is capable of producing the same result when the test on one sample is repeated on different days by different technicians using different sets of reagents. It is possible that a method is repeatable but not reproducible. Reproducible methods, on the other hand, are always repeatable. The requirement for precision is reproducibility and not repeatibility alone.

When the same test result is obtained on two or three repeated analyses of a sample, one might be tempted to think that the value is accurate. However, one can only say that the repeatibility of such an analysis is good, and nothing more. The value may or may not be accurate. The test result may be far from the true value. Even the precision may be poor. However, if accurate results are obtained again and again in an analysis, precision is achieved automatically.

The terms accuracy and precision may be a little confusing at first. To make things worse, these terms have been used more or less synonymously by many physicians and quite a few laboratorians. Though accuracy and precision are both desirable qualities of an analysis, they are not exactly the same.

MEAN

The average value of all results, calculated as follows :

$$\bar{x} = \Sigma x/N$$

where Σx is the sum of all the values, and N is the number of values.

STANDARD DEVIATION

A calculated value denoting the degree of dispersion of results about the mean. Assuming a "normal" distribution of data, 68.27% of the values will fall within ± 3 S.D. Standard deviation may be calculated by using the following equation:

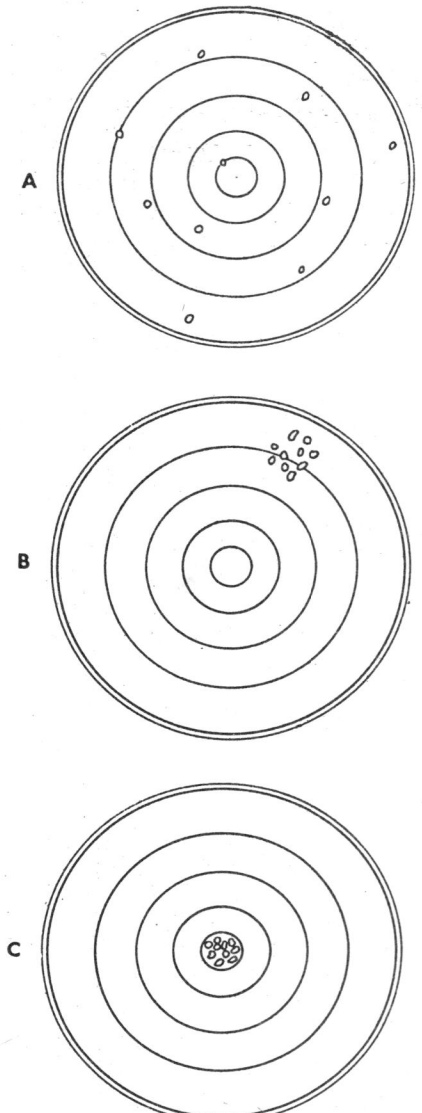

Fig. 86. Precision and accuracy of target shooting. A, shots are neither accurate nor precise. B, Shots are precise but not accurate, C, Shots are both precise and accurate.

$$S.D. = \sqrt{\frac{\Sigma(x - \bar{x})^2}{N - 1}}$$

where $(x - \bar{x})$ is the difference between the actual value and the mean value, and N represents the number of samples. Another equation that may be used and is more convenient if a calculator is available is as follows :

$$S.D. = \sqrt{\frac{N\Sigma(x^2 - (\Sigma x)^2}{N - 1}}$$

It is entirely possible to have excellent precision yet inaccurate results. This situation may be due to improper standards or reagents, even though the procedure is quite good. If, on the other hand, precision is poor, it becomes extremely difficult to obtain accurate results.

228

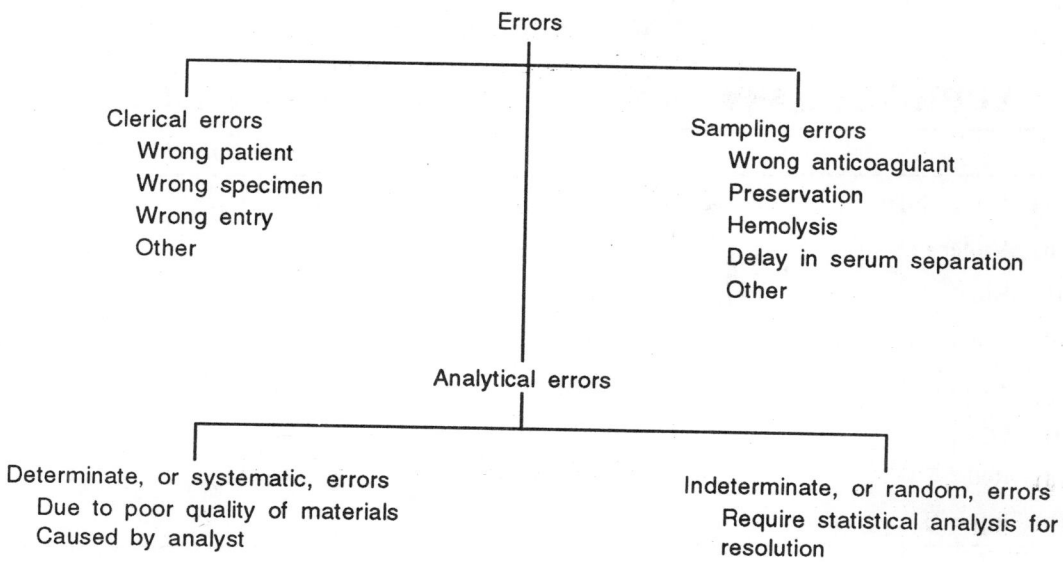

Errors

Clerical errors
    Wrong patient
    Wrong specimen
    Wrong entry
    Other

Sampling errors
    Wrong anticoagulant
    Preservation
    Hemolysis
    Delay in serum separation
    Other

Analytical errors

Determinate, or systematic, errors
    Due to poor quality of materials
    Caused by analyst

Indeterminate, or random, errors
    Require statistical analysis for
    resolution

Fig. 87. Errors in the clinical laboratory.

ANNEXURE I
APPROXIMATE WAVELENGTH OF COLOURS

			Complimentary filter
(a)	Ultra violet	< 400 mμ	—
(b)	Violet	400-450 mμ	—
(c)	Blue	450-500 mμ	Yellow or Red
(d)	Green	500-570 mμ	Red
(e)	Yellow	570-590 mμ	Blue
(f)	Orange	590-620 mμ	—
(g)	Red	620-760 mμ	Green
(h)	Infrared	> 760 mμ	—

ANNEXURE II
NOMOGRAM FOR COMPUTING RELATIVE CENTRIFUGAL FORCES

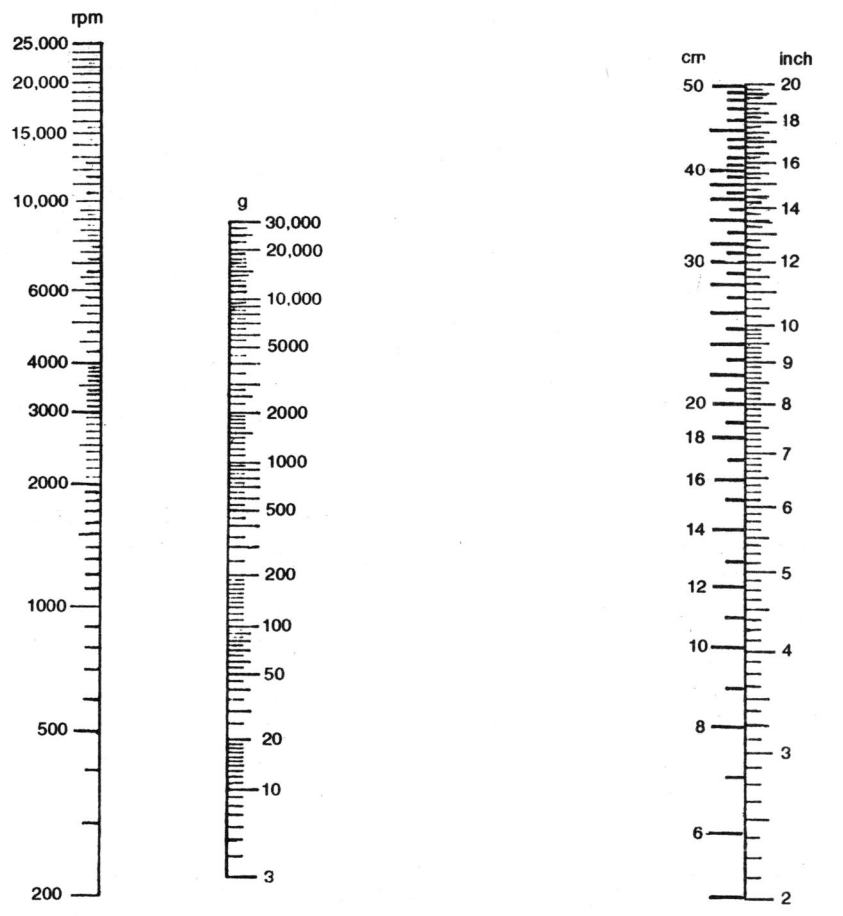

ANNEXURE III

A NOMOGRAM FOR THE MCHC

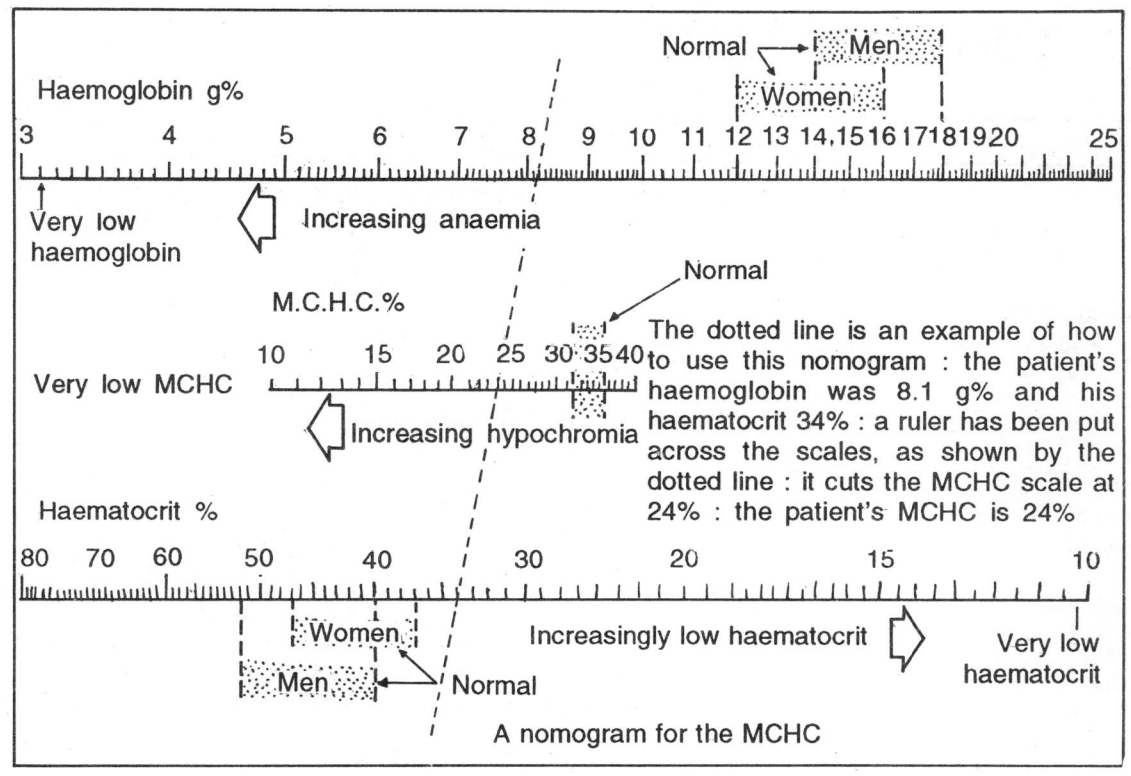

A nomogram for the MCHC

The dotted line is an example of how to use this nomogram : the patient's haemoglobin was 8.1 g% and his haematocrit 34% : a ruler has been put across the scales, as shown by the dotted line : it cuts the MCHC scale at 24% : the patient's MCHC is 24%

ANNEXURE IV

A CHART FOR THE MICROHAEMATOCRIT

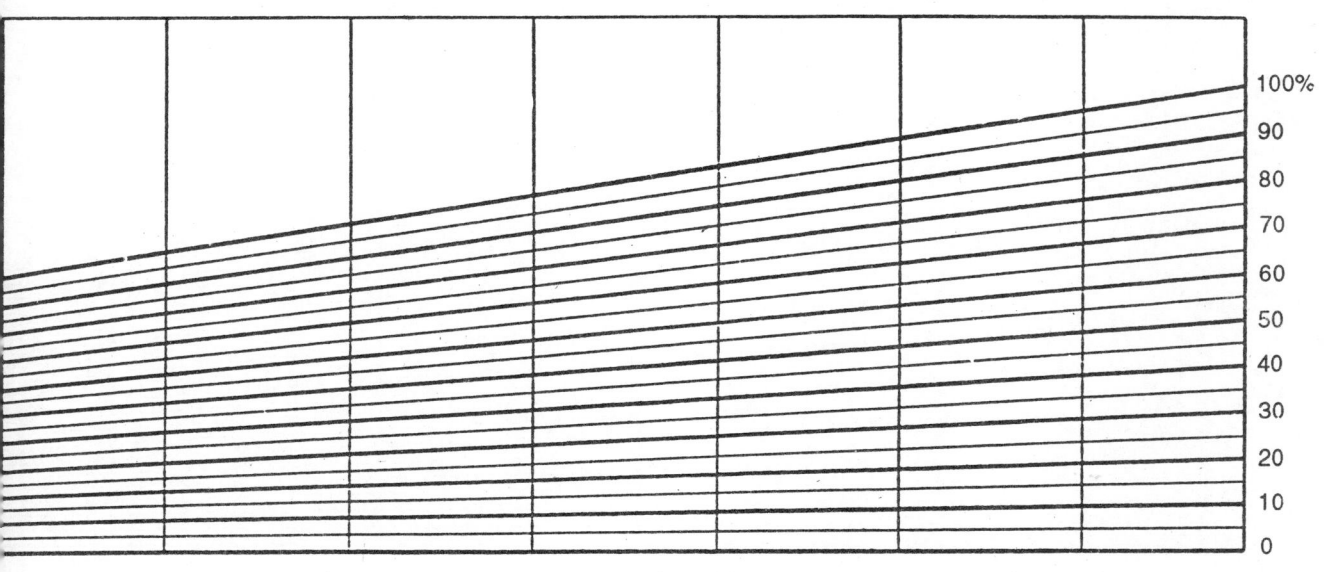

ANNEXURE V

COMMONLY USED ANTICOAGULANTS

Sl. No.	Anticoagulant	mg/ml blood	Use	Mode of action
1.	Heparin	0.2	Procedures requiring whole blood or plasma; especially useful when intact erythrocytes are desired	Inhibits conversion of prothrombin to thrombin
2.	Ethylenediamine - tetraacetic acid i.e., EDTA	1	Procedures requiring whole blood or plasma	Chelates ionic calcium
3.	Oxalates (a) Lithium (b) Sodium (c) Potassium (d) Ammonium	1-2	Procedures requiring whole blood or plasma. Causes shrinkage of cell volume, should not be used in hoematological procedures	Forms unionized calcium oxalate complex; reduces level of ionized calcium below that required for clotting
4.	Sodium citrate	5	As for oxalates	Forms unionized complex with calcium
5.	Sodium fluoride	10	Combination anticoagulant and preservative for blood glucose determination by inhibiting blood enzymes causing glycolysis; causes erythrocyte shrinkage. Combined with thymol (1 mg + 10 mg NaF) for effective control of microbial growth in stored blood samples	Forms unionized calcium fluoride complex

PREPARATION OF CERTAIN REAGENTS, ANTOCOAGULANTS PRE-SERVATIVE SOLUTIONS

Acid-citrate-dextrose (ACD) solution - 'NIH-A'

Trisodium citrate, dihydrate (75 mmol/l)	22 g
Citric acid, monohydrate (42 mmol/l)	8 g
Dextrose (139 mmol/l)	25 g
Water	to 1 litre

Sterilize the solution by autoclaving at 121°C for 15 min. Its pH is 5.4. For use, add 10 volumes of blood to 1.5 volumes of solution.

Alserver's solution

Dextrose (114 mmol/l)	20.5 g
Trisodium citrate, dihydrate (27 mmol/l)	8.0 g
Sodium chloride (72 mmol/l)	4.2 g
Water	to 1 litre

Adjust the pH to 6.1 with citric acid (c 0.5 g) and then sterilize the solution by micropore filtration (0.22 μm) or by autoclaving at 121°C for 15 min. For use, add 4 volumes of blood to 1 volume of solution.

Citrate-phosphate-dextrose (CPD) solution, pH 6.9

Trisodium citrate, dihydrate (102 mmol/l)	30 g
Sodium dihydrogen phosphate, monohydrate (1.08 mmol/l)	0.15 g
Dextrose (11 mmol/l)	2 g
Water	to 1 litre

Sterilize the solution by autoclaving at 121°C for 15 min. After cooling to c 20°C, it should have a brown tinge and its pH should be 6.9. For use in red cell survival studies add 1 volume of blood to 2 volumes of solution.

Citrate-phosphate-dextrose-adenine 9CPD-A) solution, pH 5.6-5.8

Trisodium citrate, dihydrate (89 mmol/l)	26.30 g
Citric acid, monohydrate (17 mmol/l)	3.27 g
Sodium dihydrogen phosphate, monohydrate (16 mmol/l)	2.22 g
Dextrose (177 mmol/l)	31.8 g
Adenine (2.04 mmol/l)	0.275 g
Water	to 1 litre

Sterilize the solution by autoclaving at 121°C for 15 min. For use as an anticoagulant-preservative, add 7 volumes of blood to 1 volume of solution.

Citrate-phosphate-dextrose (CPD) solution, pH 5.6-5.8

Trisodium citrate, dihydrate (89 mmol/l)	26.30 g
Citric acid, monohydrate (17 mmol/l)	3.27 g
Sodium dihydrogen phosphate, monohydrate (16 mmol/l)	2.22 g
Dextrose (142 mmol/l)	25.50 g
Water	to 1 litre

Sterilize the solution by autoclaving at 121°C for 15 min. For use as an anticoagulant-preservative, add 7 volumes of blood to 1 volume of solution.

Low ionic strength solution

Sodium chloride (NaCl) (30.8 mmol/l)	1.8 g
Disodium hydrogen phosphate (Na_2HPO_4) (1.5 mmol/l)	0.21 g
Sodium dihydrogen phosphate (NaH_2PO_4) (1.5 mmol/l)	0.18 g
Glycine (NH_2CH_2COOH) (240 mmol/l)	18.0 g
Water	to 1 litre

Dissolve the sodium chloride and the two phosphate salts in c 400 ml of water; dissolve the glycine separately in c 400 ml of waater; adjust the pH of each solution to 6.7 with 1 mol/l NaOH. Add the two solutions together and make up to 1 litre. Sterilize by Seitz filtration or autoclaving. The pH should be within the range of 6.65-6.85, the osmolality 270-285 mmol, and conductivity 3.5-3.8 mS/cm at 23°C.

Saline

Sodium chloride (NaCl) (154 mmol/l)	9.0 g
Water	to 1 litre

Trisodium citrate

($Na_3C_6H_5O_7.2H_2O$), 109 mmol/l

Dissolve 32 g in 1 litre of water. Distribute convenient volumes (e.g. 10 ml) into small bottles and sterilize by autoclaving at 121°C for 15 min.

EDTA

Ethylenediamine tetra-acetic acid, dipotassium or disodium salt	100 g
Water	to 1 litre

Allow appropriate volumes to dry in bottles at c 20°C so as to give a concentration of 1.5 ± 0.25 mg/ml of blood.

Neutral EDTA, pH 7.0, 110 mmol/l

Ethylenediamine tetra-acetic acid, dipotassium salt	44.5
or disodium salt	41.0 g
1 mmol/l NaOH	75 ml
Water	to 1 litre

Neutral buffered EDTA, pH 7.0

Ethylenediamine tetra-acetic acid, disodium salt (9 mmol/l)	3.35 g
Disodium hydrogen phosphate (Na_2HPO_4) (26.4 mmol/l)	3.75 g
Sodium chloride (NaCl) (140 mmol/l)	8.18 g
Water	to 1 litre

Heparin

Powdered heparin (lithium salt) is available with an activity of c 160 iu/mg. Dissolve it in water at a concentration of 4 mg/ml. Sodium heparin is available in 5 ml ampoules with an activity of 1000 iu/ml. Add appropriate volumes of either solution to a series of containers and allow to dry at c 20°C so as to give a concentration not exceeding 15-20 iu/ml of blood.

ANNEXURE VII

BUFFERS

(a)

Barbitone buffer, pH 7.4

Sodium diethyl barbiturate ($C_8H_{11}O_3N_2Na$) (57 mmol/l)	11.74 g
Hydrochloride acid (HCl) (100 mmol/l)	430 ml

Barbitone buffered saline, pH 7.4

NaCl	5.67 g
Barbitone buffer, pH 7.4	1 litre

Before use, dilute with an equal volume of 9 g/l NaCl.

Barbitone-buffered saline, pH 9.5

Sodium diethyl barbiturate ($C_8H_{11}O_3N_2Na$) (98 mmol/l)	20.2 g
Hydrochloric acid (HCl) (100 mmol/l)	20 ml
NaCl	5.67 g

Before use, dilute the buffer with an equal volume of 9 g/NaCl.

Barbitone-bovine serum albumin (BSA) buffer, pH 9.8

Sodium diethyl barbiturate ($C_8H_{11}O_3N_2Na$) (54 mmol/l)	10.3 g
NaCl (102 mmol/l)	6.0 g
Sodium azide (31 mmol/l)	2.0 g
Bovine serum albumin (e.g. Sigma)	5.0 g
Water	to 1 litre

Dissolve the reagents in c 900 ml of water. Adjust the pH to 9.8 with 5 mol/l HCl. Make up the volume to 1 litre with water. Store at 4°C.

(b)

Citrate-saline buffer

Trisodium citrate ($Na_3C_6H_5O_72H_2O$) (5 mmol/l)	1.5 g
NaCl (96 mmol/l)	5.6 g
Barbitone buffer, pH 7.4	200 ml
Water	800 ml

Glycine buffer, pH 3.0

Glycine (NH_2CH_2COOH) (82 mmol/l)	6.15 g
NaCl (82 mmol/l)	4.80 g
Water	820 ml
0.1 mol/l HCl	180 ml

HEPES buffer, pH 6.5

4-)2-hydroxyethyl)-1-piperazineethane sulphonic acid (100 mmol/l)	23.83 g

Dissolve in c 100 ml of water. Add a sufficient volume of 1 mol/l NaOH (c 1 ml) to adjust the pH to 6.5. If the buffer is intended for use with Romanowsky staining (p. 79), then add 25 ml of dimethyl sulphoxide (DMSO). Make up the volume to 1 litre with water.

HEPES-saline buffer, pH 7.6

HEPES (4-(2-hydroxyethyl)-1-piperazineethane sulphonic acid (20 mmol/l)	4.76 g
NaCl	8.0 g

Dissolve in c 100 ml of water. Add a sufficient volume of 1 mol/l NaOH to adjust the pH to 7.6. Make up volume to 1 litre with water.

(c)

Imidazole-buffered saline, pH 7.4

Imidazole (50 mmol/l)	3.4 g
NaCl (100 mmol/l)	5.85 g

Dissolve in c 500 ml of water. Add 18.6 ml of 1 mol/l HCl and make up the volume to 1 litre with water. Store at room temperature (18-25°C).

Phosphate buffer, iso-osmotic

(A) $NaH_2PO_4.2H_2O$ (150 mmol/l)   23.4 g/l
(B) Na_2HPO_4 (150 mmol/l)   21.3 g/l

pH	Solution A	Solution B
5.8	87 ml	13 ml
6.0	83 ml	17 ml
6.2	75 ml	25 ml
6.4	66 ml	34 ml
6.6	56 ml	44 ml
6.8	46 ml	54 ml
7.0	32 ml	68 ml
7.2	24 ml	76 ml
7.4	18 ml	82 ml
7.6	13 ml	87 ml
7.7	9.5 ml	90.5 ml

Normal human serum has an osmolality of 289 ± 4 mmol. Hendry recommended slightly different concentrations of the stock solution, namely, 25.05 g/l $NaH_2PO_4.2H_2O$ and 17.92 g/l Na_2HPO_4 for an iso-osmotic buffer.

(d)

Phosphate-buffered saline

Equal volumes of iso-osmotic phosphate buffer and 9 g/l NaCl.

Phosphate buffer, Sorensen's

66 mmol/l stock solutions :

(A) KH_2PO_4	9.1 g/l
(B) Na_2HPO_4	9.5 g/l or
$Na_2HPO_4.2H_2O$	11.9 g/l

100 mmol/l and 150 mmol/l stock solutions may be similarly prepared. To obtain a solution of the required pH, add A and B in the indicated proportions :

pH	A	B
5.4	97.0	3.0
5.6	95.0	5.0
5.8	92.8	7.8
6.0	88.0	12.0
6.2	81.0	19.0
6.4	73.0	27.0
6.6	63.0	37.0
6.8	50.8	49.2
7.0	38.9	61.1
7.2	28.0	72.0
7.4	19.2	80.8
7.6	13.0	87.0
7.8	8.5	91.5

This buffer is not iso-osmotic with normal plasma.

(e)

Tris-HCl buffer (200 mmol/l)

Tris (hydroxymethyl) aminomethane (24.33 g/l) 250 ml

To obtain a solution of the required pH add the appropriate volume of 1 mol/HCl and then make up the volume to 1 litre with water :

pH	Volume
7.2	44.5 ml
7.4	42.0 ml
7.6	39.0 ml
7.8	33.5 ml
8.0	28.0 ml
8.2	23.0 ml
8.4	17.5 ml
8.6	13.0 ml
8.8	9.0 ml
9.0	5.0 ml

100 mmol/l, 150 mmol/l, 300 mmol/l and 750 mmol/l stock solutions may be similarly prepared with an appropriate weight of tris and volume of acid.

Tris-HCl bovine serum albumin (BSA) buffer, pH 7.6, 20 mmol/l

Tris (hydroxymethyl) aminomethane (20 mmol/l)	2.42 g
EDTA, disodium salt (10 mmol/l)	3.72 g
NaCl (100 mmol/l)	5.85 g
Sodium azide (3 mmol/l)	0.2 g

Dissolve the reagents in c 800 ml of water. Adjust the pH to 7.6 with 10 mol/l HCl. Add 10 g of bovine serum albumin (e.g. Sigma) and make up to 1 litre with water.

ANNEXURE VIII

UNITS OF WEIGHT AND MEASUREMENT

Weight (unit : gram [g])

$\times\ 10^3$ kilogram (kg)

$\times\ 10^{-3}$ milligram (mg)

$\times\ 10^{-6}$ microgram (μg) (formerly γ)

$\times\ 10^{-9}$ nanogram (ng) (formerly μmg)

$\times\ 10^{-12}$ picogram (pg) (formerly $\mu\mu$g)

Length (unit : metre [m])

$\times\ 10^{-1}$ decimetre (dm)

$\times\ 10^{-2}$ centimetre (cm)

$\times\ 10^{-3}$ millimetre (mm)

$\times\ 10^{-6}$ micrometre (μm) (formerly m)

$\times\ 10^{-9}$ nanometre (nm) (formerly mm)

Volume (unit : litre [l] = dm^3)

$\times\ 10^{-1}$ decilitre (dl) (formerly 100 ml)

$\times\ 10^{-3}$ millilitre (ml) = cm^3 (formerly cc)

$\times\ 10^{-9}$ microlitre (μl) = mm^3

$\times\ 10^{-9}$ nanolitre (nl)

$\times\ 10^{-12}$ picolitre (pl) (formerly mml)

$\times\ 10^{-15}$ femtolitre (fl) = μm^3

Amount of substance (unit : mole [mol])

$\times\ 10^{-3}$ millimole (mmol)

$\times\ 10^{-6}$ micromole (mmol)

Substance concentration (unit : moles per litre [mol/l]) (formerly M)

$\times\ 10^{-3}$ millimole per litre (mmol/l)

$\times\ 10^{-6}$ micromole per litre (μmol/l)

Mass concentration (unit : gram per litre [g/l])

$\times\ 10^{-3}$ milligram per litre (mg/l)

$\times\ 10^{-6}$ microgram per litre (μg/l)

When preparing a small amount of a reagent, it is more appropriate to express its concentration per ml or dl.

ANNEXURE IX

MICROSCOPE MAGNIFICATION

Focal length (mm)	Magnification
2	$\times$ 100
4	$\times$ 40
16	$\times$ 10
40	$\times$ 4

ANNEXURE X

NORMAL REFERENCE RANGE - HAEMATOLOGY

Cell Counts

Erythrocytes

Males	4.5-6.5 million/mm³
Females	3.9-5.6 million/mm³
Children	4.5-5.1 million/mm³
(Varies with age)	

Coagulation test

Bleeding time (Template)	1-4 min
Clotting time (Lee & White)	5-8 min
Clot retraction (Macfarlane's method)	48-64%
Factor VIII and other coagulation factors	50-150% of normal
Fibrin split products (Thrombowelco)	< 10 μ mg/ml
Fibrinogen	200-400 mg/dl
Prothrombin ratio	1 : 1
Prothrombin index (Quick's one stage)	100%
Partial thromboplastin time (PTT)	20-35 sec
Prothrombin time (PT)	12.0-14.0 sec

Corpuscular values of erythrocytes

Mean Corpuscular haemoglobin (MCH)	26-34 pg
Mean Corpuscular volume (MCV)	80-96 μm³
Mean Corpuscular haemoglobin concentration (MCHC)	32-36%

Haemoglobin

Males	13.5-18.0 gms%
Females	11.5-16.5 gms%
Newborns	16.5-19.5 gms%
Children (Varies with age)	11.2-16.6 gms%
Haemoglobin foetal	1.0% of total
Haemoglobin A1c	3-5% of total
Haemoglobin A2	1.5-3.0% of total
Haemoglobin plasma	0-0.5 mg/dl
Maethemoglobin	30-130 mg/dl

Haematocrit

Males	40-54 ml/dl
Females	37-47 ml/dl
Newborns	49-54 ml/dl
Children (Varies with age)	35-49 ml/dl

Leucocytes

Total		4500-11000 mm³
Differential	Percentage	Absolute
Myelocytes	0	0/mm³
Band neutrophils	3-5	150-400/mm³
Segmented Neutrophuils	40-75%	3000-5800/mm³
Lymphocytes	20-50%	1500-3000/mm³
Monocytes	2-10%	300-500/mm³
Eosinophils	1-6%	50-250/mm³
Basophils	0-1%	15-50/mm³
Platelets		1.4-4.0 Lacs/mm³
Reticulocytes		25000-75000/mm³

ANNEXURE XI

BLOOD BIOCHEMISTRY

Albumin	3.2-5.3 gms%	Glucose PP/PL (Enzymatic)	Upto 130 mg%
Alkaline phosphatase	Upto 270 Units U/L	Inorganic phosphorus	3-4 mg%
Bilirubin (Total)	Upto 1.2 mg%	L.D.H.	Upto 240 units U/L
Calcium	9-11 mg%	Potassium	3.5-5.0 meq/L
Carbon dioxide (Total)	24-34 meq.	Proteins (Total)	6.2-7.9 gms%
Cholestrol	120-220 mg%	SGOT	Upto 40 U/L
Creatinine	1-2 mg%	SGPT	Upto 40 U/L
Gamma GT	10-50 U/L	Urea Nitrogen	5-20 mg%
Globulin		Uric acid	2-6/2-7 mg%
Glucose F (Enzymatic)	60-110 mg%		

ANNEXURE XII

NORMAL RANGE FOR SEROLOGICAL INVESTIGATIONS

ASO titre	Less than 200 IU/ml
Anti sperm antibodies (Microagglutination)	1 : 16 (Significant titre)
Anti thyroid antibody	
Antimicrosomal	Less than 1 : 100
Antihyroglobulin	Less than 1 : 100
Brucella	≥ 80 (Significant titre)
Cold agglutination test	1 : 16 (Significant titre)
Complements	
C3	71-154 IU/ml
C4	64-160 IU/ml
FDP	≥ 10 mcg/ml (Significant titre)
Immunoglobulins	
IgG	302-3218 mg%
IgM	34-430 mg%
IgA	27-350 mg%
T cell count	60-80%
B cell count	70-75%
Weli felix	≥ 80 (Significant titre)

ANNEXURE XIII

NORMAL RANGE FOR SPECIAL INVESTIGATIONS

Investigation	Normal Range	
ACTH	8 am : 10-100 pg/ml	
	4 pm : 10-80 pg/ml	
AFP	Upto 15 ng/ml	
Aldosterone	Supine position	50-194 pg/ml
	Upright position	94-338 pg/ml
	COHNS syndrome	335-940 pg/ml
Beta - HCG	For non pregnant woman & male : less than 10 mIU/ml	
CA 125	Upto 35 U/ml	
CEA	Non detectable upto 4.8 ng/ml	
CMV	More than 40 EU/ml : Positive	
	30-40 EU/ml : Equivalent	
	Less than 30 EU/ml : Negative	
Cortisol	AM : 5-25 mcg/dl	
	PM : Approx 1/2 of the AM value	
DHEA SO	Males : 18-414 ng/ml.	
	Females : 110-673 ng/ml.	
Estradiol	Post menopausal females : Undetectable - 14 pg/ml	
	Ovulating females : By day in cycle relative to LH peak	
	Follicular phase	−12 10-50 pg/ml
		−4 60-200 pg/ml
	Mild cycle	120-375 pg/ml
	Luteal phase	+250-115 pg/ml
		+12 12-115 pg/ml
Ferritin	15-300 ng/ml	
Free T4	0.8-2.0 ng/100 ml	
Folic acid	1-13 ng/ml	
FSH	Prepubertal children less than 10 mIU/ml	
	Adult males	3-15 mIU/ml
	Females:	
	Reproductive age	3-20 mIU/ml
	Midcycle peak	15-25 mIU/ml
FSH	Menopausal	30-100 mIU/ml
	Postemenopausal	30-100 mIU/ml
Growth hormone	0-7 ng/ml	
Herpese	More than 100 EU/ml	Positive
	Less than 100 EU/ml	Negative
IgE	Children	Up to 28 IU/ml
	Adult	Up to 14 IU/ml

Insulin	3-35 mIU/ml	
LH	Males	3-16 mIU/ml
	Females :	
	Reproductive age	3-20 mIU/ml
	Midcycle peak	20-90 mIU/ml
	Menopausal	40-320 mIU/ml
Prolactin	Up to 20 ng/ml	
Progestrone	Follicular phase	0.1-1.5 ng/ml
	Luteal phase	2.5-28 ng/ml
	Mid luteal phase	2.8-28 ng/ml
	Post menopausal	ND-0-7 ng/ml
	Oral contraceptives	0.1-0.3 ng/ml
	Pregnant females :	
	First trimester	9-47 ng/ml
	Second trimester	17-146 ng/ml
	Third trimester	55-255 ng/ml
17, OH, progestone	Follicular phase	0.10-0.80 ng/ml
	Luteal phase	0.27-2.9 ng/ml
PSA	0.5-6 ng/ml	
PTH	12-72.0 pg/ml	
Rubella	More than 40 EU/ml	Positive
	30-40 EU/ml	Equivocal
	Less than 30 EU/ml	Negative
T_3	70-200 ng/dl	
T_4	5.5-13 mcg/dl	
TSH	0-6.0 uu/ml	
Testosterone	Males	3-16 ng/ml
	Females	0.1-1.0 ng/ml
Toxoplasma	More than 80 EU/ml	Positive
	40-80 EU/ml	Equivocal
	Less than 40 EU/ml	Negative
Vitamin B_{12}	200-900 pg/ml	

NORMAL RANGE FOR SPECIAL BIOCHEMICAL INVESTIGATIONS

24 Hr faecal fat	If the daily fat excretion is more than 5 gms/24 hrs. then fat malabsorption is occuring
Ceruloplasmin	0.20 to 0.55 O.D. change
CPK	24-195 U/L
CPK-MB fraction	Up to 8% of total CPK
D-Xylose in urine	For 5 gms of X-xylose more than 1-2 gm/5 hrs.
Foetal Hb	
New born	70-90% of Hb
1 month	50-75% of Hb
2 month	25-60% of Hb
3 month	10-35% of Hb
6 month	Up to 8% of Hb
1 year	Up to 2% of Hb
Fructosamine	205-295 µmol/L
Glucose 6 phosphate dehydrogenase	8.6-17.4 IU/gm of Hb

240

Glycosylated Hb by column	4.4-6.6% of Hb
Methaemoglobin	Less than 1% of total pigment
Microalbuminuria	Urinary albumin excretion between 20 μg/min to 200 μg/min
Serum ammonia	25-94 μg/dl
Serum amylase	40-200 SU/100 ml
Serum copper	60-165 μg/dl
Serum iron	60-150 μg/dl
Serum total iron binding capacity	270-380 μg/dl
Serum magnesium	1.9 to 2.5 mg%
Serum magnesium (24 hrs.)	0.05 to 0.20 gm/24 hrs.
Urinary amylase	500-5000 SU/24 hrs.
Urinary calcium	Up to 250 meq/24 hrs.
Urinary chloride	Up to 140 meq/L
Urinary chloride	Up to 200 meq/24 hrs.
Urinary creatinine	1-2 gms/24 hrs.
Urinary 17 ketogenic steroids	6-20 mg/24 hrs.
Urinary oxalic acid	15-50 mg/24 hrs.
Urinary phosphorus	Up to 1.5 gms/24 hrs.
Urinary potassium	Up to 45 meq/L
Urinary Potassium	Up to 70 meq/24 hrs.
Urinary sodium	Up to 130 meq/L
Urinary sodium	Up to 200 meq/24 hrs.
Urinary uric acid	300-500 mg/24 hrs.
Urinary Vma	1.7-7.1 mg/24 hrs.

ANNEXURE XIV

BLOOD GAS - NORMAL RANGE

pH	7.27 to 7.44
pCO_2	31 to 42 mm of Hg
Base excess blood	+2 to -2
Total CO_2	22 to 25 mmol/l
Bicarbonate (Actual)	24 to 26 mmol/L
pO_2	85 to 95 mm of Hg
Oxygen saturation	96 to 100%
Potassium	4.4 to 5.0 meq/L

ANNEXURE XV

NORMAL REFERENCE RANGE-SERUM PROTEINS

Total protein	6.2 to 7.9 gm%
Albumin	3.2 to 5.3 gm%
Globulin	
Alfa-1 globulin	0.1 to 0.4 gm%
Alfa-2 globulin	0.4 to 1.2 gm%
Beta globulin	0.5 to 1.1 gm%
Gamma globulin	0.5 to 1.69 gm%

ANNEXURE XVI

NORMAL REFERENCE RANGE - LIPID PROFILE

Total cholesterol	120-220 mg%
Serum triglycerides	40-140 mg%
HDL cholesterol	32-55 mg%
LDL cholesterol	Up to 160 mg%
VLDL	Up to 35 mg%
LDLC/HDLC ratio	Up to 4.5
TC/HDLC ratio (Risk Ratio)	M - upto 4.97
	F - upto 4.66
Esterified cholesterol	60-80% of total
Total lipids	400-1000 mg%

ANNEXURE XVII

NORMAL REFERENCE RANGE - CSF

Test	Normal for C.S.F.	Test	Normal for C.S.F.
Quantity	Clear	Count W.B.C.	1-5 per cmm
Appearance	Colourless	R.B.C.	Nil
Colour	Nil	Differential counts	
Deposit	Absent	Lymphocytes	Predominates
Proteins	15-40 mg%	Polymorphonuclears	(0-10%)
Globulin	Negative		
Chlorides	119-129 Meq/Litre		
Glucose	40-80 mg%		

INDEX